# Osteopathy Is in the Blood

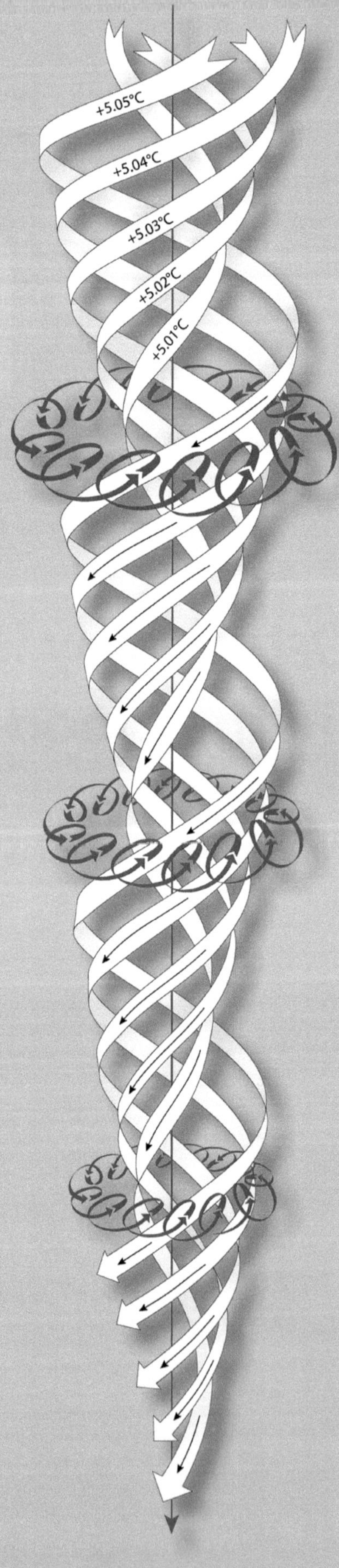
+5.05°C
+5.04°C
+5.03°C
+5.02°C
+5.01°C

# Osteopathy Is in the Blood

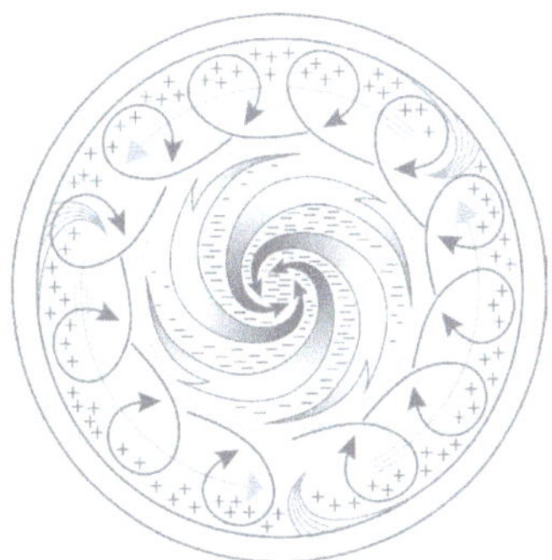

## The Science and Clinical Application of the *Rule of the Artery*

**Maxwell Fraval**

THE PROMISE
OSTEOPATHY'S PROMISE TO CHILDREN

**Disclaimer:** This book is intended solely for educational and informational purposes. The content within is not a substitute for professional medical advice, diagnosis, or treatment. Readers should consult their healthcare provider with any questions regarding a medical condition or treatment. The publisher, authors, and contributors are not responsible for any adverse effects or consequences arising from the use of any suggestions, preparations, or procedures discussed in this book.



Published by Osteopathy's Promise to Children
3706 Ruffin Rd., San Diego, CA 92123
Website: www.the-promise.org

Library of Congress Control Number: 2024925236
Title: *Osteopathy Is in the Blood: The Science and Clinical Application of the Rule of the Artery*
Author: Maxwell Fraval
Subjects: Osteopathy, Clinical Applications of the Rule of the Artery

ISBN:
979-8-9917420-0-9 (softcover)
979-8-9917420-1-6 (hardcover)

Printed in the United States of America

Book and cover design by Lubosh Cech (www.luboshcech.com)

First Edition

*Guiding Thought*

~

*In the wave*
*Lies the secret*
*Of creation*

~

Walter Russell

# Contents

# Foreword

*"The rule of the artery and vein is universal in all living beings, and the Osteopath must know that, and abide by its rulings, or he will not succeed as a healer."*[1]

What wisdom from the founder of Osteopathy, Andrew Taylor Still, DO! And what wisdom abounds about "the rule of the artery" in *Osteopathy Is in the Blood.* The osteopaths from Australia and New Zealand (ANZ) who developed and teach the work contained here practice an elevated brand of clinical Osteopathy based on concepts of anatomy and function that stretch our conventional paradigm. They follow the truth of this advanced line of thinking (just as Dr. Still followed the truth in first developing Osteopathy) along many, varied paths that lead to profound, mind-bending, and yet practical discoveries for osteopathic diagnosis and treatment. These teachers are among those leading the way in a burgeoning current of new thought that is elevating osteopathic understanding. In attending their courses, my whole osteopathic perspective enlarged, both microscopically and universally.

I first learned about their Rule of the Artery course when Maxwell Fraval invited me to Australia to present my curriculum and help him and his colleagues teach their "summer school" to osteopathic students. For years, this faculty has performed a very special duty: enriching the standard curriculum in Australia's osteopathic teaching institutions for the students interested in digging deeper into the cranial concept, originated by William G. Sutherland. At that course, all was going smoothly for me until lunch when the conversation turned to such topics as the *heart is not a pump*, the *blood conveys several types of essential information* not just nutrients such as oxygen and glucose, and the *vasculature acts as a fulcrum during development* of the body. Yes, these people were blowing my mind.

Upon returning home, I spoke with Dr Rachel Brooks, who had a longstanding connection with members of the ANZ faculty. We agreed that our country acutely needed this information, and so we invited them to teach in the United States. After launching the US courses with Rachel in 2017 and then annually teaching with these remarkable osteopaths, I learned new ways to perceive subtle palpatory cues to diagnose and treat osteopathic dysfunctions. I made a surprising leap in my palpatory skill, not knowing that I needed to or could. I discovered palpable physiological phenomena that I didn't know existed or didn't imagine I could feel. Indeed, my whole osteopathic perspective enlarged.

I was also gratified to learn that my book, *Interface*,[2] had filled in a blank spot in their understanding. Their exposition of the fact that the heart delivers multiple varieties of information through the vasculature to the cells had a missing segment in the chain of information transfer, specifically from the blood capillaries to the parenchymal cells, that is, through the interstitium. I had developed a hypothesis, first expressed in *Interface*, that the extracellular fluids actively convey **life** from the capillaries to otherwise inert structures, like connective tissue fibres involved in extracellular structural support and physiological functions, as well as cell membranes and intracellular proteins that determine the rate of cellular metabolism.[3] [For a brief synopsis of my hypothesis describing the interstitium and the transfer of information, see the Appendix, p. 253]

Several years after my trip to Australia, I am excited we have this presentation of their work that extends the legacy of this ANZ faculty. Whether one has taken the Rule of the Artery course or not, this book will be an invaluable reference for its readers. I am proud to be able to endorse the work of these ANZ osteopaths that enriches the world with a new perspective, a new discipline, a forever-giving paradigm for healing through Osteopathy. I celebrate with these colleagues and friends their opus, *Osteopathy Is in the Blood*, an expansive source of instruction and insight for the subtle and profound work of future osteopaths.

**R. Paul Lee, DO, FAAO, FCA, DABMA**
Author, *Interface: Mechanisms of Spirit in Osteopathy*

1. A.T. Still, *The Philosophy of Osteopathy* (Kansas City: Hudson-Kimberly Pub. Co., 1899), 153.

2. R. Paul Lee, *Interface: Mechanisms of Spirit in Osteopathy* (Portland: Stillness Press, 2005).

3. R. Paul Lee, "The Living Matrix: A Model for the Primary Respiratory Mechanism," *Explore* 4 (2008): 374–8, https://cranialosteopathy.com/wp-content/uploads/2017/03/livingmatrix.pdf.

# Acknowledgements

*By Maxwell Fraval, with deep gratitude to all who have helped to birth, develop, teach, and evolve our understanding of The Rule of the Artery.*

This book owes its existence to many people.

Foremost, I am deeply grateful for the tremendous support I have received from my wife, Asmaniah, starting from the very first day I understood that osteopathy was my life's work. Because of Asmaniah's support, I have been able to dedicate time to: learning from the "old masters"; engaging in ongoing research and collaborations; teaching here in Australia and overseas; and following my dream of discovering what it was "the old doctor" had been shown. Asmaniah was always there to support me and to nurture our six beautiful children. This book is the culmination of a 40-year journey that would not have been possible without Asmaniah by my side. Thanks as well to my family who encouraged me to write this book.

Grateful thanks also go to:

*Michael Solano* for his years of dedicated research and collaboration. His critical thinking, keen observations, insightful clinical applications, and effective teaching have moved the understanding of the *Rule of the Artery* forward in so many ways.

*Rachel Brooks* for her helping hand at the start of this book and for consistently being there at the vital points along the way.

*Donna Stewart*, the chief editor, for her enormous effort and support that made this book possible, contributing her considerable passion and skills to the project. We appreciate the many hours she spent obtaining the beautiful images in the book; her editing acumen, her many helpful suggestions, and for her collaboration with the skilled medical editor, *Audrey Lusher*.

*Paul Lee* for his inspiration and for his thoughtful, critical, and helpful review of the manuscript.

*Brian Freeman* for the invaluable mentorship he offered to Michael and those involved in the Rule of the Artery teaching. With the courage and determination of a pioneer he generously gave us the knowledge and vision needed to bring about significant relief from suffering in our patients.

*Alistair Moresi, Cate McDonald, Prue Eddie, Julie Streckfuss, and Ben Stringer* for their essential contributions to the manuscript.

*Beth Ann Levendoski* and *Osteopathy's Promise to Children* for seeing the value in our work and for the generous support given.

*Hugh France* for his fine embryology illustrations.

*Lubosh Cech* for bringing his creative and artistic skills to this project, particularly for his efforts to optimise the quality of each and every image.

# Introduction

## *Our* Rule of the Artery *Journey*

In the 1980s, a group of us who were young osteopathic practitioners from Australia and New Zealand, were singularly struck by Dr Rollin Becker's most emphatic injunction to let the involuntary mechanism[1] (an expression of the primary respiratory mechanism) do the work. Later, in the 1990s, following our discovery of Viktor Schauberger's work, a study group formed that included Maxwell Fraval, Anthony Norrie, Pili Munoz, George Stylian, Dion Kulak and Michael Solano. We went on to run our first Rule of the Artery course in 2001 and with varying faculties have continued to present the course since, both nationally and internationally. In 2006 we published an article in the *Journal of Holistic Healthcare* that provided an overview of our work.[2]

### Sources of Inspiration and Guidance

We very much acknowledge that in writing this book, we are standing on the shoulders of giants. Drs Still, Sutherland and Becker have been our mentors to whom we have recurrently returned for inspiration.

***Rollin E. Becker***: Dr Becker told us that the involuntary mechanism is far more intelligent than each of us as practitioners, and it can provide us with profound information about the state of the body we investigate with "thinking, feeling and knowing touch."[3] Dr Sutherland, likewise, referred to "a potency, an intelligent potency, that is more intelligent than your own human mentality" and instructed us that it could be depended upon "to do the work for you. In other words, don't try to drive the mechanism through any external force."[4]

We have done our best to follow this injunction and, over many years, have come to recognise that, apart from our developing sense of the difference between the tissues that our mentors talked about (bone, membrane, ligament, fascia, central nervous system and cerebrospinal fluid), there was another component that had its own clear pattern in many ways and recurred frequently during treatments: the perception of the function of the heart and the vasculature.

Dr Becker spoke more than once about recognising the difference between palpation and perception. Whereas palpation "is the process of feeling an object in or on the body to determine its size, shape, firmness, or location",[5] perception "is the organisation, identification, and interpretation of sensory information in order to represent and understand the environment."[6] Furthermore, "It is not the passive receipt of these signals, but is shaped by learning, memory, expectation, and attention."[7,8]

Dr Becker described the perceptual experience by using the metaphor that we commonly experience as drivers of motor cars. When driving, our feet never touch the ground; however, we have a very accurate perception of the car in space and in relation to the road and other cars, whether they are parked or moving. In our work, we have used palpation and perception in equal measure, using our knowledge and experience to inform our osteopathic medical perceptions.

***Viktor Schauberger***: Our lightbulb moment occurred when reading about the work of naturalist Viktor Schauberger, which is described in this book in Chapter 1, and his work has underpinned our ongoing quest. Schauberger was a self-taught scientist (like Einstein was self-taught) and a brilliant inventor whose deductions offer startling insights for osteopaths. Callum Coats' book on Viktor Schauberger, *Living Energies*,[9] was gifted to us by our osteopathic friend, Steve Porter, who wrote, encouragingly, on the inside cover, "Keep on making statements that switch on lights!"

***Virginia Farnum***: We benefited from the 50 years of clinical experience of the only remaining American osteopathic physician in Australia, Dr Virginia Farnum, who completed her training at the American School of Osteopathy in Kirksville, Missouri (now known as A.T. Still University), the founding college of osteopathy.

Her father, Dr C. Edward Farnum, trained as an osteopath at the Kirksville school at the time that Dr Andrew Taylor Still was living there. Dr Virginia Farnum felt strongly that many osteopaths in

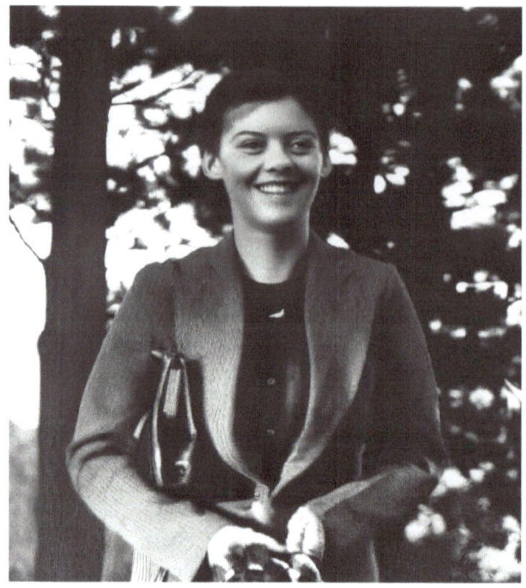

**Dr Virginia Farnum—the last American DO in Australia.**

the profession had forgotten about the importance of arterial function within the osteopathic paradigm. "Osteopathy is in the blood", she said most forcefully.

***Brian Freeman***: In 2005, Michael Solano was gifted a copy of Erich Blechschmidt's *The Ontogenetic Basis of Human Anatomy*, which was edited and translated by Dr Brian Freeman, a professor of anatomy and embryology. Recognising the importance of this work, but finding the concepts difficult to comprehend, Michael reached out to his fellow Australian, Dr Freeman, who was pioneering a view of embryology not widely accepted by the medical profession. The biodynamic approach he promoted spoke directly to our osteopathic reasoning, and he became a very important source of knowledge and support.

Dr Still, Dr Freeman and those who practice Osteopathy share a fundamental principle of wholeness. Dr Freeman taught us that to compartmentalise the human body contradicts the wisdom of the embryo, which demonstrates wholeness at every stage of growth and at different levels of complexity.

Many osteopaths have learned to apply this biodynamic principle of growth and development in their diagnosis and treatment, benefitting their patients with this understanding of the living connections between cells, organs, and tissues.

***R. Paul Lee***: In 2005, Anthony Norrie drew our attention to Dr R. Paul Lee's book *Interface: Mechanisms of Spirit in Osteopathy.*[10] We have drawn upon Dr Lee's deep insight of Dr Still's philosophy of osteopathy and his meticulous and detailed exposition and referencing of the latest research on the connective tissue matrix and its bioelectric structure and function, providing a communication network that is ubiquitous within the body. We quickly saw how Dr Lee's work provided the basis for explaining how Dr Still's concept of the heart imbuing the blood with knowledge passes via the connective tissue matrix to every cell of the body. [For a valuable synopsis of his work, see the Appendix, p. 253.]

***Andrew Taylor Still***: Finally, we believe that many within our profession have lost sight of the fact that Dr Still constantly talked about osteopathy as a philosophy that embraced the whole body and affirmed its innate ability to heal, maintain, and sustain itself. Dr Still's insight was that "the body of man was God's drug-store and had in it all liquids, drugs, lubricating oils, opiates, acids, and antacids, and every sort of drug that the wisdom of God thought necessary for human happiness and health."[11]

Following his initial insight, Dr Still spent many years searching for a way to engage with, support, and optimise that innate ability of the body. In addition to his work and studies as a physician, Still was also trained in mechanical engineering and was an avid student of philosophy, cosmology, theology, and Nature. The structural and philosophical combination of these and other studies resulted in a highly effective bio-energetic approach to medicine using processes that have been difficult to fully articulate. We believe physics offers some of the answers to unravelling the way to engage the **Health** that is to be found in the body.

One of Dr Still's earliest students, Dr Carl McConnell, who was losing his sight before being treated by one of Dr Still's sons, Dr Charlie Still, remarked:

> "The osteopathic approach is so fundamentally different from that of any other method, that one should make a determined effort not to let symptomatic and laboratory features confuse the issue. This is not implying that they contain no merit. But we should be cognisant of the fact that it is the interpretation of 'chemical man' that may gain the ascendancy and unduly warp judgement. Of course these interpretations have a relative value, but their role should not be one of usurpation; instead, one of helpful suggestion in the final evaluation. For if not thus viewed and utilised, the underlying osteopathic concept will be distorted. Of course, organic chemistry is a great big fact. So is organic physics…in unified man. Nothing is more striking in existing physiological texts than many 'gaps' of knowledge and the lack of structural (*biological*) physics."[12]

We are coming into an era when the ability to understand, measure, and work with the submolecular or electronic and photonic aspects of body function will enable us, as osteopathic practitioners, to apply Dr Still's philosophy more fully. As Nobel laureate Dr Szent-Györgyi suggested, "There are four dimensions with which the biologist must be concerned: macroscopic (anatomy), microscopic (cells), molecular (proteins), and sub-molecular or electronic. Biology readily followed physics into the first three, but took practically no cognisance of the fourth; it stopped at the molecular level."[13]

So here we are. This book comes out of our clinical experience and is an attempt to draw upon scientific support for our clinical observations.

## Endnotes

1. William Garner Sutherland, *Teachings in the Science of Osteopathy* (Indianapolis: Sutherland Cranial Teaching Foundation, 1990).

2. Munoz, "The Heart–More Than Just a Pump," *Journal of Holistic Healthcare* 3, no. 3 (August 2006): 10.

3. Sutherland, *Teachings,* 140, 187, 195.

4. Sutherland, *Teachings,* 14.

5. Wikipedia, s.v. "Palpation," last modified September 15, 2022, https://en.wikipedia.org/wiki/Palpation.

6. Daniel Schacter, *Psychology* (New York: Worth Publishers, 2011).

7. Richard Gregory, "Perception" in *The Oxford Companion to the Mind* (New York: Oxford University Press, 1987), 598–601.

8. Douglas A. Bernstein, *Essentials of Psychology* (Cengage Learning), 123–4.

9. Callum Coats, *Living Energies: An Exposition of Concepts Related to the Theories of Viktor Schauberger* (Dublin: Gil Books, 2001).

10. R. Paul Lee, *Interface: Mechanisms of Spirit in Osteopathy* (Portland: Stillness Press, 2005).

11. A.T. Still, *Autobiography of Andrew Taylor Still* (Kirksville, MO: A.T. Still, 1908), 182.

12. Carl McConnell, "Osteopathic Art – IV," *Journal of the American Osteopathic Association* 34 (March 1935): 319–20.

13. James Oschman, *Energy Medicine in Therapeutics and Human Performance* (Oxford: Butterworth Heinemann, 2003), 33.

Chapter One

# Osteopathy Is in the Blood

"In the year 1874," stated Dr A.T. Still, "I proclaimed that a disturbed artery marked the beginning to an hour and a minute when disease began to sow its seeds of destruction in the human body. That in no case could it be done without a broken or suspended current of arterial blood, which by nature was intended to supply and nourish all nerves, ligaments, muscles, skin, bones, and the artery itself. He who wishes to successfully solve the problem of disease or deformities of any kind in all cases without exception would find one or more obstruction in some artery, or some of its branches."[1]

This excerpt from Still is well known to osteopathic practitioners, as is his statement that "the rule of the artery is absolute, universal, and it must be unobstructed, or disease will result."[2]

What is less commonly known is that Still thought of the heart in a very particular way that is quite different from the conventional medical perspective. He said: "The heart, the fountain of life, is the organ in the human body which imparts the attributes of life and knowledge to the blood so that it can proceed correctly with all its work."[3] The more we pondered Still's statement that the heart imparts **knowledge** to the blood, the more impressed we were with it; it has become a cornerstone of our work.

In attempting to develop a coherent paradigm, we have frequently drawn upon embryology as the basis for understanding the ongoing dynamic between structure and function. As you will see in later chapters, we have drawn heavily upon the insights and understandings of embryologist Erich Blechschmidt in Germany and Brian Freeman in Australia.

Professor Blechschmidt was a German anatomist and embryologist. He wrote more than 120 scientific papers, wrote many books and atlases, and studied more than 200,000 serial sections of embryos in order to understand the dynamics of growth. His work made significant contributions to our understanding of the biomechanics of growth movements. The biomechanical influences of growth occur alongside many other processes that involve biochemistry, physics, and molecular biology. Growth cannot be understood without an understanding of all of the processes and how each process creates the whole. Where Still said that "all parts of the whole obey one eternal law of life and motion," Blechschmidt said:

> "Body systems do not exist in reality. It is always impossible to define where one system ends and the next starts. The body functions as a whole and it is only as a whole that we should attempt to com-

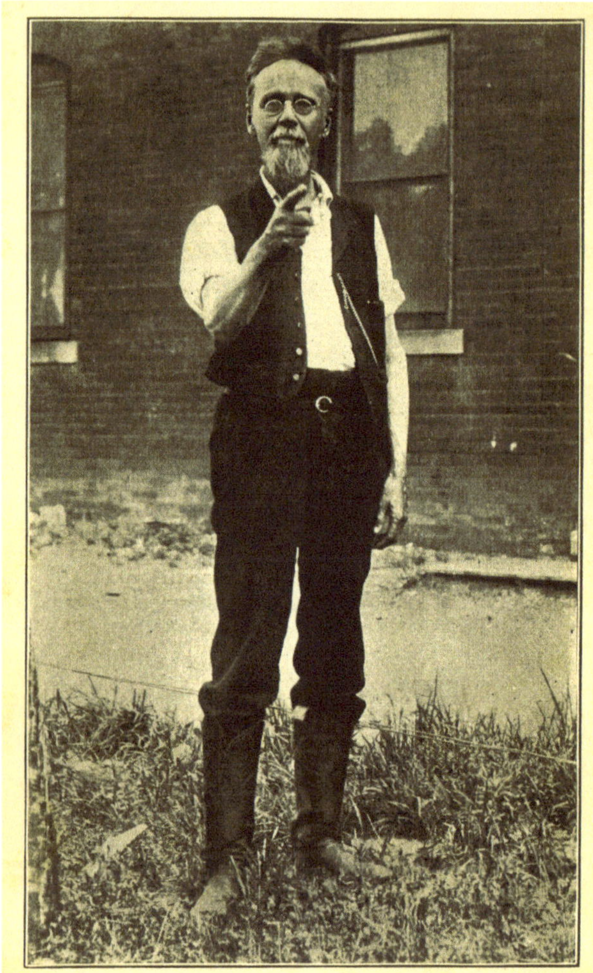

**Dr Still Points the Way.** Museum of Osteopathic Medicine, Kirksville, MO [cat#: 2010.02.1587].

prehend it. The context of the whole in relation to the part and the part relating to the whole."[4]

Dr Brian Freeman, a retired associate professor of anatomy from the University of South Wales, edited and translated a book by Blechschmidt. This book, *The Ontogenetic Basis of Human Anatomy,* and Freeman's lectures helped us understand how the genes and environment interact in the development of human form and emphasises—more than anything else, **function** precedes **form**. Raymond F. Gasser, who co-authored *Biokinetics and Biodynamics of Human Differentiation* with Blechschmidt, summarised these principles in his preface to the 2012 edition of their book:

> "Dr. Blechschmidt reasoned that because forces cause all movements (e.g., pushes and pulls), they must be generated within the embryo as its organs and tissues grow at varying rates. Since the cell membrane is extremely thin and very flexible, he concluded that the shape of cells reflects the external forces acting on them, and he discovered that certain tissues form in regions where specific, three-dimensional forces act on the tissues."[5]

Still, Schauberger, Sutherland, Becker, and Blechschmidt all had the ability to "see" what is in nature and then to translate it into a science-based description.

As we struggled to understand what we were palpating and **perceiving**, an insight occured as a result of being gifted that book on the work of Schauberger, who spent his life attempting to understand the inherent and intrinsic attributes of water. Schauberger came to understand that water has a natural tendency to move in a vortical pattern and optimally gave expression to that pattern at a certain temperature (+4°C). As we looked at the diagram in the book on Schauberger's work (Figure 1.1), it struck us that we were seeing in visual form what we had been perceiving in so many of our patients during diagnosis and treatment.[6]

This diagram demonstrates that water flows in a vortical pattern **and** also carries charge, and this electrical phenomenon, together with the related magnetic field, was central to our perceptual experience. As we began to consider how this might relate to blood flow, we also began to question the standard conventional model of the heart as a pump and how Still's observation of the heart imparting knowledge to the blood might give rise to a different view.

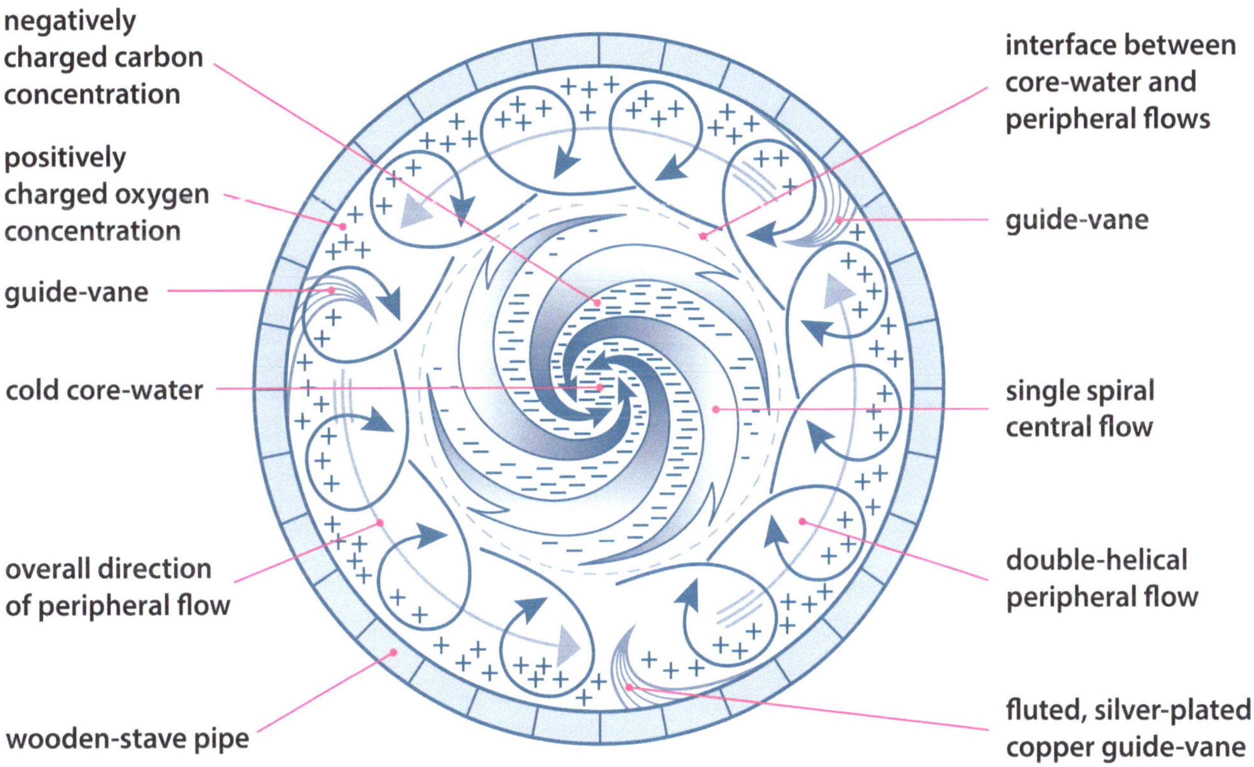


**Figure 1.1 – Flow Dynamics of the Double-Spiral Pipe.** Diagram recreated from *Living Energies* by Callum Coats—fluid flow in a pipe carries **charge.**[7]

Interestingly, M. Beraia and G. Beraia recently described the electrical and magnetic effects of blood flow in a research report from Tbilisi State Medical University:

> "The electric impulse from the heart initiates an oscillating electric field around the charged cells/particles and an emerging repulsing electromagnetic force, based on the electroacoustic phenomena, promotes the blood flow, in addition to the pulse pressure from the myocardial contraction. Blood conduces mechanical, electromagnetic waves of different frequencies and transmits energy/information to implement the spontaneous chemical processes in the human body."[8]

So, in terms of our perception, the electrical component gives a sense of direction while the magnetic component gives a sense of thickness or power.

We found that Rudolf Steiner, a contemporary of Schauberger, believed that the heart was much more than just a pump. Steiner questioned the pump model, pointing out that the vascular network is 95,000 km long and, with blood viscosity being five times greater than water, a daily pumping requirement of 8,000 L would result in a work equivalence of lifting 50 kg over 1.3 km each day. All this is to be done by a pump—the heart—which has an average weight of 300 g.[9]

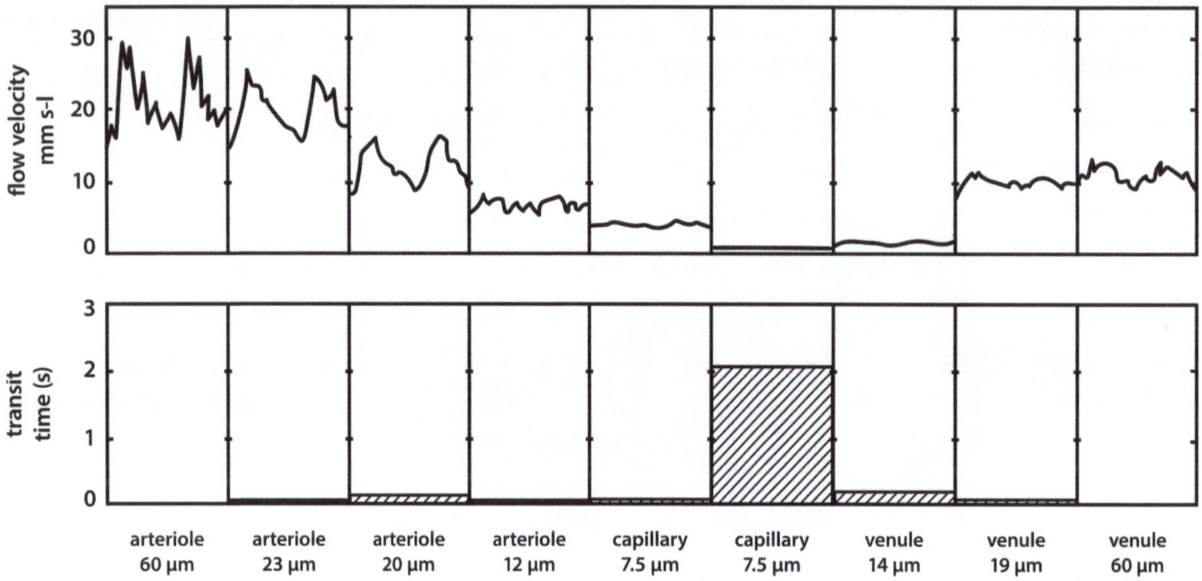


**Figure 1.2 – Flow of Peripheral Blood.** The flow of blood on the outermost periphery. Flow pulsations are evident in both the arterioles and the venules. They are caused by spontaneous pulsation of the arterioles and venules (so-called vasomotion) at frequencies of 0.5 to 20 per minute and have nothing to do with the cardiac cycle. In the actual capillary bed (centre of chart), these pulsations decrease dramatically, to less than 5% of the average flow (after 7). The slow transit time in capillaries no longer relates to the cardiac cycle. Reprinted with permission from Holdrege.[11]

The pump model is also flawed by virtue of the fact that the circulatory system is not a closed system but an open one. Figure 1.2[10] shows how high velocity with consequent low transit time in the arterial system is not matched in the massive capillary bed, which has a slow transit time and low-flow velocity.

The pulsations in the capillary bed decrease dramatically while the transit time increases. Thus, this is not a "closed system" with a pump linked by a return pipe of fixed diameter equal to the outflow diameter.

Central to Schauberger's thought was a concept of suction in relation to fluid flow. In this concept, flow is relatively frictionless, whereas in a pressure pumping system, friction is generated because the force applied to the fluid has to overcome an initial resistance and the pressure increases before flow.

The work of Gerald Pollack, author of *The Fourth Phase of Water*, and Stephanie Seneff, senior research scientist at the Massachusetts Institute of Technology's Computer Science and Artificial Intelligence Laboratory, have considerably enhanced our understanding of the biophysics of circulation. Pollack and Seneff explain the electromagnetically based charge interaction between the red blood cells as they flow in a structured fluid medium.[12,13] The charge on the red blood cells interacts with the charge of the epithelial wall of the capillary bed as the basis for a gradient-driven and frictionless flow of blood in the arteries, arterioles and capillary beds.[14]

Interestingly, blood velocity has been found to peak **before** pressure in the aorta. Additionally, it has been found that left ventricular pressure is translated into aortic positive pressure only in the first half of systole, and then it reverses.[15]

This finding means that aortic pressure is greater than ventricular pressure in the second half of ventricular ejection, which in turn suggests that blood continues to flow out against a pressure gradient. Momentum flow based around vortical motion provides an answer if we look at the vortical flow diagram (Figure 1.3) to see how this can occur.

The SphygmoCor is an instrument that measures central blood pressure and vascular pliability, or the degree of vascular stiffness, present. It is used primarily to help physicians tailor treatment for patients with conditions such as heart failure, renal disease, chronic obstructive pulmonary disease, or diabetes. What the SphygmoCor has also shown is that, **in health,** negative pressure occurs in the aorta; in other words, the blood is being sucked along.[16]

Something else to consider is the shape of the aorta. Its shape suggests that it ought to function like a Bourdon gauge, a mechanism used for measuring pressure, or a curved tube that, when subjected to pressure, straightens. For example, your water hose may have a curved shape when it lies on the ground, but when the tap is turned on, the hose straightens out. However, the curve of the aorta increases during systole; it does not straighten. This implies a negative pressure, which of course runs counter to the pressure pump model.[17]

Marinelli highlighted "stable vortex flow patterns behind the cusps of the mitral and tricuspid valves as confirmed by Taylor and Wade".[18,19] Marinelli also pointed out that "Brecher conducted an experiment on dogs that demonstrated a region of continuous negative pressure in the ventricle by observing the continuous flow of Ringer's solution from a vessel outside the heart through a cannula positioned in the left ventricle via the atrial auricle."[20]

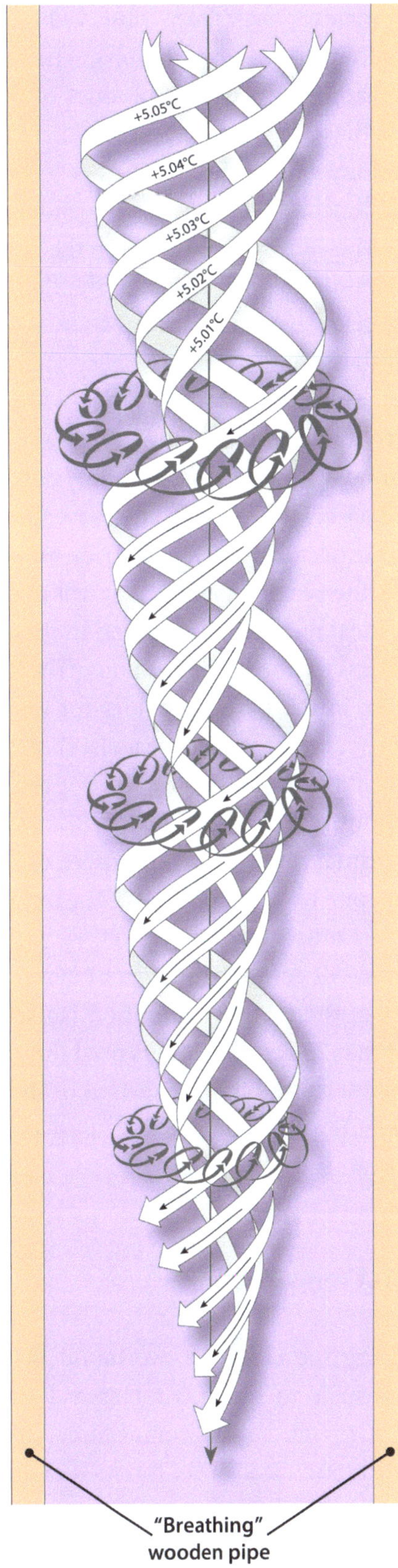


**Figure 1.3 – The Double Spiral Vortex.** This diagram, taken from *Living Energies*, shows vortical/longitudinal motion as well as helical flow as water spirals outward towards the periphery. Recreated from Coates.[21]

These vortexes have been observed using cine imaging, doppler imaging, and magnetic resonance velocity mapping.[22] Another product of the vortical flow is that the substances in blood are not scattered randomly. In vortical flows, it is observed that heavier objects migrate to the centre and lighter objects to the periphery. This occurs in the blood, with the red blood cells in the core of the flow and the lighter platelets peripheral to the core. A sleeve of plasma is found at the very periphery of the vessel.

Interestingly, at the end of systole, 40% of ventricular volume remains. If the heart was a truly efficient pump, which it would certainly need to be to achieve the workload referred to above, then at rest we would expect to see 100% ejection efficiency.

We see the residual ventricular volume as part of the vortical mechanics for blood in the ventricle that is necessary for flow continuity. The retention of a vortex in the blood provides for an ongoing suction process that we believe assists both the output blood flow as well as the lower pressure systemic venous return[23] (see Chapter 8).

If the primary or even sole purpose of the heart is a pump, one would expect all of the oxygen to be used to fuel muscular activity. Yet, we find that at rest, of the 250 cc/min (of oxygen) available to it, only 10% of the total consumption is used by the heart. Of that 25 cc/min, 20% is used for basal metabolism, 5% is used in the exertion of the beating heart, and 70% (more or less) is used in the creation of heat.

## The Spiral Template

In reviewing the literature, we found that spiralling is intrinsic to blood. At Harvard University in the 1930s, John Lewis Bremer filmed his observations of blood circulation in chick embryos before the valves of the heart formed. Bremer filmed the beating embryonic heart in which the already "spiralling blood is boosted by the pulsating heart without creating turbulence in the blood. This suggests that the momentum transfer occurring between the heart and the blood is in phases."[24]

It appears that somehow the heart senses the motion of the blood and responds to it with a spiralling impulse the same as the velocity of the blood, thereby combining blood and heart momenta, "as movement without applied pressure is movement with momentum."[25]

In addition, Pomerance and Davies[26] noted the inherent spiralling of the blood in an embryo that never formed a heart. The fetus lived to term in utero, but the baby was tragically stillborn and disfigured. Thus, Marinelli et al determined "that the blood is not propelled by pressure, but rather moves with its own biological momentum and with its own intrinsic flow pattern."[27–29]

Bremer described "two streams of spiralling blood with different forward velocities in the heart of the single tube stage embryo."[30,31] Nevertheless, Marinelli et al noted that the blood had "a definite direction of flow within the conduits and moves without an apparent propelling mechanism" and that the streams "spiral around their own longitudinal axes and around each other"[32] similar to the way in which Viktor Schauberger envisaged.[33]

Vortices are interesting phenomena. They require a gas-filled space within fluid to exist. This seems absurd when talking about blood because of the potential for an air embolism in such a situation. However, in each 100 cc of blood there is 0.3 mL of dissolved oxygen, 2.6 mL of dissolved carbon dioxide, and 1 mL of nitrogen. The dissolved oxygen is considered a physiologically significant amount in cases of extreme anaemia. Blood flowing within the vessels forms a composite vortex, which is made up of solids including red blood cells, plasma cells, and platelets. Liquid and soluble gases are maintained in a stable form by the centripetal flow at the centre of the vortex.

Because the water in the blood is structured and negatively charged, it is able to carry a richer concentration of oxygen than bulk water—the higher the charge, the greater the capacity to load oxygen.[34] This is discussed in greater detail in Chapter 3: Water: Flow and Function.

So, if the heart is not solely a pump, then what more does it do? We suggest that when the heart begins to function on day 22 of its embryological development, it enhances the blood's momentum and the complexity of its spiralling impulses.

The heart imparts knowledge to the blood in part by imprinting a pressure wave in it. It does this by spiralling the blood in the left ventricle, which initiates vortical motion and the code (or knowledge and information), which is maintained peripherally by the vessel walls. The code, discussed more fully in Chapter 5, is a complex of sound waves (phonons), pressure waves, electrons and photons. We see the spiralling of the blood and its complex vortical patterns as a way of maintaining this information over distance and of maintaining coherence.

As a muscular organ, the heart produces a magnetic field that is 5,000 times more powerful than that produced by the brain.[35] However, corollary to that, research carried out by John and Beatrice Lacey at the National Institutes of Health in the United States showed that about 65% of the cells of the heart are neurons like those found in the brain. So the heart has both magnetic and electrical qualities as previously described by Beraia and Beraia.

In fact, J. Andrew Armour referred to these neurons as "the little brain in the heart" as seen in Figures 1.4 through 1.8.[36] In his monograph, Armour describes the neuronal cooperation across numerous regions necessary for cardiovascular stability and efficiency. In addition, he examines how the cardiac nervous system impacts heart disease and discusses recent research regarding the complex neuronal processing and memory capabilities of the intrinsic cardiac nervous system. This research

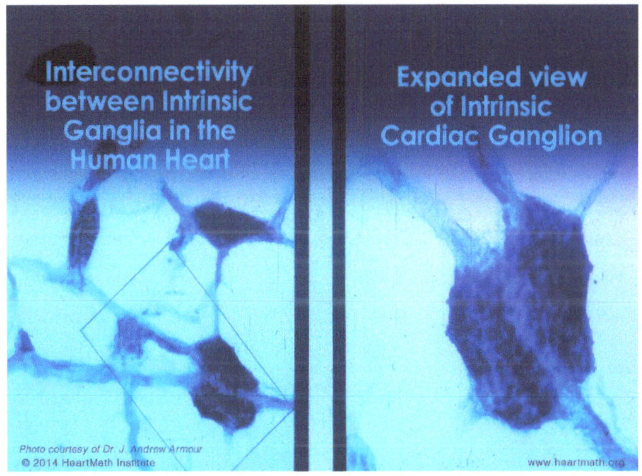


**Figure 1.4 – Interconnectivity Between Intrinsic Cardiac Ganglia in the Human Heart.** The thin light-blue structures in the image on the left are multiple axons coursing between and connecting the ganglia. The image on the right is a further magnified view of the ganglia shown in the rectangular box in the image on the left.

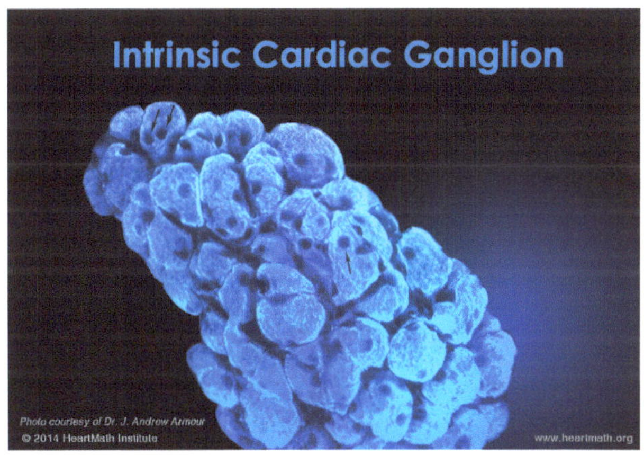


**Figure 1.5 – Intrinsic Cardiac Ganglia Magnified.** This highly magnified view of a cardiac intrinsic ganglia was taken with a confocal microscope, which is able to take images layer-by-layer and then build a three-dimensional image. Ganglia are made up of groups of nerve cells (somata) that exist outside of the brain and spinal cord. Each of the smaller circular structures shown is the cell body of an individual neuron.

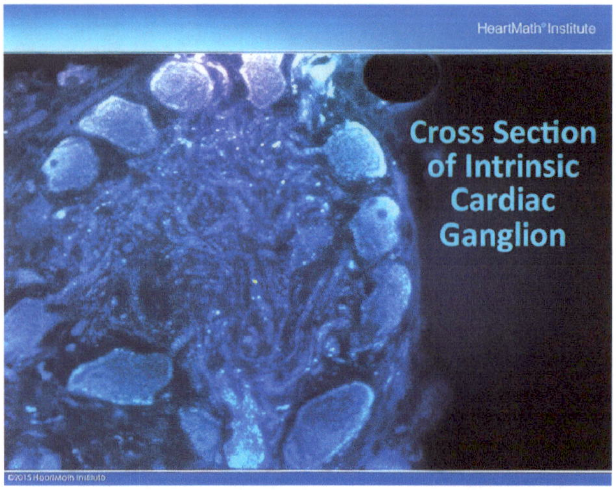


**Figure 1.6 – Intrinsic Cardiac Ganglia Cross Section.** This image represents a cross-section through an intrinsic cardiac ganglion. In the centre, there is a mass of dendrites that interconnect individual neurons. This structure is ideal for an independent neural processing unit.

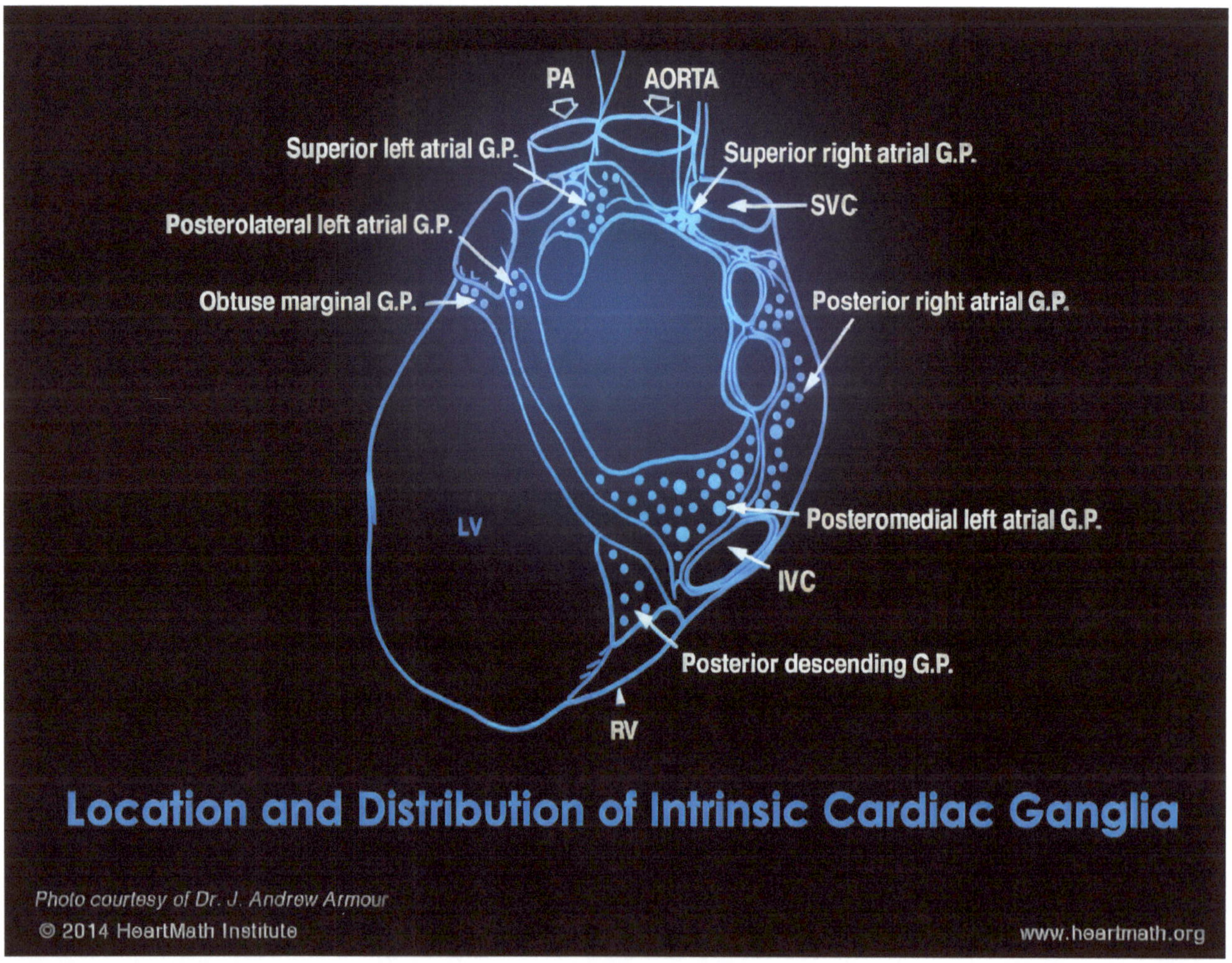


**Figure 1.7 – Location and Distribution of Intrinsic Cardiac Ganglia.** Note how the cardiac ganglia or ganglionated plexi (G.P.) are distributed particularly around the orifices of major vessels. Abbreviations: IVC = inferior vena cava; PA = pulmonary artery; RV = right ventricle; SVC= superior vena cava.

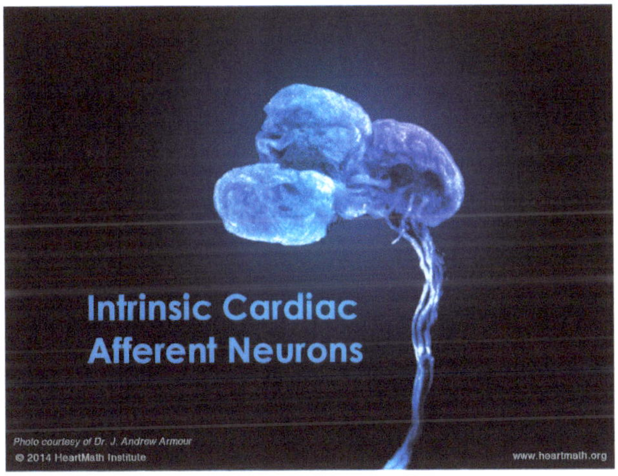


**Figure 1.8 – Intrinsic Afferent Cardiac Neurons.** This image was taken with a confocal microscope. An afferent neuron is one that sends information to another neuron. These sensory neurons detect the local mechanical and biochemical changes that occur in cardiac tissue. They send this information to the rest of the intrinsic cardiac nervous systems and, in many cases, to the brain. So there is two-way signalling, both efferent and afferent. This would describe an efferent function.[38]

suggests an ability for the heart-brain to act independent of the central nervous system—that it can process information and make decisions without information being transmitted outside itself. According to Armour, this research reveals "the newly emerging view of the heart as a complex, self-organised system that maintains a continuous two-way dialogue with the brain and the rest of the body."[37]

In addition to imprinting pressure waves, the heart appears to imprint knowledge to the blood in various other ways. The central nervous system contains information on how body homeostasis should be maintained. There is thus an ongoing moment-to-moment communication between the brain and "the little brain in the heart." It appears to us that the heart imprints the regulatory information provided to it by the central nervous system into the oxygenated blood using four methods:

- by imprinting information directly into the haemoglobin;
- by sound in the form of phonons travelling through the blood matrix;
- by electrical conduction (electrons) in the blood conductance, which can be increased by increases in adrenalin; and
- by photons being absorbed and released by various factors in the blood.

These processes convert the ongoing information from the central nervous system into dynamic inputs to be used by cells. This information is received by cells from the oxygenated blood detailing maintenance of homoeostasis, including temperature (as discussed in Chapter 7: The Heart as a Generator), oxygenation, toxicity, pH levels, osmotic balance and ion and sugar levels, to name a few. In deoxygenated blood, this includes the regulation of cell division, functioning and information from organelles, and all cellular feedback about the cells' activity.

Within a single beat of the heart, all cells in the body have the message of how that person is doing. This feat comes not from the rapid rate of flow through the arterial system but rather from the electrical charge passing through the blood (which is an excellent conductor) and from the heart sounds generating phonons and photons, which carry information.[39] The heart then receives information on how the body is functioning through the (de)oxygenated blood, and this information is fed back to the central nervous system. The central nervous system can then modify its instructions in light of what is actually happening in the body. Information from the atmosphere is gathered in the lungs and transported to the heart and the brain. These processes allow the body to adapt chemically to new conditions.

Once the blood has been imprinted by the heart and carried to the capillary bed, the paravasal plasma mantle, also described in the literature as the perivascular space, allows entrainment between the pattern within the capillary and from the paravasal plasma mantle via the extracellular matrix (ECM) to the cell. Figure 1.9, which was extracted from an article by Hauk,[40] shows how it is possible for information within the capillary to be entrained with the mantle and then to pass in the pre-lymphatic paths between the gel and sol islands, moving through the matrix towardss the cells. With the recent focus on the lymphatics of the brain, it appears that the perivascular space is the same as the paravasal plasma mantle.[42–44] The paravasal mantle facilitates the movement of oxygen, minerals and nutrients, electrical charge, photons, and phonons into the extracellular matrix. The fine details of both the physics and chemistry in this wonderfully coherent extracellular system are reviewed in detail in

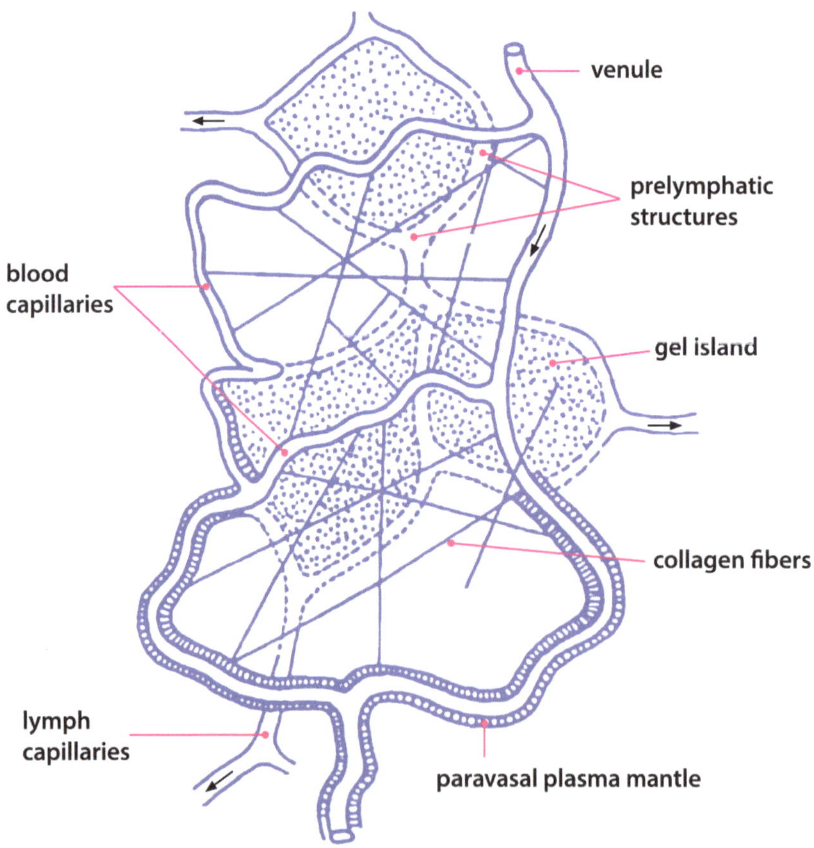


**Figure 1.9 – Outer Peripheral Circulation.**[41] The colloidal medium of the extracellular matrix alternates between a gel-like, island-forming state and a sol-like channel-forming state. Here, the barrier function with regard to the blood is not morphologically determined but is accomplished through flow processes, the so-called paravasal plasma mantle and intervasal edge flow, which interact with the blood clotting system.

Chapter 5: The Fascia and the Code, which covers the recent work of Hachisu and Yoshimura, who, in using the more sophisticated laboratory equipment available to them, were able to demonstrate sol and gel islands side by side in the extracellular matrix.

In *Energy Medicine in Therapeutics and Human Performance*, Physiologist, Cellular Biologist and Biophysicist James Oschman gives a wonderful summary of the importance of the fascia or extracellular matrix:

> "The connective tissue is the most abundant component of animal matter and forms the bulk of the animal body. The overall form of the body, as well as the architecture and mechanical and functional properties of all its parts, are largely determined by the local configuration and properties of the connective tissue. All of the systems of the body – the circulation, nervous system, musculoskeletal system, digestive tract, and the various organs – are ensheathed in and partitioned by connective tissue. The connective tissue forms a continuously interconnected system throughout the living body. All movements of the body as a whole and of its smallest parts, are created by tensions carried through the connective tissue fabric. It is a liquid crystalline material and its components are semiconductors, properties that give rise to many remarkable properties. One of the semiconductor properties of connective tissue is piezoelectricity, from the Greek, meaning 'pressure electricity.' Because of piezoelectricity, every movement of the body, every pressure or tension anywhere, generates a variety of oscillating bioelectric signals or micro currents and other kinds of signals that will be described later. These signals are precisely characteristic of those tensions, compressions, and movements. Because of the continuity and conductivity of the connective tissue, these signals spread through the tissues. Due to the continuity with cell interiors, these micro currents also are conducted into cells. If the parts of the organism are cooperative and coordinated in their functioning and every cell knows what every other cell is doing, it is due to the continuing and signalling properties of the connective tissue."[45]

Oschman reviewed the scientific basis for information transfer within the extracellular matrix.[46] He highlighted the following contributions:

- In 1941, Nobel laureate Szent-Györgyi suggested that the proteins in the body act as semiconductors:[47] "If a great number of atoms be arranged with regularity in close proximity, as for example in a crystal lattice, single valency electrons cease to belong to one or two atoms only, and belong instead to the whole system. A great number of molecules may join to form energy continua, along which energy, namely excited electrons, may travel a certain distance."[48] Many studies have shown that organic systems have semiconductor properties and elucidated the mechanisms by which these properties are acquired and regulated in living systems.[49–52]
- Becker researched the properties of the connective tissue surrounding nerves, which is called the perineurium. Becker found that the perineural tissues were sensitive to magnetic fields.[53]
- Frölich's work showed that "all parts of the living matrix set up vibrations that move about within the organism, and are radiated into the environment."[54,55]
- Pienta and Coffey discriminate between the vibrations within the matrix; its continuity within tissue, combined with its qualities of piezoelectricity and coherence, make it the perfect system for the specific transfer of information to cells throughout the organism.[56]

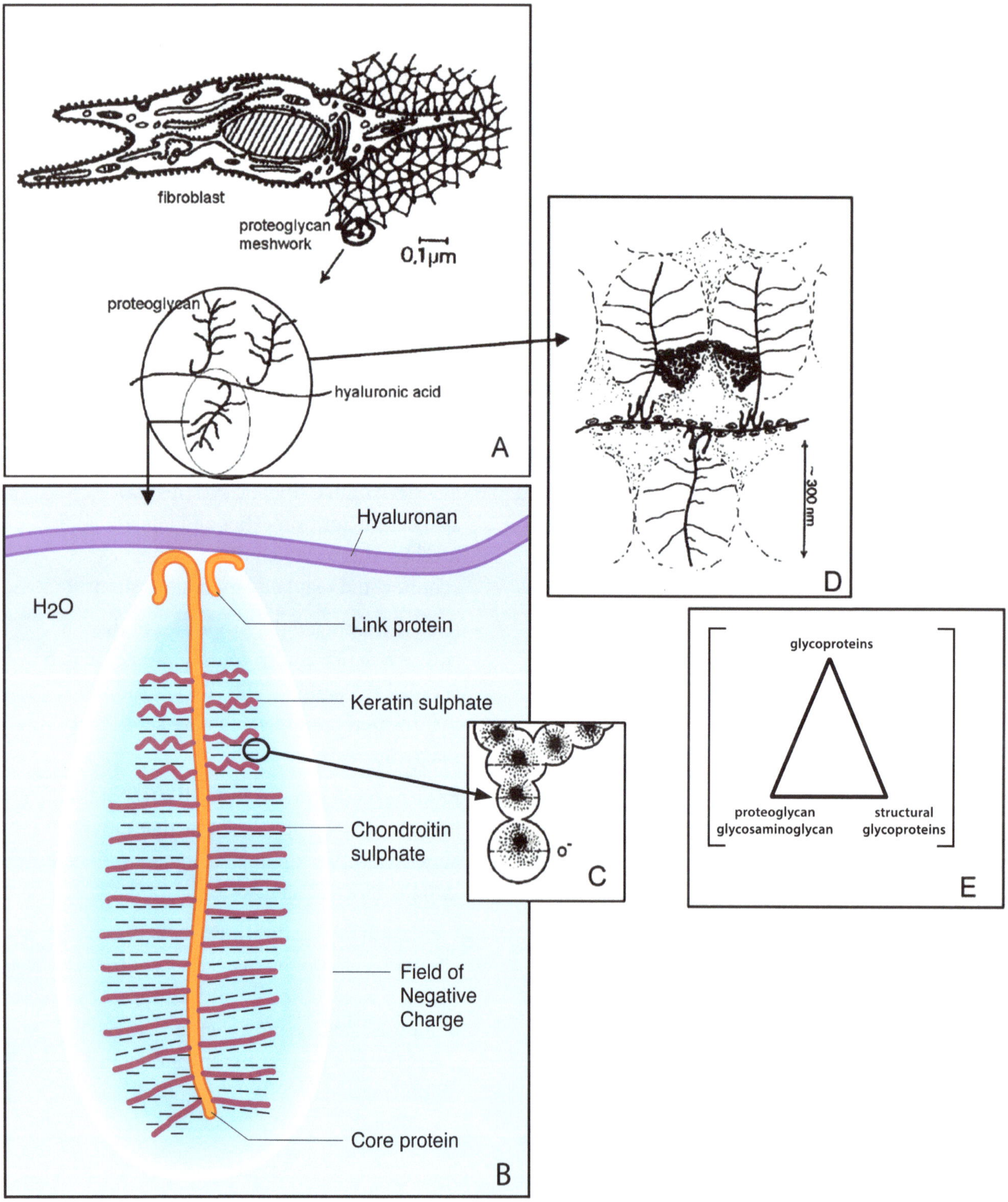


Original artwork by Raychel Clemma.

**Figure 1.10 – Examining the Extracellular Matrix.**[59–61] Details of the extracellular matrix: (A) The fibroblast is embedded in the proteoglycan meshwork, together with details of the ways the proteoglycan hands attach to hyaluronic acid. The cervical region represents one "matrisome" and is enlarged below in (B). The matrisome is a repeating proteoglycan and unit consisting of the core protein linked to hyaluronan and glycosaminoglycan sidechains: the glycosaminoglycans stand out straight from the proteoglycan backbones, and the adjacent chains repel each other to form an arrangement like the bristles of a brush. The result of the charge density is a strong field, or "domain," of negative charge. (C) Detail of the origin of the negative charges in the glycosaminoglycan molecules. The dots represent the distribution of electrons in the atoms. From Ling.[62] (D) Detail from (A) shows inclusive packing of proteoglycans (matrisomes) within tissues. The dotted lines depict the "domains" of the individual proteoglycan and molecules. The double arrow shows the exchange of water and ions between the matrisome and the extracellular fluids. (E) A single matrisome unit within a bracket. This structure is repeated again and again (n is an extremely large number) to form a continuous ground substance reaching into every part of the organism. Images reprinted with permission from James Oschman and R. Paul Lee.[63] Figures A, D and E were originally published in Pischinger's book on matrix regulation.[64]

Oschman later published a review of charge transfer in the extracellular matrix[57] and provided a helpful image summarising the physiology of charge transfer (Figure 1.10).[58]

In his article "Charge Transfer in the Living Matrix," Oschman stated that "Pischinger's work and that of his colleagues demonstrated more than any other that the extracellular matrix is not an inert filler substance or a passive mechanical filter, lying between the capillaries and the cells. Instead, the matrix is a dynamic, vibrant and alive component of the organism with vital roles in the moment-by-moment operations of virtually all physiological processes."[65]

In his book *The Extracellular Matrix and Ground Regulation: Basis for a Holistic Biological Medicine*, Pischinger noted that "Recent research has demonstrated that the matrix components are actually semi-conducting liquid crystals, materials known to have a variety of remarkable properties for the transmission, storage, and procession of information involved in regulation."[66]

Nordenström made a substantial contribution to understanding the physiology of the extracellular matrix (ECM), which is more extensively discussed in Chapter 5. He referred to the vascular-interstitial closed circuit (VICC) as one specific biologically closed electrical circuit system.[67] Nordenstrom's observations led him to the conclusion that, in addition to existing descriptions of mechanical flow, the blood flowing in the circulation also carried charge. It is this charge that provides the ability for bidirectional ion transport to occur. The VICC is powered and influenced both by the natural and inherent charge energy that produces electromotive force (electrophoresis) and by current disturbances resulting from injury (dielectrophoresis).

Nordenström reported that the ion transfer across the capillary wall resulted in a grouping or aggregation of ions in the adjacent matrix that he referred to as *ionars.**

This grouping of ions produces oscillating calcium concentrations that move through the ECM as calcium ion waves, which sets up an electric potential and results in water being cyclically picked

* An electrophoretic-dielectrophoretic system – in electrophoresis – is a technique used to separate DNA, RNA, or protein molecules based on their size and electrical charge. An electric current is used to move the molecules through a gel or other matrix. Dielectrophoresis occurs when a polarisable particle is suspended in a non-uniform electric field. The electric field polarises the particle, and the poles then experience a force along the field lines, which can be either attractive or repulsive according to the orientation on the dipole. Since the field is non-uniform, the pole experiencing the greatest electric field will dominate over the other, and the particle will move.

up and released as the polymers (glycosaminoglycans and proteoglycans) polymerise and depolymerise. This process frees bound water in the gel and changes its viscosity to promote the movement of fluids and nutrients towards the cells where the charged Ca++ moves. The evidence for sol and gel islands is reviewed in Chapter 5, including the research work of Hachisu and Yoshimura, who, in using the more sophisticated laboratory equipment available to them, demonstrated alternating sol and gel islands in the extracellular matrix.[69]

At the level of cellular function, Oschman highlighted two discoveries. The first discovery was by Mark Bretscher at Cambridge University in England, who found proteins on the surface of cells that connect the interior of the cell with its exterior surroundings. This led to the recognition that integrin molecules connect every cell's cytoskeleton with not only neighbouring cells but also with the "surrounding extracellular connective tissue matrix that pervades the body."[70]

The second discovery was from Berezney and colleagues,[71] from Johns Hopkins University, who found that there are also "connections across the nuclear envelope that join the cytoskeletal matrix with the nuclear matrix."[72]

Oschman recognised that these two discoveries demonstrated that there is a continuous molecular fabric within the body that extends throughout the entire organism.

The research referred to by Oschman, together with the research of others, particularly Lee and Nordenström, suggest a mechanism for information transfer from the capillary bed to cells. This mechanism is how the knowledge or information from the heart, once imprinted on the blood, is passed to the cells.

## Clinical Examples From Artificial Heart Recipients

The lack of variability in artificial hearts became an important factor in how disturbed artificial heart recipients were. The monotony of a heart beat at a rate that is constant and unchanging is in stark contrast to one that is constantly changing with changes in activity level and the social environment of the person concerned.[73] A sudden, unexpected event results in an increase in the heart rate, whereas the largo in a classical piece of music results in a slowing rate. Thus, the lack of heart rate variability in an artificial heart results in a disconnect between the external and internal milieu, impacting homeostasis.

There have been various attempts since the 1980s to develop an artificial heart. In 1984, a plastic-titanium heart was put into a number of recipients. The longest early survivor lived 620 days. However, these patients experienced various symptoms and adverse effects, including strokes, infections, high fevers, and deep depression.

These symptoms suggest that the heart is involved in arterial wall dynamics because the normal or usual vortical flow does not occur. The immune response (due to cardiac allograft vasculopathy, which is complex, with immunological and nonimmunological factors contributing) and psychoemotional states result from the disconnect of emotionally charged events not being registered in any way by the artificial heart.[74] The first recipient of the Jarvik-7 artificial heart, dentist Barney Clark, was described by his wife as having "experienced periods of despondency and repeatedly asked to die or be killed". His wife said that he had suffered a significant loss of personality and it was as though "he was walled up within himself". The wife of transplant recipient Bill Schroeder, a retired United States Air Force sergeant, made similar remarks—her husband didn't seem himself, often was barely willing to speak and was weepy and depressed.[75]

In his book *The Heart's Code*, Pearsall reviewed many anecdotes of people who had received heart transplants. After studying the effects reported by heart transplant recipients, Pearsall came to the conclusion that the heart "has a voice, and speaks to us if we will listen".[76] He concluded from his many interviews that the heart has something like a memory.

One of the most telling stories is of the recipient who started to hear a word repeated over and over in his head. When eventually a meeting was arranged between the recipient and the donor's widow, the widow revealed that the word is a secret code word she and her deceased husband used when they had made up after having had an argument. The code word was "copacetic" and meant that now everything was okay between them. The couple, driving in the car together, had been having a blazing row† when the accident occurred in which the husband was killed. His heart was very insistent in getting a message to his wife to tell her that even though they had been fighting at the time of his death, everything was "copacetic".[78]

The heart has long been associated with our emotional life. British cardiologist Peter Nixon published extensively on the *effort syndrome* and the importance of our ability to make adaptations related to the performance-arousal curve.[79–81] He has found that adapting well when performance is poor, despite high arousal levels, means appropriate withdrawal and re-setting of goals. Psychosocial qualities associated with people who adapt well include good mothering, feelings of being competent and in control, and feelings of being secure, well-loved, satisfied with achievements, appreciated and supported. Nixon found that in a healthy subject, performance increases with arousal as there is sufficient energy available and the system is in constant regeneration. If the subject is stressed, every increase reduces performance. Fit individuals have high curves whereas unfit subjects have flatter curves, which suggest quicker exhaustion.

Our language and inheritance speaks to us of an intuitive understanding and recognition of the fact that the heart imparts knowledge to the blood that impacts our feeling of the intuitive world: our food likes and dislikes, smells we are affected by, music that inspires us, people we like or dislike, and so on. It is not surprising, then, that English is replete with references to the heart: heartache, heartbreaking, heartless and heartfelt, heart-rending and pulling the heartstrings; being hearty or warm-hearted; and having a heart-to-heart conversation.

## Applications to Osteopathic Practice

Earlier in this chapter, we discussed the impact of Schauberger's work in our palpation and perception epiphany regarding osteopathic treatment's ability to influence charge-carrying blood and the vortical nature of blood flow, which occurs as a result of suction rather than pressure.

In reviewing the work of Marinelli and colleagues, we were impressed by their argument that the role of the heart in health was not a mechanical pump. The diagram in Figure 1.2 impresses on us the fact that the transit time in the capillary bed is considerably longer than elsewhere and the flow velocity is correspondingly low. This is consistent with flow resulting from suction, but it poses a problem for the pressure-pump model, which is: what is the pump that takes 80% of the blood back to the heart?

Think of a bicycle tyre that has been filled with water. You place your foot on one point of the tube. To one side is the arterial blood, arriving eventually at the capillary. On the other side is the start of the venous blood (which contains **80%** of the blood

† A very loud and angry argument.

in the body), which flows back to the heart. If the blood slows to a trickle, it does not appear to be the heart's pumping action that is responsible for the return of the venous blood from the cells at the periphery back to the heart. Where is the pump or motive force for the venous return? We know that the muscular contraction of the muscles in the extremities exerts considerable influence on venous return.[82] We also know that the valves in the veins ensure that the flow is unidirectional, carrying the blood back to the heart.

What of the great vessels, carrying blood back to the heart? We know from our work on patients with low back pain that breathing greatly influences venous return. When the roughly 8 trillion cells in the lungs are recruited, during deep breathing, we can feel them draw blood out of the valveless lumbar veins back to the heart, thereby reducing lumbar congestion.

Bremer's research of the embryonic cardiovascular system tells us that "the blood is not propelled by pressure; rather, it moves with its own biological momentum and with its own intrinsic flow pattern."[83] It is that innate embryological flow that we, as osteopathic practitioners, can attune ourselves to and use in effective treatment. The recognition of this innate pattern of flow led to the question of what the function of the heart is in health. If the heart enhances the blood's momentum and the complexity of its spiralling impulses, why does it do that?

Armour's reference to "the little brain in the heart" and the complex neuronal processing and

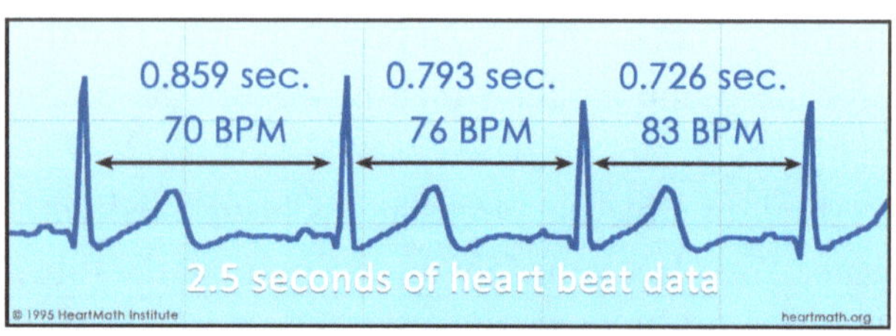


**Figure 1.11 – Heart Rate Variability.** Image courtesy of the HeartMath® Institute (www.heartmath.org).

memory capabilities of the intrinsic cardiac nervous system" raise interesting possibilities for the processing situations in which a person may experience shock.[84] We know from the research from the HeartMath Institute that subjects shown an image that is shocking will react cardiovascularly just before or at the moment the image is shown. But not only may the heart cause a reaction in the moment, it can also cause a shift in heart rate variability, which is illustrated in Figure 1.11.[85]

An adverse shift in heart rate variability may result in a long-term change in a person's resilience and behavioural flexibility.

## Making The Code

*As a man thinketh in his heart, so is he; as a woman thinketh in her heart, so is she.* (Proverbs 23:7)

In his writing, Still clearly thought about the body primarily from the point of view of the spirit and mechanics (physics): "As an electrician controls electric currents, so an Osteopath controls life currents and revives suspended forces."[86] We have understood his view to mean that the heart imparts the *Breath of Life* and knowledge to the blood as part of that overall view that physics is important in biological systems.

It appears to us that the heart communicates with both the brain and the body as a whole in a number of ways. There is the neurological communication that was referred to earlier in this chapter regarding neurotransmitters that have been found in the brain that have also been found in the heart.[87]

Furthermore, we saw that if a biological organism can use and store energy, then it must operate by known physical principles and cellular structures must exist that allow for the storage and utilisation of that energy. In the words of Dr Still, life "must have definite arrangements by which it can be united and act with matter."[88] Biophysical research has shown that electromagnetic energy plays crucial roles in determining the form, organisation and functions of biological structures "through self-organising liquid crystal molecules and through the activation of biochemical reactions."[89] For example, Beraia and Beraia refer to "the electric impulse from the heart, which initiates an oscillating electric field around the charged particles, and an emerging, repulsing electromagnetic force, that, based on the electroacoustic phenomena, promotes the blood flow, in addition to the pulse pressure from the myocardial contraction."[90]

Hahn and Schwartz described mechanotransduction in blood vessel physiology and how endothelial cells respond to stretch, changes in pressure, and flow rates. They referred to the way in which the cytoskeleton has an important role in endothelial cell responses to shear stress. There are also luminal membrane responses that directly experience shear stress, which may also mediate flow responses.[91]

In 2020, Ikeya and Woodward made a discovery so stunning even *Forbes* featured an article on it. Science writer David Bressan explained that "In the living cells of animals with magnetoreception, proteins called cryptochromes are thought to be … magnetic field sensitive molecules. Cryptochromes are a class of photoactive pigments found in plants and animals. When they absorb light, they emit an electromagnetic signal. Based on this property, researchers believe that they are also sensitive to magnetic fields". He went on to highlight how in 2020, "for the first time ever, a team of researchers at the University of Tokyo directly observed cryptochromes responding to magnetic fields in a living cell".[92,93]

Our understanding of embryonic morphogenesis is dependent on recognising and comprehending how biological systems self-assemble consistent, highly complex, four-dimensional patterns on many scales. The role of tensile forces in this process is beginning to be appreciated. The role of electromagnetic fields and radiation in physics remains largely neglected by molecular embryology.

In order to continue advancements in our molecular approaches to understanding form and function in the post-genome era, we need to combine our knowledge from the sciences of genetics, biophysics and physiology within the context of living organisms. In his article "Bioelectromagnetics in Morphogenesis", Levin argued that current research suggests that bioelectromagnetic phenomena may act as a morphogenetic mediator in embryonic development.[94]

Levin refers to well-known aspects of bioelectromagnetics. These aspects include "detection of physiological electric and magnetic fields via SQUID,[95] light,[96,97] ionizing radiation,[98] and claims of human disorders caused by exposure to fields of technological origin (extremely low frequency and microwave fields)".

In addition, Levin found "Many properties of biological systems, such as polarity, long-range spatial order, and positional information are present in the physics of electromagnetic fields",[99–102] and that "there is suggestive evidence that endogenous direct current electric fields, magnetic fields, and ultraweak photon emission are part of the medium by which information flows in biological systems."[103–105]

We believe that information distribution occurs neurologically; biochemically; through photons, phonons and electrons; as well as through high-speed pressure waves generated by the ventricle. By the time the blood from a particular systolic event leaves the heart via the aorta, the pressure wave from that same systolic event has already reached the feet.

All the molecules of the body and their chemical bonds are constantly vibrating at a specific rate — like a signature tune. This innate resonance gives these components the ability to both emit and absorb electromagnetic and sound energy. According to quantum theory, an atom or a molecule pos-

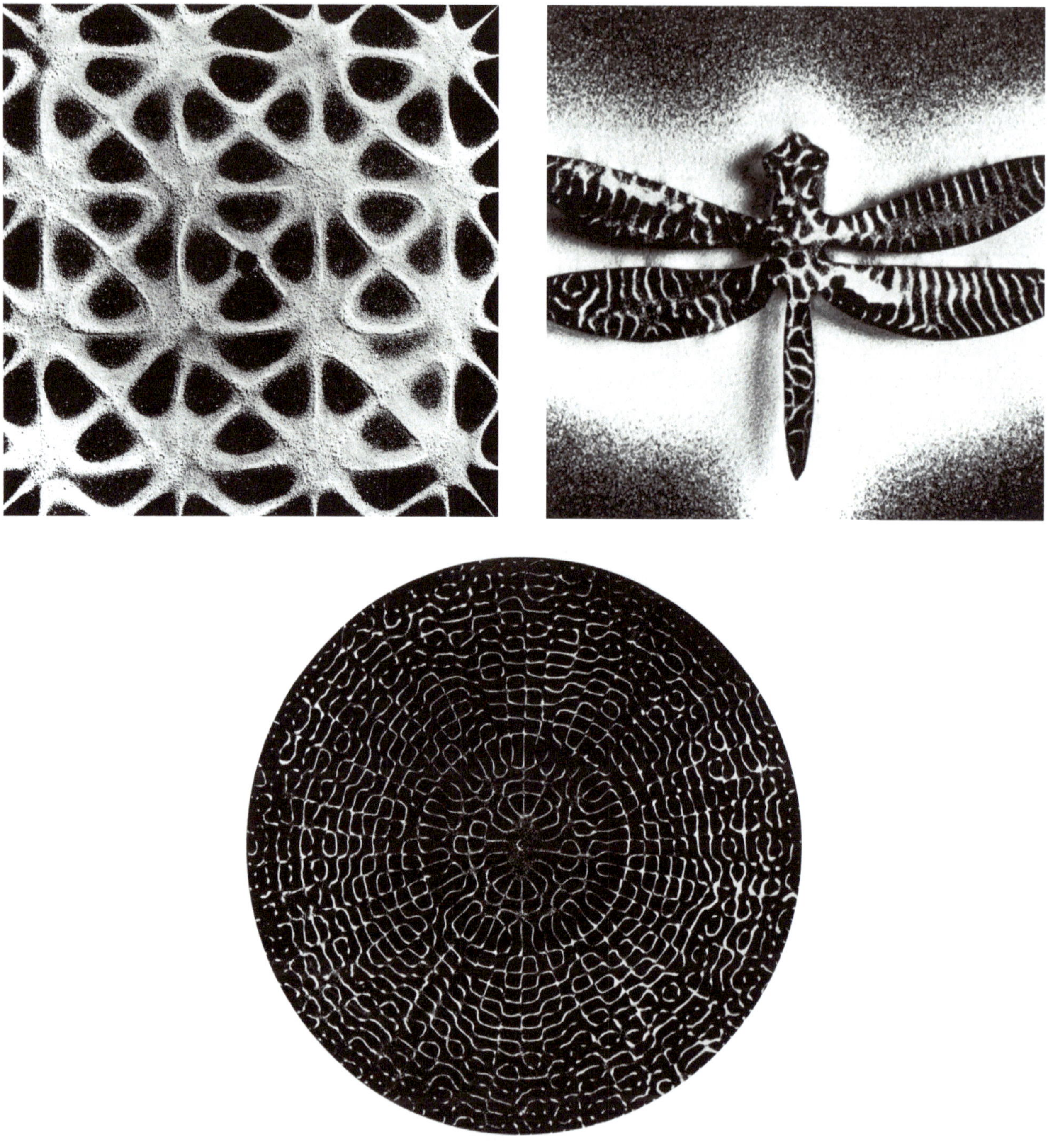

**Figure 1.12 –** Striking images from Hans Jenny's book *Cymatics: A Study of Wave Phenomena and Vibration.*[109]

sesses the properties of both a particle and a wave. When two waves come together they may interact with each other and produce an interference pattern or pressure wave; such patterns are able to hold information.

A phonon is a collective excitation in a periodic, elastic, or crystalline arrangement of atoms or molecules in condensed matter, such as solutes, in some liquids. It represents an excited state in the quantum mechanical quantisation of the modes of vibrations of elastic structures of interacting particles.

All sound, in fact all forms of vibrational energy, can be mathematically considered as a superposition or nesting of pure sine waves, even though the representative complex wave of an object vibrating at multiple frequencies is no longer audible. A complex wave can be broken up into individual sine waves with distinct frequencies by using Fourier transformation.

Physician and natural scientist Hans Jenny spent more than 14 years experimenting with and meticulously documenting the generative power of sound and the myriad ways that wave phenomena arise from its pulsations. His extensive body of work, which he called *cymatics* (from the Greek *kyma*, or "wave"), helped define a branch of physics that had been observed since Pythagoras' time but had never been sufficiently articulated.

In the film about his work, *Cymatics Soundscapes: Bringing Matter to Life With Sound*, we are told that events "do not take place in a continuous sequence, in a straight line, but are in a continual state of constant vibration, oscillation, undulation and pulsation", and this vibration influences the formation and expression of everything, from the smallest molecule to the vast ocean.[106]

Much of Jenny's research focused on the study of sound as an organising principle. Figure 1.12 presents three striking examples of his experiments using quartz sand randomly strewn on a steel plate and then vibrated by audible sound frequencies, which Jenny referred to as *piezoelectric excitation*. The particles settle at nodal, or still points in the vibrating dynamic, and distinct patterns form. Changes in frequency and amplitude result in changes in patterns, each pattern demonstrating a unique physical representation of these influences. In these examples, each experiment is on a type of smooth-surface plate. Modulating the frequency and/or amplitude distinctly alters the structure of the image. Patterns form no matter the shape of the plate, as you can see in the following images, though in shapes such as the dragonfly "planar and axial symmetry enter as factors".[107] In this film, titled *Amazing Resonance Experiment* (https://www.youtube.com/watch?v=wvJAgrUBF4w), you can watch as, in a matter of seconds, these images flow from one remarkable form to another as different frequencies are applied.‡ You may also use your phone to scan the following QR code:

The shape and orientation of red blood cells affect the sound energy in the blood they flow through, with certain shapes and orientations leading to a loss of sound energy because they swing, glide, and "parachute through" the vessel and have an effect on health.[110–112] Recently, experimental work at the Australian National University demonstrated the

‡ Jeff Volk, who first published the English translations of Hans Jenny's work in *Cymatics: A Study of Wave Phenomena and Vibration,* in 2001, is preparing an updated and expanded edition to include new translations and new research from advancements spawned by Jenny's work in the fields of physics, conceptual mathematics, morphology, embryology and evolutionary theory. You can learn more at www.cymaticsource.com.

link between mechanical distortion and metabolic changes in whole mammalian cells.[113]

Oschman described how "waves of mechanical vibration, moving through the living matrix, produce electrical fields and these same electrical fields can produce mechanical vibrations. Phonons are electromagnetic waves in a piezoelectric medium." All movements of the body as a whole, or any part, are created by tensions that are carried through connective tissues. Connective tissue is a liquid crystalline material and one of its properties is that it behaves like a semiconductor. One of the qualities of semiconductors is piezoelectricity, which means that pressure can give rise to electricity and electricity can produce a vibration.[114]

Additionally, the heart, "through hormones, neurotransmitters, and 'subtle quantum energies,' exerts at least as much control over the brain as the brain exerts over the heart."[115] Lacey and Lacey suggested there is evidence that the heart neurohormonally calls for a constant environmental update from the brain in order to organise the energy of the body.[116] For example, the hormone atrial natriuretic factor (ANF) was first isolated in 1983 and found to be produced by the contraction of the muscular heart. ANF was discovered to have widespread effects on tissues, including blood vessels, kidneys, and adrenal glands. ANF also affects a large number of regulatory regions in the brain, including the thalamus, hypothalamus, pituitary gland, pineal gland, limbic system, and immune system.[117]

Since 1983, more work has been done and further peptides have been identified. The brain natriuretic peptide (BNP) was identified soon after ANF. Whereas ANF is produced in the atria of the heart, BNP is produced in the ventricles.[118] The systemic biological effects of BNP are peripheral vasodilatation, increased natriuresis and diuresis, and inhibition of the sympathetic nervous system and the renin–angiotensin–aldosterone system.

Soon after the discovery of BNP, C-type natriuretic peptide (CNP), heart-produced vessel dilator (HPVD), and calcitonin-gene related peptide (CGRP) were discovered. In 2020, Kozlowski showed that HPVD also has the ability to inhibit the growth of cancer cells in the pancreas.[119]

The pineal gland regulates melatonin production, which regulates our sleep/wake cycle, the ageing process and general energy levels. ANF is a powerful vasodilator and is involved in the homeostatic control of body water, sodium, potassium and adipose tissue. The discovery that the natriuretic peptides play a role in lipid mobilisation within human white adipose tissue, skeletal muscle fat oxidation, and dissipation of energy in brown adipose tissue all point to the fact that the natriuretic peptides are possibly associated with glucose homeostasis, fatty acid metabolism, and insulin sensitivity.[120–122]

ANF is released by the atrial myocytes in the atria in response to high blood volume. It acts to reduce the water, sodium and adipose loads on the circulatory system, thereby reducing blood pressure.[123] CGRP reacts synergistically with nitric oxide to cause vaso-relaxation and to protect the arteries from atherosclerosis, coronary artery disease and stroke. [§,125,126]

Stress can induce BNF production, which results in the production of beta amyloid precursor protein. This protein is neuroprotective in neurones found both in the brain and the heart and particularly protective of the hippocampus.[127]

BNF and CNP are present in the cerebrospinal fluid and affect both pituitary and hypothalamic function. CNP has a direct influence on adrenal function. The attributes of learning, memory, and exploratory activity when faced with a new

§ Nitric oxide dilates blood vessels, raising blood supply and lowering blood pressure. Conversely, it helps protect tissues from damage due to low blood supply. Also a neurotransmitter, nitric oxide acts in the nitrergic neurons active on smooth muscle, which is abundant in the gastrointestinal tract and erectile tissue.

environment requires the engagement of the hippocampus, and ANF, CNP, and BNF all strongly impact hippocampal function.[128]

Armour also pointed out that the cell type known as "intrinsic cardiac adrenergic cells"[129–132] synthesise and release the catecholamines norepinephrine and dopamine. This might provide the basis for explaining Howard Shifke's assertion that "a change of heart" (a change of emotional patterns) resulted in the resolution of his Parkinson's symptoms.[133] More recently, it has also been found that the heart secretes oxytocin, the "love" or "bonding hormone." Oxytocin has been shown to influence lactation, cognition, tolerance, adaptation, complex sexual and maternal behaviours as well as the learning of social cues and the establishment of enduring bonds. Remarkably, McCraty and Tomazino found that "concentrations of oxytocin in the heart are as high as those found in the brain."[134,135]

Those "subtle quantum energies" referred to by Lacey and Lacey echo both Drs Still and Sutherland. Sutherland compared it to the phenomenon of lightning: "Do you know anything about sheet lightning? You see its manifestation all through the cloud, but it doesn't touch the cloud. I want you to see this invisible 'liquid light', or the breath of life as sheet lightning and a transmutation; the sheet lightning all through the nerves not touching the 'copper tube.'" The "copper tube" is described by Sutherland as being similar to a coaxial cable. The transmutation is what Still pointed to in the early days as "nerve force." He was trying to put across this understanding using the example of the electrical force, or the electrical "juice", that runs along the wire. "That signal that runs along has to have a track to run on."[136] In part, Sutherland seemed to be referring to the perineural semiconductor communication system, which is mentioned earlier in this chapter.

Our focus here is on the liquid light to which Sutherland refers. Virtual particles, including virtual photons (infinite information in virtual waveforms, including what Sutherland referred to as the breath of life) compose the zero point field. They emit real photons randomly. Real photons are involved in quantum electrodynamics (QED), the principle of physics that describes how electrons and photons interact. Photons carry infinite information (a principle of physics). They pass on information through interactions with electrons (and everything else). Photons are the language of electrons.

The charge of the electrons takes the information baton from the photons, through QED (photons and electrons), and is represented in the body by the electrons contained in the helical waves in the blood, which also represent the palpable Traube-Hering waves.[137] Waves carry charge (electrons). So, the light speed of photons has been reduced to the speed of sound; electrons in fluid waves. This is the transmutation spoken of by Sutherland with specific references to the coaxial cable; this is how the breath of life stimulates an oscillation of fluid; this is the palpable oscillation of direct current that Oschman described in *Energy Medicine*.

Then, these electrons in the helical waves of the blood pass the baton to the calcium ions waiting in the ECM next to the capillaries and collect as ionars (Nordenström) into EMF-producing waves that generate from the EMF of the helical waves delivered by the blood in the capillaries (Nordenström[138] and Pischinger[139]). It is almost more about the relationship between elements than the elements themselves. Calcium waves are the next intermediary that deliver information to the ECM and embedded cells.

The information (calcium ion concentration) dissolves the gel to allow nutrients, another form of information, to be delivered. The metabolic activity in the cell is stimulated by the calcium ions binding to the integrins in the plasma membrane, which pass on the information in the form of the increased activity of enzymes located on the cytoplasmic fibres

(Ingber), as well as the diffusion of glucose and oxygen to the mitochondria for the production of adenosine triphosphate (ATP).

It is also likely that the Traube-Hering waves (helical waves in the blood flow) are harmonics of the pulse pressure of the blood from heart activity and from cerebral blood flow picking up the oscillation of charge in the brain and cerebral spinal fluid. As Still said, the heart and brain work together to deliver life to the cells.

Fritz-Albert Popp was a theoretical biophysicist and one of the pioneers whose research highlighted the importance of light within the body. In the 1970s, he taught radiology with a focus on the interaction of electromagnetic radiation on biological systems at the University of Marburg in Germany. Popp had been examining benzo[a]pyrene, the polycyclic hydrocarbon known to be one of the most lethal carcinogens to humans. As part of his examination, he illuminated the benzo[a]pyrene with ultraviolet light and discovered that it had an unusual optical property.

The substance absorbed the ultraviolet light, then re-emitted it at a completely different frequency. In effect, benzo[a]pyrene is a chemical that doubles as a biological frequency scrambler. Its near relative benzo[e]pyrene, another polycyclic hydrocarbon, is virtually identical in every way to benzo[a]pyrene save for tiny alterations in its molecular makeup. This slight difference in one of the compound rings allowed light to pass through unaltered, rendering it harmless to humans.

Popp then performed his test on 37 other chemicals, some of which were cancer-causing. In the experiments on the carcinogenic compounds, the ultraviolet light was absorbed, the frequency altered and then re-emitted. Additionally, Popp found that the carcinogens reacted only to light at a specific wavelength: 380 nm. After searching through research, Popp found reports of "photo repair", which means that a cell, including its DNA, can be almost wholly destroyed and then be almost entirely repaired by a very weak intensity of UV light at 380 nm. Popp then found reports of 380 nm being the most effective wavelength of UV light for triggering auto-repair, the same wavelength that the carcinogens had a "scrambling" effect on. Popp inferred that the carcinogens must have an adverse effect upon auto-repair processes driven by light that was naturally present in the body and was essential to the innate ability of the body to repair itself. Popp therefore concluded light must be a major control factor of the biological organism.[140–142]

When Popp presented his findings to a conference at the German Cancer Research Centre, which assumed that a weak light of 380 nm is being produced in the body, he was challenged because the current wisdom at the time was that there was no light occurring within the body. Popp then recruited Bernhard Ruth, an experimental physicist, who built a photomultiplier (EMI 9558QA selected type d) that enabled him to count individual photons being emitted. Ruth's photomultiplier picked up photons being emitted from cucumber seedlings, which Ruth initially thought must have something to do with chlorophyll.

Ruth then grew potato seedlings in the dark so that they could not undergo photosynthesis. Nevertheless, when placed in the photomultiplier, these potatoes registered a high intensity of light.[143] Popp called this phenomenon *biophoton emission*. He said that "Biophoton emission is a general phenomenon of living systems. It concerns low luminescence from a few up to some hundred photons-per-second per square-centimeter surface area. At least within the spectral region from 200 to 800 nm. The experimental results indicate that biophotons originate from a coherent (or/and squeezed) photon field within the living organism, its function being intra- and inter- cellular regulation and communication." Popp went on to show that DNA emits and receives coherent light. The fact that the light is coherent establishes the possibility of having a communication system; it is like a subatomic telephone network.[144–146]

Mae-Wan Ho studied with Popp and extended his work, as did many others. In particular, Ho was able to show that microtubules are able to act as liquid light guides for the transfer of information within the cell and onward to the extracellular matrix.[147] Ho reported that she obtained "...an image of single *Drosophilia* embryos...(that) indicate that the light is emitted over the entire embryo, though certain areas may be emitting more strongly than others at different times".[¶,149] It was initially suggested that the ultraweak luminescence, or biophoton emission, was an oxidatively driven production of light with an emission spectrum ranging from 200 nm to 700 nm.

## Applications to Osteopathic Practice

As osteopathic practitioners, we need to be aware that the heart communicates with both the brain and the body as a whole in a number of ways. In his book, *The Heart's Code*, Pearsall draws attention to the stories of heart transplant patients where they experienced peculiar changes to their habits or preferences, such as developing tastes for foods they never used to eat, developing changes in their taste for music, or other personality variations that were completely out of character. This heart's code is active and influential in all our patients.

As osteopath practitioners, listening to the body, as Dr Rollin Becker encouraged us to do, we increasingly become aware that all forms of vibrational energy can be considered as a superposition or nesting of pure sine waves. This linking of the macro with the micro is the insight Irving Dardik provides in his recent book *The Nature of Nature*.[150] It shows how waves can affect other waves and how quantum theory can become a part of our understanding of Still's philosophy of the body as a single unit of function with all parts related and affecting each other.

This is also why we feel such kinship with James Oschman's writing where he describes "waves of mechanical vibration, moving through the living matrix, producing electrical fields and these same electrical fields producing mechanical vibrations. Phonons are electromagnetic waves in a piezoelectric medium."[151]

These fascial mechanical vibrations or waves are vital in normal function. As Korr points out in *The Physiological Basis of Osteopathic Medicine,* we notice one soldier out of step.[152] This can be a fascial wave that is "out of step" with the tissues surrounding it. As we achieve balanced ligamentous or membranous tension, the fascial wave that is "out of step" progressively fades and disappears. When this happens, we have a momentary opportunity to perceive the difference between a focal mechanical vibration that is dysfunctional and the normal physiology expressed by the fascia as a whole.

Popp is one of the pioneers whose research highlighted the importance of light within the body. Many osteopathic practitioners experience perceiving light in the course of their osteopathic practice. Until very recently there has been great reticence about discussing these perceptions and their significance. Ho referred to the fascia, or ECM, as "liquid light guides," which, together with the cytoskeleton, form a network like a subatomic telephone system linking all parts of the body. It is in the fascia that Dr Still saw the river of life running. "By its action we live," he said, "and by its failure we wither and die."

¶ Drosophila melanogaster, known colloquially as the fruit fly, remains one of the most commonly used model organisms for biomedical science.

## Chapter 1 Endnotes

1. A.T. Still, *Autobiography of Andrew Taylor Still* (Kirksville, MO: A.T. Still, 1908), 182.

2. Still, *Autobiography*, 182.

3. A.T. Still, *Osteopathy: Research and Practice* (Kirksville, MO: A.T. Still, 1910), 318.

4. Erich Blechschmidt, *Ontogenetic Basis Human Anatomy: A Biodynamic Approach to Development From Conception to Birth* (Berkeley, CA: North Atlantic Books, 2004).

5. Erich Blechschmidt and Raymond F. Gasser, *The Biokinetics and Biodynamics of Human Differentiation: Principles and Applications* (Berkeley, CA: North Atlantic Books, 2012).

6. Alick Bartholomew, *Hidden Nature: The Startling Insights of Viktor Schauberger* (Edinburgh: Floris Books, 2003), 158.

7. Callum Coats, *Living Energies: An Exposition of Concepts Related to the Theories of Viktor Schauberger* (Dublin: Gil Books, 2001).

8. M. Beraia and G. Beraia, "Energy/Information Dissipation and Blood Flow in the Human Body," *Cardiology Research and Reports* 3, no. 2 (April 2021), https://doi.org/10.31579/2692-9759/017.

9. Heinrich Brettschneider, "The Polarity of Centre and Periphery in the Circulatory System," in *The Dynamic Heart and Circulation,* ed. Craig Holdrege (Fair Oaks, CA: The American Waldorf School of North America, 2002), 34.

10. P. Gaethens, "Mikrozirkulation," in *Krieslaufphysiologie*, ed. R. Busse (Stuttgart, Germany: Thieme Verlag, 1982), 70–103.

11. Craig Holdrege, *The Dynamic Heart and Circulation* (Fair Oaks, CA: The Waldorf Schools of North America, 2002), 34, 40.

12. Gerald H. Pollack, *The Fourth Phase of Water: Beyond Solid, Liquid, and Vapor* (Seattle: Ebner & Sons, 2013).

13. Stephanie Seneff, "The Mineral Power of Your Body's Electrical Supply," *TEDx Talk* (November 15, 2016), www.youtube.com/watch?v=fDWEVXhaydc.

14. Stephanie Seneff et al., "A Novel Hypothesis for Atherosclerosis as a Cholesterol Sulfate Deficiency Syndrome," *Theoretical Biology and Medical Modelling* 12, no. 9 (May 2015), https://doi.org/10.1186/s12976-015-0006-1.

15. Ralph Marinelli et al., "Rotary Motion in the Heart and Blood Vessels: A Review," *Journal of Applied Cardiology* 6 (1991): 421-431.

16. Jonathan P. Mynard et al., "Measurement, Analysis and Interpretation of Pressure/Flow Waves in Blood Vessels," *Frontiers in Physiology* 27 (August 2020), https://doi.org/10.3389/fphys.2020.01085.

17. Mynard et al., "Measurement, Analysis and Interpretation."

18. Ralph Marinelli et al., "The Heart Is Not a Pump: A Refutation of the Pressure Propulsion Premise of Heart Function," *Frontier Perspectives* 5, no. 1 (1995): 15–24.

19. D.E.M. Taylor and J.D. Wade, "Pattern of Blood Flow in the Heart," *Cardiovascular Research* 7, no. 1 (January 1973): 14–21, https://doi.org/10.1093/cvr/7.1.14.

20. Gerhard A. Brecher, "Experimental Evidence of Ventricular Diastolic Suction," *Circulation Research* 4 (September 1956): 513–18.

21. Coats, *Living Energies.*

22. Peter A. Stonebridge, "Three-Dimensional Blood Flow Dynamics: Spiral/Helical Laminar Flow," *Methodist DeBakey Cardiovascular Journal* 7, no. 1 (January-March 2011): 21–6, http://doi.org/10.14797/mdcj-7-1-21.

23. Kevin Dann, "The Spiralist," *The Public Domain Review,* August 5, 2021, https://publicdomainreview.org/essay/the-spiralist.

24. J.L. Bremer, "The Presence and Influence of Two Spiral Streams in the Heart of the Chick Embryo," *American Journal of Anatomy* 49, no. 3 (January 1932): 409–40. https://doi.org/10.1002/aja.1000490305.

25. Ralph Marinelli et al., "The Heart Is Not a Pump: A Refutation of the Pressure Propulsion Premise of Heart Function," *Front Perspect.* 5 (1995): 15-25.

26. Ariela Pomerance and Michael J. Davies, *The Pathology of the Heart* (London: Blackwell Scientific Publications), 538–9.

27. Marinelli et al., "The Heart is Not a Pump."

28. Leon Manteuffel-Szoege, "Remarks on Blood Flow," *Journal of Cardiovascular Surgery* 10 (1969): 22-30.

29. P.A. Stonebridge and C. M. Brophy. "Spiral Laminar Flow in Arteries?" *The Lancet* 338, no. 8779 (November 1991): 1360–61, https://doi.org/10.1016/0140-6736(91)92238-W.

30. Bremer. "The Presence and Influence of Two Spiral Streams in the Heart of the Chick Embryo."

31. Stonebridge and Brophy, "Spiral Laminar Flow in Arteries?"

32. Marinelli et al., "The Heart is Not a Pump."

33. Alick Bartholomew, *Hidden Nature: The Startling Insights of Viktor Schauberger* (Edinburgh: Floris Books, 2003), 158.

34. Ralph Marinelli et al., "The Heart is Not a Pump: A Refutation of the Pressure Propulsion Premise of Heart Function," *Frontier Perspectives* 5, no. 1 (1995): 15–24.

35. Ali M. Alshami, "Pain: Is It All in the Brain or the Heart?" *Current Pain and Headache Reports* 23 (2019): 88, https://doi.org/10.1007/s11916-019-0827-4.

36. J. Andrew Armour, *Neurocardiology: Anatomical and Functional Principles* (Boulder Creek, CA: HeartMath Institute, 2019), e-book.

37. Armour, *Neurocardiology: Anatomical and Functional Principles.*

38. HeartMath Institute, *Science of the Heart: Exploring the Role of the Heart in Human Performance*, accessed October 14, 2022, https://www.heartmath.org/research/science-of-the-heart/heart-brain-communication/.

39. Gary E. Schwartz, "Energy Cardiology: A Dynamical Energy Systems Approach to Integrating Conventional and Alternative Medicine," *Advances in Mind Body Medicine* 12, no. 4 (1996): 4–24.

40. G. Hauk, "Physiologische Aspekte der Hämorheologie," *Hämostaseologie* 4, no. 1 (1984): 9–12.

41. Heinrich Brettschneider. "The Polarity of Centre and Periphery in the Circulatory System," in Craig Holdrege, ed., *The Dynamic Heart and Circulation* (Fair Oaks, CA: The Waldorf Schools of North America, 2002), 40.

42. Tsutomu Nakada et al., "Aquaporin-4 Functionality and Virchow-Robin Space Water Dynamics: Physiological Model for Neurovascular Coupling and Glymphatic Flow," *International Journal of Molecular Sciences* 18, no. 8 (August 2017): 1798.

43. Alan W.J. Morris et al., "Vascular Basement Membranes as Pathways for the Passage of Fluid Into and out of the Brain," *Acta Neuropathologica* 131, no. 5 (May 2016): 725–36.

44. Eva Syková and Charles Nicholson. "Diffusion in Brain Extracellular Space," *Physiological Reviews* 88, no. 4 (October 2008): 1277–340.

45. James Oschman, *Energy Medicine in Therapeutics and Human Performance* (Oxford: Butterworth Heinemann, 2003), 61.

46. James L. Oschman, "Charge Transfer in the Living Matrix," *Journal of Bodywork and Movement Therapies* 13, no. 3 (July 2009): 215–28.

47. A. Szent-Györgyi, "The Study of Energy in Biochemistry," *Nature* 148 (1941): 157–9.

48. A. Szent-Györgyi, "Towardss a New Biochemistry," *Science* 93, no. 2426 (June 1941): 609–11, https://doi.org/10.1126/science.93.2426.609.

49. Felix Gutman and Lawrence E. Lyons, *Organic Semiconductors* (New York: John Wiley & Sons, 1981), 492-504.

50. D.D. Eley, *Organic Semiconducting Polymers,* ed. J.E. Katon (London: Edward Arnold, 1968), 259–95.

51. L.I. Bugoslavski and A.V. Vannikov, *Organic Semiconductors and Biopolymers* (New York: Plenum Press, 1970).

52. E.O. Forster and A.P. Minton, *Electric Properties of Biopolymers: Proteins in Physical Methods in Macromolecular Chemistry,* vol. 2., ed. B. Carroll (New York: Marcel Dekker, 1972), 185–344.

53. Robert O. Becker, "Evidence for a Primitive DC Electrical Analogue System Controlling Brain Function," *Subtle Energies* 2, no. 1 (1991): 71–88.

54. H. Frölich, "Bose Condensation of Strongly Excited Longitudinal Electric Modes," *Physics Letters* 26, no. 9 (1968): 402–3.

55. Herbert Frölich H, ed., *Biological Coherence and Response to External Stimuli* (Berlin: Springer Verlag, 1988).

56. K.J. Pienta and D.S. Coffey, "Cellular Harmonic Information Transfer Through a Tissue Tensegrity Matrix System," *Medical Hypotheses* 34, no. 1 (January 1991): 88–95.

57. Oschman, "Charge Transfer in the Living Matrix," *Journal of Bodywork and Movement Therapies* 13, no. 3 (July 2009): 215–28.

58. Original artwork by Raychel Clemma.

59. R. Paul Lee, *Interface: Mechanisms of Spirit in Osteopathy* (Portland: Stillness Press, 2005).

60. James Oschman, *Energy Medicine: The Scientific Basis* (Edinburgh: Elsevier, 2016), 172–3.

61. James L. Oschman, "Charge Transfer in the Living Matrix," *Journal of Bodywork and Movement Therapies* 13, no. 3 (July 2009): 215–28.

62. Gilbert Ning Ling and R.B. Lindsay, "A Physical Theory of the Living State: the Association-Induction Hypothesis," *Physics Today* 16, no. 12, (1963), 72–74.

63. Lee, *Interface.*

64. Alfred Pischinger, *The Extracellular Matrix and Ground Regulation: Basis for a Holistic Biological Medicine,* ed. Hartmut Heine, trans. Ingeborg Eibl, 2004 English ed. (North Atlantic Books, 2007).

65. James L. Oschman, "Charge Transfer in the Living Matrix," *Journal of Bodywork and Movement Therapies* 13, no.3 (July 2009): 215–28.

66. Alfred Pischinger, *The Extracellular Matrix and Ground Regulation: Basis for a Holistic Biological Medicine,* (North Atlantic Books, 2007), 12.

67. Björn E.W. Nordenström, "Impact of Biologically Closed Electric Circuits (BCEC) on Structure and Function," *Integrative Physiological and Behavioural Science* 27, (1992): 285–303.

68. See footnote on page 13.

69. Sei Hachisu and Shigekuni Yoshimura, "Optical Demonstration of Crystalline Superstructures in Binary Mixtures of Latex Globules," *Nature* 283 (1980): 188–9.

70. Oschman, *Energy Medicine in Therapeutics and Human Performance.*

71. R. Berezney et al., "Nuclear Matrix and DNA Replication," in *The Nuclear Envelope and the Nuclear Matrix*, ed. Gerd G. Maul (New York: Alan R. Liss, 1982), 183–97.

72. James L. Oschman, "Foreword and Special Contribution: The Living Matrix," in *Energy Medicine East and West,* ed. David Mayor and Marc S. Micozzi (Churchill Livingstone, 2011), x-xix, https://doi.org/10.1016/B978-0-7020-3571-5.00032-9.

73. Fred Shaffer, Rollin McCraty, and Christopher L. Zerr, "A Healthy Heart Is Not a Metronome: An Integrative Review of the Heart's Anatomy and Heart Rate Variability," *Frontiers in Psychology* 5, (September 2014): 1040, https://doi.org/10.3389/fpsyg.2014.01040.

74. Josef Stehlik et al., "Honoring 50 Years of Clinical Heart Transplantation," *Circulation* 137, no. 1 (January 2018): 71–87, https://doi.org/10.1161/CIRCULATIONAHA.117.029753.

75. Charles Siebert, *A Man After His Own Heart* (Danvers: Crown Publishing, 2004).

76. Paul Pearsall, *The Heart's Code* (New York: Broadway Books, 1998).

77. See footnote on page 15.

78. Pearsall, *The Heart's Code.*

79. Peter G.F. Nixon, "The Human Function Curve. With Special Reference to Cardiovascular Disorders: Part I," *Practitioner* 217, no. 1301 (November 1976): 765–9, 935–44.

80. Peter G.F. Nixon, "An Appraisal of Thomas Lewis' Effort," *Syndrome Quarterly Journal of Medicine* 88 (1995): 741–7.

81. Maxwell Fraval, Anu Norrie, and Pilar Munoz, "The Heart — More than Just a Pump," *Journal of Holistic Healthcare*, 3, no. 3 (August 2006): 10-14.

82. Etain A. Tansey et al., "Understanding Basic Vein Physiology and Venous Blood Pressure Through Simple Physical Assessments," *Advances in Physiology Education* 43, no. 3 (September 2019): 423–9, https://doi.org/10.1152/advan.00182.2018.

83. J.L. Bremer, "Presence and Influence of Spiral Streams in the Heart of the Chick Embryo," *American Journal of Anatomy* 49, no. 3 (January 1932): 409–40.

84. Armour, *Neurocardiology.*

85. "Your Heart's Changing Rhythm," The Science of HeartMath, accessed November 8, 2023, https://www.heartmath.com/science/.

86. Still, *Autobiography.*

87. Armour, *Neurocardiology.*

88. A.T. Still, *The Philosophy of Osteopathy* (Kansas City: Hudson-Kimberly Pub. Co., 1899).

89. Michael Levin, "Bioelectromagnetics in Morphogenesis," *Bioelectromagnetics* 24, no. 5 (July 2003): 295–315.

90. Beraia and Beraia, "Energy/Information Dissipation."

91. Cornelia Hahn and Martin A. Schwartz, "Mechanotransduction in Vascular Physiology and Atherogenesis," *Nature Reviews Molecular Cell Biology* 10, no. 1 (January 2009): 53–62, https://doi.org/10.1038/nrm2596.

92. David Bressan, "Scientists Observe Cells Responding to Magnetic Fields for the First Time," *Forbes*, January 28, 2021, https://www.forbes.com/sites/davidbressan/2021/01/08/scientists-observe-cells-responding-to-magnetic-fields-for-first-time/.

93. Noboru Ikeya and Jonathan R. Woodward, "Cellular Autofluorescence is Magnetic Field Sensitive," *PNAS* 118, no. 3 (January 2021): e2018043118, https://doi.org/10.1073/pnas.2018043118.

94. Levin, "Bioelectromagnetics in Morphogenesis."

95. Rollin McCraty, *Science of the Heart: Exploring the Role of the Heart in Human Performance* (Boulder Creek, CA: HeartMath Institute, 2001), 20.

96. G. Albrecht-Buehler, "Surface Extensions of 3T3 Cells Towardss Distant Infrared Light Sources," *Journal of Cellular Biology* 114, no. 3 (August 1991): 493–502.

97. Guenter Albrecht-Buehler, "Cellular Infrared Detector Appears to Be Contained in the Centrosome," *Cell Motility and the Cytoskeleton* 27, no. 3 (1994): 262–71, https://doi.org/10.1002/cm.970270307.

98. L. Zecca, P. Ferrario, and G.D. Conte, "Activation of Immune System by Pulsed Magnetic Fields After G-ray Irradiation," in *Transactions of the First Annual Meeting*, vol. 4 (Bioelectrical Repair and Growth Society, 1981).

99. R. Nuccitelli, "Transcellular Ion Currents: Signals and Effectors of Cell Polarity," *Modern Cell Biology* 2 (1983): 451–1.

100. E.J. Lund, "Experimental Control of Organic Polarity by the Electric Current. III. Normal and Experimental Delay in the Initiation of Polyp Formation in Obelia Internodes," *Journal of Experimental Zoology* 37, no. 1 (January 1923): 69–87.

101. R.P. Bajpai, P.K. Bajpai, and D. Roy, "Ultraweak Photon Emission in Germinating Seeds: A Signal of Biological Order," *Journal of Bioluminescence and Chemiluminescence* 6, no. 4 (October 1991): 227–30.

102. Mary E. O'Connor, Richard H. Bentall, and John C. Monahan, *Emerging Electromagnetic Medicine* (New York: Springer-Verlag, 1990).

103. Arthur A. Pilla and Marko S. Markov, "Bioeffects of Weak Electromagnetic Fields," *Reviews of Environmental Health* 10, no. 3–4 (July 1994): 155–69.

104. Mae-Wan Ho, Fritz-Albert Popp, and Ulrich Warnke, eds., *Bioelectrodynamics and Biocommunication* (NJ: World Scientific Pub. Co., 1994).

105. Levin, "Bioelectromagnetics in Morphogenesis."

106. *Cymatics: Soundscapes and Bringing Matter to Life With Sound,* directed by Hans Jenny (MACROmedia Publishing, 2006).

107. Hans Jenny, *Cymatics: A Study of Wave Phenomena and Vibration*, rev. ed. (MACROmedia Publishing, July 2001).

108. See footnote on page 19.

109. Jenny, *Cymatics.*

110. Dmitry A. Fedosov, Matti Peltomäki, and Gerhard Gomppe, "Deformation and Dynamics of Red Blood Cells in Flow Through Cylindrical Microchannels," *Soft Matter* 10, (2014): 4258–67.

111. A.S. Ahuja and R.E. Hendee, "Effects of Particle Shape and Orientation on Propagation of Sound in Blood," *Journal of the Acoustical Society of America* 63 (1978): 1074–80.

112. M.J. Cruz and J.F. Garcia-Diego, "Dielectrophoretic Motion of Oblate Spheroidal Particles: Measurements of Motion of Red Blood Cells Using the Stokes Method," *Journal of Physics D: Applied Physics* 31 (1998): 1745–51.

113. Philip W. Kuchel and Dmitry Shishmarev, "Accelerating Metabolism and Transmembrane Cation Flux by Distorting Red Blood Cells," *Science Advances* 3, no. 10 (October 2017): eaao1016, https://doi.org/10.1126/sciadv.aao1016.

114. James L. Oschman, *Energy Medicine in Therapeutics and Human Performance* (Oxford: Butterworth-Heinmann, 2003).

115. Joseph Chilton Pearce, *Evolution's End: Claiming the Potential of Our Intelligence* (San Francisco: Harper, 1992).

116. Beatrice C. Lacey and John I. Lacey, "Two-Way Communication Between the Heart and the Brain," *American Psychologist* 33, no. 2 (February 1978): 99–113, https://doi.org/10.1037//0003-066x.33.2.99.

117. Charles B. Clayman, ed., *The American Medical Association Encyclopedia of Medicine* (Random House, 1989): 142–3.

118. A.M. Richards et al., "Brain Natriuretic Factor: Regional Plasma Concentrations and Correlations with Haemodynamic State in Cardiac Disease," *British Heart Journal* 69, no. 5 (May 1993): 414–7. https://doi.org/10.1136/hrt.69.5.414

119. Michael R. Kozlowski and Roni E. Kozlowski, "A Novel, Small Peptide With Activity Against Human Pancreatic Cancer," *American Journal of Cancer Research* 10, no. 5, (May 2020): 1356–65.

120. Max Lafontan et al., "Control of Lipolysis by Natriuretic Peptides and Cyclic GMP," *Trends in Endocrinology & Metabolism* 19, no. 4 (May-June 2008): 130-7.

121. Stefan Engeli et al., "Natriuretic Peptides Enhance the Oxidative Capacity of Human Skeletal Muscle," *The Journal of Clinical Investigation* 122, no. 12 (December 2012): 4675–9.

122. K. Verboven et al., "Natriuretic Peptides in the Control of Lipid Metabolism and Insulin Sensitivity," *Obesity Reviews* 18, no. 11 (November 2017): 1243–59.

123. Eric P. Widmaier, Herschel Raff, and Kevin T. Strang, *Vander's Human Physiology,* 11th ed. (McGraw-Hill, 2008), 291, 509–10.

124. See footnote on page 20.

125. Gregory J. Dusting, "Nitric Oxide in Coronary Artery Disease: Roles in Atherosclerosis, Myocardial Reperfusion and Heart Failure," *EXS* 76 (1996): 33-55, https://doi.org/10.1007/978-3-0348-8988-9_3.

126. Gregory J. Dusting et al., "Nitric Oxide in Atherosclerosis: Vascular Protector or Villain?" *Clinical and Experimental Pharmacology & Physiology* 25 (1998): S34–41, https://doi.org/10.1111/j.1440-1681.1998.tb02298.x.

127. James P. Herman, "Neural Pathways of Stress Integration," *Alcohol Research* 34, no. 4 (2012): 441–447.

128. Rachael D. Rubin et al., "The role of the hippocampus in flexible cognition and social behavior," *Frontiers in Human Neuroscience* 8 (September 2014): 742, https://doi.org/10.3389/fnhum.2014.00742.

129. J. Andrew Armour, "Intrinsic Cardiac Neurons," *Journal of Cardiovascular Electrophysiology* 2, no. 4 (August 1991): 331–41, https://doi.org/10.1111/j.1540-8167.1991.tb01330.x.

130. J. Andrew Armour, *Neurocardiology: Anatomical and Functional Principles* (Boulder Creek, CA: Institute of HeartMath, 2003).

131. J. Andrew Armour, "Potential clinical relevance of the 'littlebrain' on the mammalian heart," *Experimental Physiology* 93 (2008): 165–76.

132. J. Andrew Armour and G.C. Kember, "Cardiac Sensory Neurons," in *Basic and Clinical Neurocardiology*, eds. J. Andrew Armour and Jeffrey L. Ardell (New York: Oxford University Press, 2004), 79–117.

133. Howard Shifke, *Fighting Parkinson's...and Winning: A Memoir of my Recovery From Parkinson's Disease* (CreateSpace, 2017).

134. Rollin McCraty and Dana Tomasino, *The Coherent Heart: Heart-Brain Interactions, Psychophysiological Coherence, and the Emergence of System-Wide Order,* Publication no. 06-022 (Boulder Creek, CA: HeartMath Research Center, Institute of Heart Math, 2006).

135. Marc Cantin and Jacques Genest, "The Heart as an Endocrine Gland," *Clinical and Investigative Medicine* 9, no. 4 (1986): 319–27.

136. William Garner Sutherland, *Teachings in the Science of Osteopathy* (Indianapolis: Sutherland Cranial Teaching Foundation, 1990).

137. R. Paul Lee, personal communication.

138. B.E.W. Nordenström, "Impact of Biologically Closed Electric Circuits (BCEC) on Structure and Function," *Integrative Physiological and Behavioural Science* 27 (1992), 285–303.

139. Alfred Pischinger, *The Extracellular Matrix and Ground Regulation: Basis for a Holistic Biological Medicine* English ed. (North Atlantic Books, 2007).

140. Fritz-Albert Popp, *Biologie des Lichtes* (Hamburg: Verlag Paul Parey, 1984).

141. E. Cadenas, "Biological Chemiluminescence," *Journal of Photochemistry and Photobiology* 40 (1984): 823.

142. Janusz Slawinski, "Luminescence Research and Its Relation to Ultraweak Cell Radiation," *Experientia* 44 (July 1988): 559.

143. B. Ruth and F.A. Popp, "Experimental Investigation of Ultra-weak Photon Emissions in Biological Systems," *Zeitschrift fur Naturforschung* 31c, no. 11-12 (1976): 741-5.

144. M. Rattemeyer, F.A. Popp, and W. Nagl, "Evidence of photon emission from DNA in living systems," *Naturwissenschaften* II (1981): 572-3.

145. F.A. Popp and J.J. Chang, "The Physical Background and the Informational Character of Biophoton Emission," in Jiin-Ju Chang, Joachim Fisch, and Fritz-Albert Popp, eds., *Biophotons.* (Dordrecht: Springer, 1998), https://doi.org/10.1007/978-94-017-0928-6_18.

146. E. Sassaroli, Y. Srivastava, J. Swain, and A. Widom, *Macroscopic Quantum Coherence Proceedings of the International Conference,* (Singapore: World Scientific, 1998).

147. Mae-Wan Ho et al., "Organisms as Polyphasic Liquid Crystals," *Bioelectrochemistry and Bioenergetics* 41, no. 1 (October 1996): 81–9.

148. See footnote on page 23.

149. Mae Wan Ho, "The Rainbow and the Worm," *The Physics of Organisms* (Singapore: World Scientific Publishing Company, 1993), 131.

150. Irving Dardik, *The Nature of Nature: The Discovery of SuperWaves and How It Changes Everything* (Rodale Books, 2017).

151. James L. Oschman, "Charge Transfer in the Living Matrix," *Journal of Bodywork and Movement Therapies* 13, no. 3 (July 2009): 215–28.

152. Irvin M. Korr, Keith A. Buzzell, and Elliot Lee Hix, *Physiological Basis of Osteopathic Medicine* (New York: Postgraduate Institute of Osteopathic Medicine and Surgery, 1970).

# Chapter Two

# The Embryology of Breathing and the Mediastinum

*"All parts of the whole obey one eternal law of life and motion."*[1]
– Andrew Taylor Still

In the quote above, Dr Still emphasised the importance of understanding the parts of the body in relation to the whole and how all of these parts obey the eternal law of life and motion. In this chapter, we introduce the biodynamic approach to embryology and human development, which requires a very different way of thinking. It involves a paradigm shift to understand the concepts of biodynamic growth and the processes of life.

The way the embryo grows, that is, the embryo's growth dynamics, precede and prepare more complex movements and future functions. For example, in an 8-week-old embryo, 3 cm long, the anatomy required for the development of adult breathing is present. These growth dynamics are a blueprint for practitioners to understand and use in diagnosis and treatment and represent the individualised construction and repair manual for each person.

In this chapter, the lungs are used to illustrate the principles of biodynamics and to explain the function and form of the mediastinum with help from the late Prof Erich Blechschmidt and Prof Brian Freeman.

In his 2023 lecture "The Heart Arises at the Transverse Confluence of Two Tubes, not from their Lengthwise Fusion", Freeman explained, "It is important to know that…there are two umbilical veins arising along the flanks of the embryo and that these veins already convey a flow of nutrients from the future placenta via the connecting stalk to the bulges of the growing brain, long before the heart itself arises. This is an important point: *flow precedes the heart*."[2] This observation is just one example of how flow or function precedes the formation of structure.

Before exploring the embryological development of the vasculature, mediastinum and the heart, it is valuable to consider why studying intrauterine growth, especially from the biodynamic model developed by Blechschmidt, is helpful beyond an academic interest. The concepts discussed go beyond the process of formation to include later biomechanical influences on health and the evolution of disease processes, as well as exploring connections of how the work of the practitioner can support the restoration of healthy tissue function.

A fundamental principle is that movement is not only an essential expression or consequence of life, but is also integral to the whole process of embryological development and ongoing homeostatic processes beyond the womb into the outside world. Essentially, what is being proposed is that the movements expressed through formation are the same movements associated with the maintenance and expression of health throughout life.

The fertilised cellular organism, the conceptus, moves without muscles, and movement is required to act as part of the interface between the internal and external world. Without movement there are no messages being passed to and from the cell, no nutrition being ingested or waste products being formed. Without motion present, the homeostatic processes stall and growth ceases.

Through metabolism and cell multiplication, lots of fluid is created. It has its own movement, which in turn helps shape the development of cells into the more structured and recognised form. This fluid (in conjunction with the shape changes of the cells themselves) exerts biomechanical forces on surrounding cells, impacting their shape and growth. Asymmetry of cell structure is observable at the very first cellular division, as one cell is always a little bit closer to the nutritional source. That cell will swell faster, exert more pressure, and multiply earlier than the cell receiving slightly less. This fundamental principle shows that asymmetry is normal from the beginning and the practitioner can apply this knowledge by not aiming for symmetry in order to achieve healthy function in the patient.

A common misunderstanding in embryology is to focus exclusively on the growth of differentiating cells. The fluids and their inherent motion are integral to development. Fluid surrounding the cells contains information via biochemical markers, hormones, and nutrition (such as oxygen and essential vitamins and minerals), as well as biomechanical forces such as shearing or pressure. The information in these processes continues to facilitate and stimulate formation of the whole, from inside the conceptus to the embryo, from the local cellular fluid movements of the fallopian tube and uterus, all the way through to the formation of the placenta and amniotic fluids.

## Genetics

Most embryological texts describe the biochemical and genetic factors contributing to development of anatomy and physiology. Indeed, it explains why, when there are critical aberrations in the genetic code, anatomical and or physiological functions are affected. While this understanding is useful and genetics are an essential part of the process, it does not explain the complexity of why a pluripotent stem cell turns into a bone cell, such as an osteoblast, or part of the liver, such as a hepatocyte. The biodynamic model not only provides a framework in which to explain why this can occur, but the fundamental processes occurring also go a long way to explaining the how and why stem cells can stimulate healing and regeneration in the fully formed human.

All cells of the developing embryo have the same genetic material. Thus, the genes do not solely determine what the cell is going to become; likewise, genetic determinism can no longer explain how different cells in living tissues form. Additionally, embryological development can be adversely impacted by outside factors, particularly those that can cross via the maternal blood supply and placenta, such as some infections, heavy metals, medications, alcohol or toxic drugs.

Humans are influenced by the environment to which they are exposed, so much so that it is now recognised that environmental and lifestyle factors play a bigger role in maintaining health or stimulating development of disease than the genetic code. One of these key factors is movement, not only how much and what type of exercise a person performs (gross motion), but also local tissue motion.

One of the most important things we have to understand is how the cell differentiates in the context of the whole. The biodynamic approach to embryology demonstrates that the context of the cell, where a particular cell happens to be, will influence the shape, the structure and the function of that particular cell.

Blechschmidt emphasised that there is flow and function before there is anatomy and that all anatomy is a crystallisation of function. He described the genes as responding to the cellular environment and specifically how they are influenced by the cell membrane. Information is transferred through the cytoplasm to the nucleus and then the nucleus, as a reservoir of information, responds to the cell membrane. This view of cell function represents a paradigm shift and is coincident with the awareness of the importance of epigenetics. It is central to the biodynamic approach to embryology.

As mentioned, differentiation is driven from the outside to the inside and then back to the outside. In this chapter, we apply these principles to the development of the lungs and the mediastinum. Specifically, we draw attention to the embryological development of the cavities, the development of the diaphragm and the fascial continuity between everything.

Blechschmidt maintained that genes do not contain any pattern of later differentiation—that genotype does not determine phenotype. Genes are constants in metabolism. All normal cells of the conceptus have the same chromosomes, yet they differentiate in different ways. As mentioned earlier, a pluripotent stem cell can develop into an osteoblast or a hepatocyte. The extragenetic information from the extracellular matrix and glycocalyx and from the external physical environment and biochemical factors act upon the cell-limiting membrane, then the cytoplasm and onto the nucleus, then back to the cell membrane. The genes are points where external stimuli are applied and consequently always have **reactive** functions.

A metaphor for this process would be planting two seeds side by side that each grow into a tree. They start to grow and appear similar but their development is influenced by the soil and the nutrients they receive, which is closer to water and the winds to which they are subject. They are genetically identical but they are responding to influences from the outside; the genes are a reference point that respond to these outside influences. As Blechschmidt put it:

> In other words, the description of the concurrent development of position (topogenesis), outer form (morphogenesis) and cell structure (tectogenesis) requires a knowledge of the kinetics or movements that occur at each of these levels, i.e. topokinetics, morphokinetics and tectokinetics.[3]

Blechschmidt and Gasser were emphatic about the embryo, writing:

> "[T]he early human embryo is master of the whole geometry that it applies to itself. It is never mistaken about any angular sum, and it is never deceived in any surface to volume ratio. It never sets an intersecting point on the wrong site and is master of every physical as well as chemical reaction.... Thus, everyone could be enlightened from the abilities of the young embryo, but it is impossible to deduce its originality from scientific findings... body systems do not exist in reality. It is always impossible to define where one system ends and the next starts."[4]

Freeman was a student of Blechschmidt and was equally emphatic about not using the word *systems*. Instead, he talks about functions—arterial and venous and vascular—because talking in terms of systems restricts the perception and consequently the palpation of tissues. (Of note, G.D. Hulett, Still's nephew, who taught osteopathic practice when Still was still at the American School of Osteopathy,

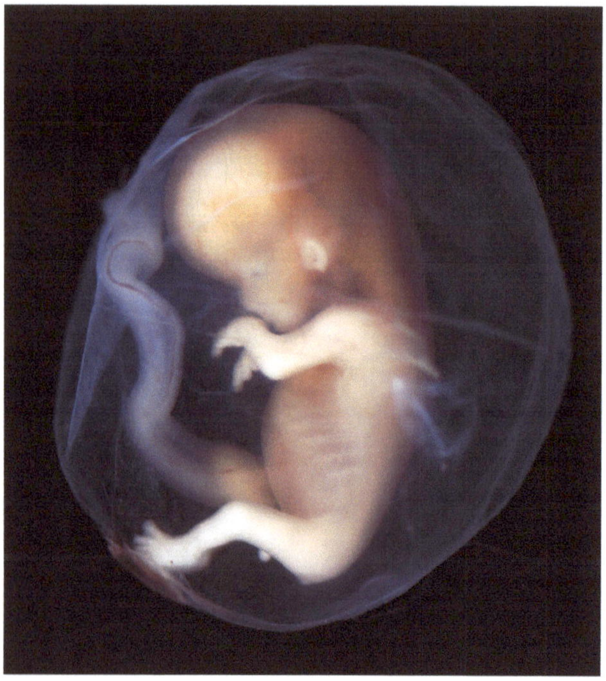

**Figure 2.1 – Embryo at 9-10 Weeks.**

maintained that function precedes structure.[5])

This continuity of all living tissues is emphasised in the image of the embryo in Figure 2.1. The developing embryo is seen folding toward the heart as the neural tube is folding into extension. Within the dural membranes there is condensation of the future cranial bones. This intramembranous bone formation can be understood in terms of the biomechanical tensions occurring within these growth movements. In this model of bone formation, the tensions in the growth movements of the dura squeeze and twist some of the water out of the intracellular and extracellular spaces, similar to squeezing water out of a wet towel. The hydroxyapatite crystals of the future bones form in the squeezing and drying environment. This image provides an example of how cells differentiate in the context of where they are in three dimensions and how they respond to the biokinetics of movement, the fourth dimension.

In a sagittal section of a cadaver (Figure 2.2), the cranial and cervical fascia can be tracked from the periosteum and superior sagittal sinus into the spinal canal and anterior fascia. Any apparent space is deceptive because all the blood and fluids have been removed and replaced by preservatives.

After studying how the kinetics of those changes related to the way they grow, Blechschmidt taught that the body functions as a whole and "it is only as a whole that we should attempt to comprehend it."[7] The results of his study can be seen at the University of Göttingen, where an exhibit of 64 large-scale reproductions of these embryos depict growth and development in three dimensions.[8]

Observing ensembles of cells in embryonic development revealed consistent rates for the conversions performed by the embryo. The cells had a purpose to them and the vasculature was an important part of what guides that purpose/trajectory. Blechschmidt observed the extent to which tissues moved, which enabled him to derive the rates of growth of different tissues. He observed that the proximity of tissues to their nutrient

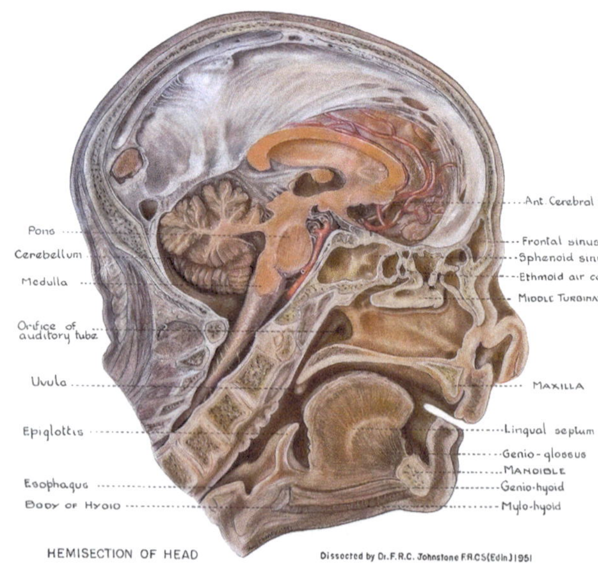


**Figure 2.2 – Skull Cross-section.** Continuity of all tissues: these are living connections. Reprinted from Cheney.[6]

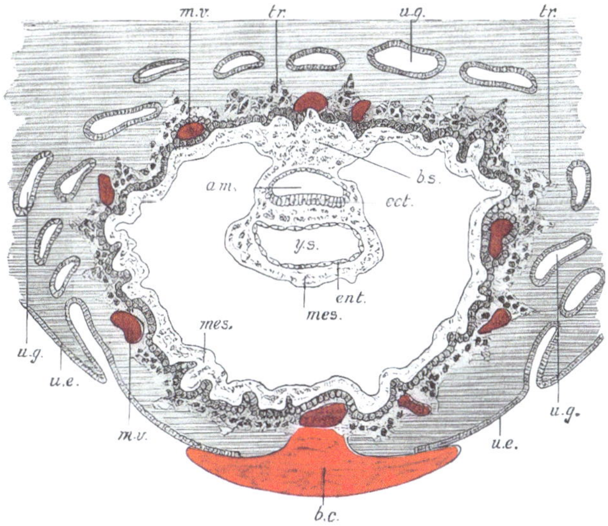


**Figure 2.3 – Section of the Ovum.** Diagram of a section through the ovum embedded in the uterine decidua. (After Peters.) Abbreviations: am., amniotic cavity; b.c., blood clot; b.s., body stalk; ect., embryonic ectoderm; ent., entoderm; mes., Mesoderm; m.v., maternal vessels; tr., trophoblast; u.e., uterine epithelium; u.g., uterine glands; y.s., yolk sac.[10]

source powerfully influenced the development and growth rates of the embryo, as illustrated in Figure 2.3. The ectoderm is the fastest-growing layer in the early embryo simply because it is closer to the maternal tissues.[9]

Growth is a function and growth in nature has spiral forms. In fact, the spiral is the most common form found in nature. We find spiral forms in snail shells, pine cones, flowers, hurricanes, galaxies and DNA. The photograph in Figure 2.4 is symbolic of so many of the principles we are attempting to elucidate. You can imagine the forces that have sculpted this magnificent tree; the predominant winds that have twisted the branches and trunk, and how the leaves and branches have grown and orientated to the movement of the sun. Most relevant for this book, the flow of nutrients is organised by the respiration of the leaves and the evaporation of water. Nutrients and water are sucked from the soil up into the tree. The movement of these nutrients is organised by metabolic activity and the flow is in response to demand.

Growth movements represent physiological momentum between supply and demand. Living tissues develop metabolic gradients toward themselves and wastes flow away from them following nutrient and waste gradients. Cells with high metabolic activity create nutrient gradients toward themselves and cells with high demand for oxygen and water develop an osmotic potential, which is more powerful than less metabolically active tissues. The cells of the neural tube, the future brain, have great proximity to the maternal tissues and grow more quickly and exhibit higher metabolic activity in the developing embryo as they do in the future adult. This process is just like a hungry newborn sucking to satisfy its hunger and its rapidly developing body and brain.

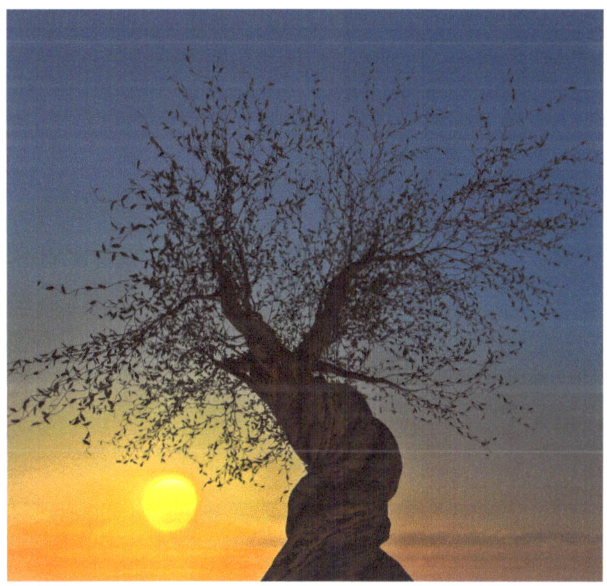

**Figure 2.4 – Growth in Spiral Form.** An ancient tree twists and strives for the sky.

## Growth Torsions

Asymmetry is also a feature of nature, and asymmetrical growth is seen on the growth torsions of the embryo. There are rhythmical twisting motions of the upper part of the embryo to one side as the lower part of the embryo twists to the opposite side. These growth movements explain many of the features of the adult form. For example, this gradual torsion to the left and then to the right explains the anatomy of the concentric fibres of the intervertebral disc; they also explain the mesenchymal twisting that is responsible for the internal oblique muscles of the torso and the external oblique muscles forming in the opposite twisting direction. There are thousands of these growth torsions as the embryo lengthens, widens, flexes and extends. As these movements contribute to the maturation of the embryo, they can be understood simply as the biomechanical kneading of the mesenchyme by the growth forces exerted by tissues that have different growth rates (Figure 2.5).

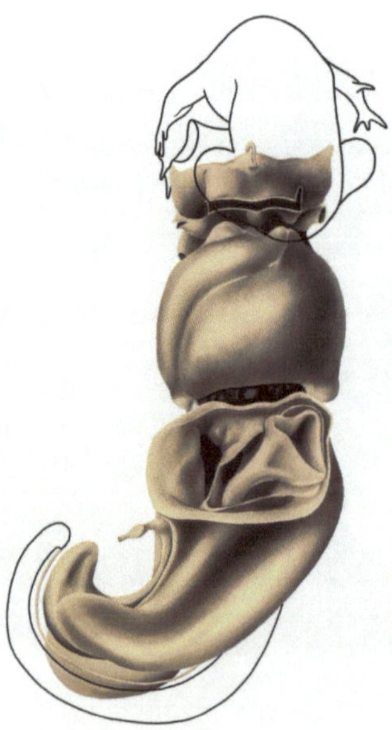

**Figure 2.5 – Growth Torsions of the Growing Embryo.** Illustration by Hugh France.

One of the best examples of this growth sculpting of the mesenchyme is the early flexion of the neural tube to compress the mesenchyme, which eventually forms the interorbital ligament. This interorbital ligament represents mesenchyme that was squeezed by folding in the longitudinal/sagittal plane and therefore grows more slowly than surrounding tissues and acts as a fulcrum for the tethering of the orbits, which eventually orientate in the forward direction (Figure 2.6).

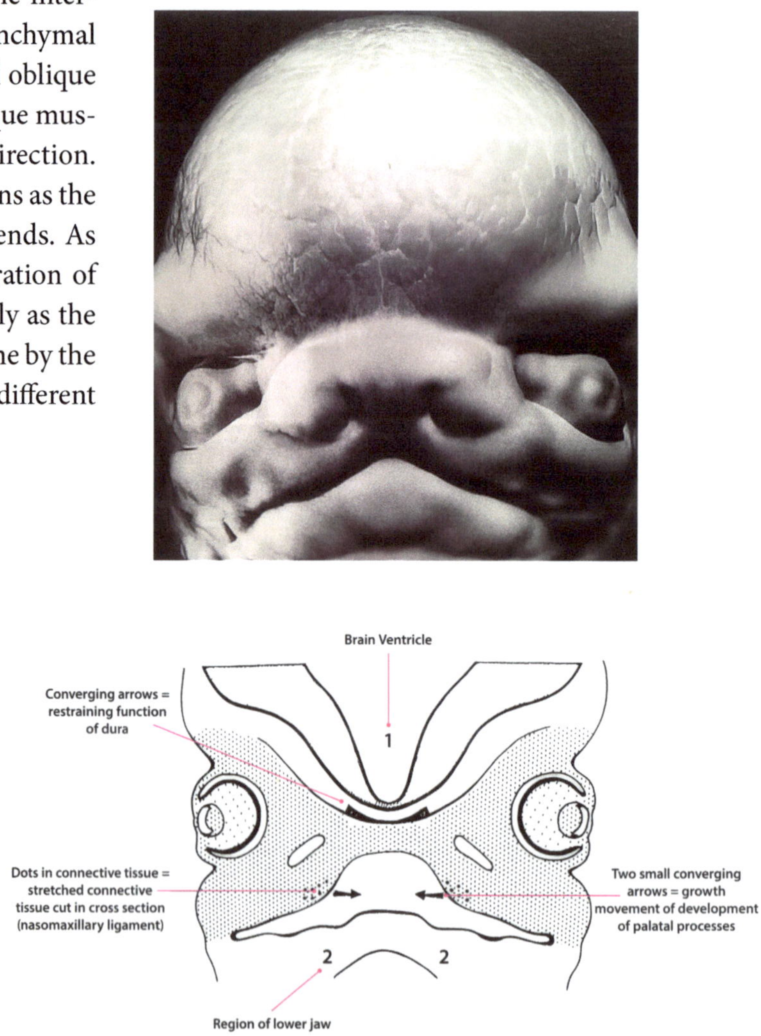


**Figure 2.6 – Blechschmidt's Images of the Interorbital Ligament.** Three-dimensional image (top) and illustration (bottom) of the interorbital ligament from Blechschmidt. [11, 12]

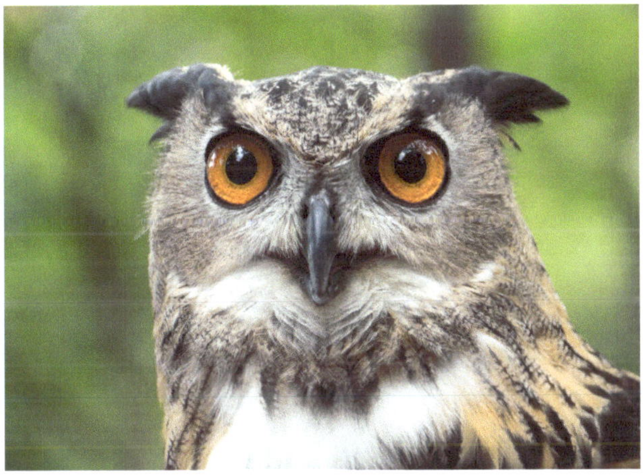

**Figure 2.7 – Eurasian Eagle-Owl.** Rehabilitated Eurasian eagle-owl (Bubo bubo) at Raptor Fest, Central Park, New York City, NY, USA. (wikimedia.org)

Freeman gave a wonderful example of one species of bird that forms an interorbital ligament that anchors the eyes front and centre rather than laterally, like most other birds, during the development of its neural tube: the owl (Figure 2.7).

For us, as osteopaths, the detailed knowledge of embryological biodynamics provides us with a guidebook. The biomechanics of embryology explain how tissues form and repair.

In addition to proximity-opportunity growth mentioned earlier, embryonic tissues that metabolise a little faster than others are going to draw more nutrients toward them. In the early embryo, one of the important dynamics is the hunger for nutrients of the developing neural tube, which draws and organises blood flow toward it.

In early embryonic development, many mesenchyme cells are pluri-potential cells, and the development of the early vasculature is an important way to understand why function precedes anatomy. In this case, the function of flow precedes the development of the early blood vessels. As nutrients start to trickle through the early mesenchymal cells, some of the cells are caught up in the flow and move with the flow of water and nutrients toward the areas where there is more metabolic activity. As growth and metabolic activity increases, the flow increases in the group and the mesenchyme deepens. An analogy for this process would be trickles of water developing into streams, as shown in Figure 2.8.

The sand represents the mesenchymal cells and, where there is a trickle of water, a small shallow groove develops. As the flow increases, so does the depth of the groove. Mesenchymal streaming is an important part of the embryological organisational process.

Take the experience of a few cells that happen to be adjacent to the flow. The tiny undifferentiated cells, which are spherical and supple, experience flow adjacent to their membranes, and the shape of the membrane changes as it is squeezed and elongated by the pressure of the flow. The cell starts to become a little longer and a little narrower, and the shape of the nucleus also changes. This cell may become an endothelial cell, which forms the wall of an early blood vessel. This is an example of a biosculpting process.[13]

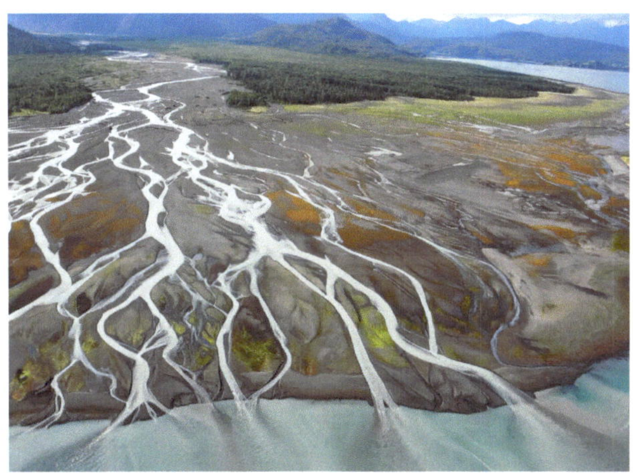

**Figure 2.8 – Trickles in the Sand Developing Into Streams on the Alaskan Shoreline.** National Oceanic and Atmospheric Administration. Photo credit: Alaska Shorezone.

## Blood Vessels as Restraining Structures and Fulcra

The vascular tissues have a restraining influence on the tissues they supply and are therefore formative in their effect on the embryological process. Blechschmidt believed that all endothelial cells, which line vascular structures, develop with the flow of nutrients parallel to their membranes. This is "**parmeation**" of nutrients, which explains why they function and grow at a lower metabolic rate. As Blechschmidt and Gasser noted, "....nutritive substances move faster along the wall of larger vessels. They do not leave the vessel but instead move along the endothelium (parmeate)."[14]

When the flow is relatively perpendicular to the cell membrane, there is the **permeation** of nutrients—diffusion moves through the membrane. The growth rate of this segment of vessels is therefore comparatively slow. The retarded lengthening of the vascular stems manifests itself as a restraining function in respect to more intensely growing tissues that have profuse capillaries. Therefore, Blechschmidt's investigations indicate that the increased bending of the embryo during the fourth and fifth weeks is probably correlated to the restraining function of the embryonic dorsal aortae.

Since the nervous and vascular systems are connected by tissue, the brain appears to be bridled by the relative shortening of the dorsal aortae that lie close to the neural tube. As soon as the aortae tether the ventral aspect of the expanding brain, the brain bends in a concave manner over the heart, which is very large in this period. The position of the bending is in accordance with the position of the aortic tethering. As the bending occurs, the ectoderm and endoderm on the ventral side of the embryonic head and neck regions undergo characteristic foldings, establishing the arching folds (pharyngeal arches), as illustrated in Figure 2.9.

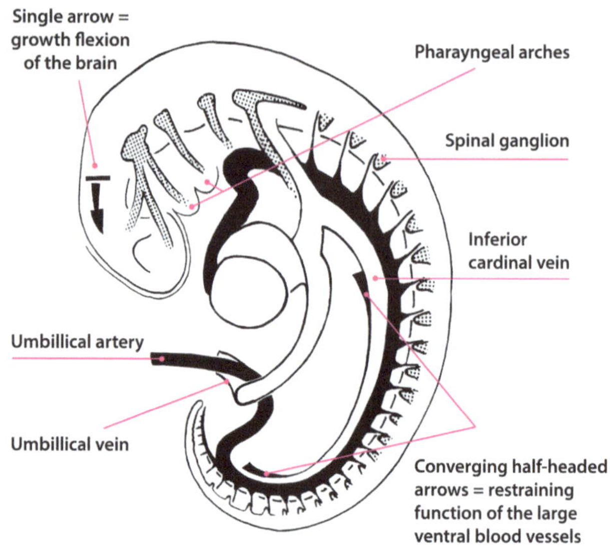


**Figure 2.9– Development of the Pharyngeal Arches.** From *The Ontogenetic Basis of Human Anatomy* by Erich Blechschmidt, translated by Brian Freeman, published by North Atlantic Books and Pacific Distributing, copyright © 2004 by Traute Blechschmidt. Reprinted by permission of North Atlantic Books.[15]

In Blechschmidt's words, "These dorsal branches of the aortae function, as do all blood vessels, as restraining structures. They hold on to the growing neural tube just as though they were cords, so that the embryo bends forward as it grows."[16]

In the documentary series Flight: The Genius of Birds,[17] scientists captured the mesenchymal streaming that occurs in a chick embryo. In one clip from the series, you can watch the gradual condensation of the notochord and the somites, the developing neural tube, and the neuropore closing as the neural tube matures. Most of this occurs before the heart starts beating. You can view the video clip at https://www.youtube.com/watch?v=-Ah-gT0hTto or scan the following QR code:

The streaming of nutrients occurs before the heart has formed and it is because of the function of flow that the heart forms. The heart absorbs and conducts the flow of blood and increases the complexity. The conventional model describes the heart as a pump, propelling nutrients to the cells. However, this model of the heart is too simple, as the heart is more than a pump. This topic is discussed in more depth in Chapter 4: The Embryology of the Heart.

The metabolic respiration of living cells involves the assimilation and dissimilation of nutrients and byproducts. It is important to understand that every cell expands and recedes with metabolic inspiratory and expiratory movements and every cell has internal circulation. This metabolic respiratory movement occurs at a cellular level and at a systemic level. Two cells enclosed within a living membrane share these metabolic and respiratory movements as do billions of cells enclosed within our skin.

This systemic metabolic respiratory motion of the whole was described by Dr William Garner Sutherland as *primary respiration*. He described it as primary because it comes before thoracic respiration and it proceeds and prepares the embryo for adult breathing. This is why understanding the embryology of breathing and how it precedes and prepares the embryo for adult breathing patterns is crucial to our understanding of function and form as osteopaths.

Venous structures have slightly more restraint than arteries because the endothelial cells of veins grow even more slowly than those in the arteries. This restraint is a reflection of the slightly slower flow rate in the veins, which exert less pressure.

In Figure 2.10, note how closely aligned the jugular vein is with the sinus transversus (posterior attachment of the tentorium cerebelli) and the sphenoparietal sinus (within the anterior dural girdle), which become part of the reciprocal tension membrane. The jugular vein and in fact all venous structures are embedded and continuous with the cranial dural and periosteal membranes.

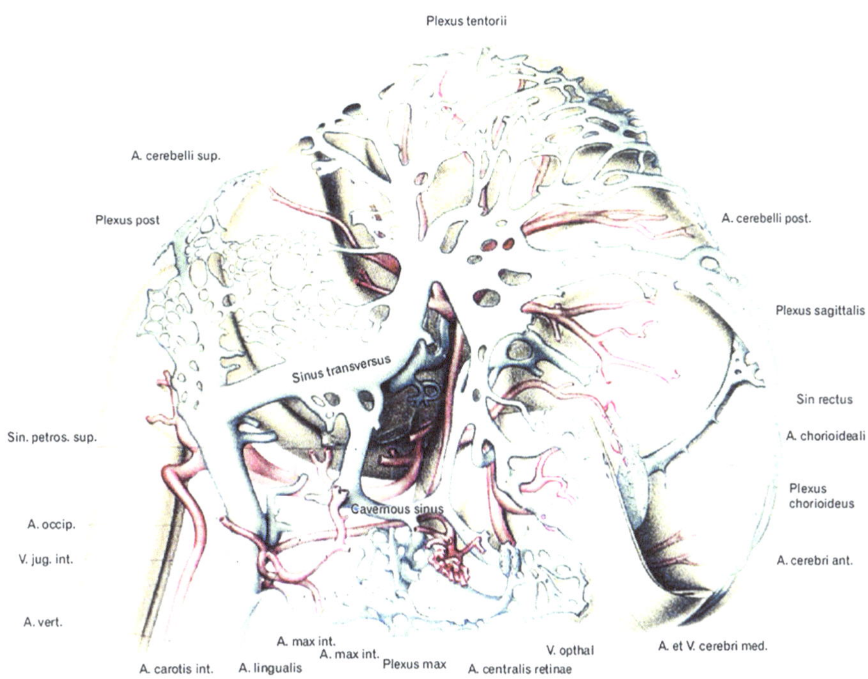


**Figure 2.10 – The Meningeal Compartment.** The main vessels of the meningeal compartment of a 50-day-old embryo as drawn by George Streeter in 1918.[18] Reprinted from Marín-Padilla.[19]

As illustrated in Figure 2.11, vascular development occurs in relation to the demand of the tissues it supplies, and the spacing of the vessels is precise to meet the demands of the tissues. Capillaries must be within 150 µm of every cell for cells to be viable.

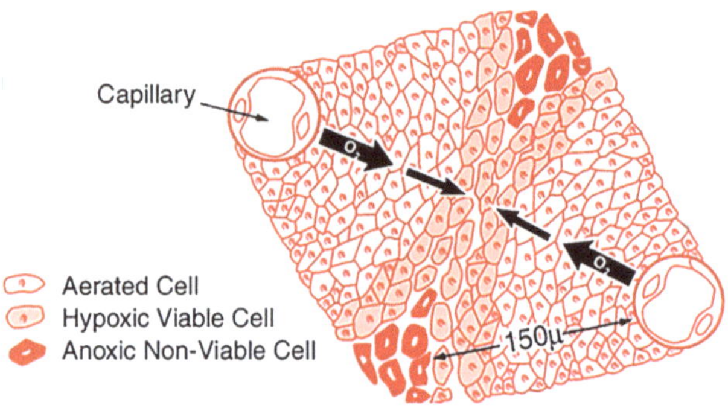


**Figure 2.11– Oxygen Diffusion Through Tissue.** Oxygen diffuses an average of 150 microns from the capillary at 37°C in living tissue. Beyond 150 to 200 microns, cells are anoxic and nonviable, whereas cells at the periphery of this radius are hypoxic but viable. As a consequence, the vascular system develops in such a way that it continuously adapts the supply of oxygen and other nutrients to the needs and morphology of the brain. Reprinted with permission from Springer under Creative Commons CC-BY 4.0 licence.[20]

In choosing the words "rule of the artery," Dr Still was not random[21]; he thought deeply and spent many years in dissection and in the observation of nature before putting pen to paper. Rules can be interpreted as guides, and a ruler can be interpreted as a tool used to measure or as someone who is in charge. All of these interpretations apply to the "rule" of the artery and vein.

## Growth Breathing

By the end of the second month of gestation, early in the third month, the 30-mm embryo has developed everything that is required for breathing.

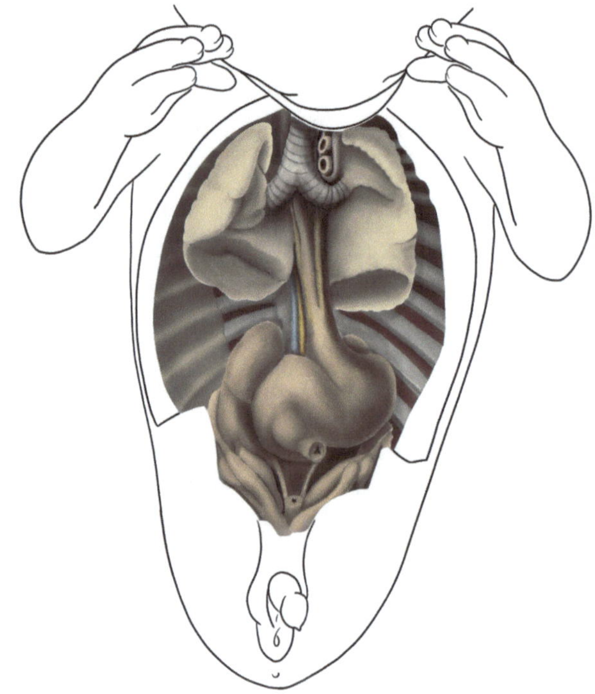

**Figure 2.12 – Organs of Respiration in a 3-Month-Old Embryo (30 mm).** Illustration by Hugh France.

As shown in Figure 2.12, early in the third month of gestation, there are the three lobes of the right lung, the slightly straighter trachea on that side, and the bifurcation of the trachea, asymmetrical in relation to the two lobes on the left (the liver has been removed to illuminate these aspects of the superior mediastinum). All gross anatomy is in place by the end of the second month.

In Figure 2.13, in the transverse section in the left image, where the lungs are developing, there are two little lung buds. The right image depicts a 4-week-old embryo. There is an endodermal tube, and structures are shown growing from the endodermal tube.

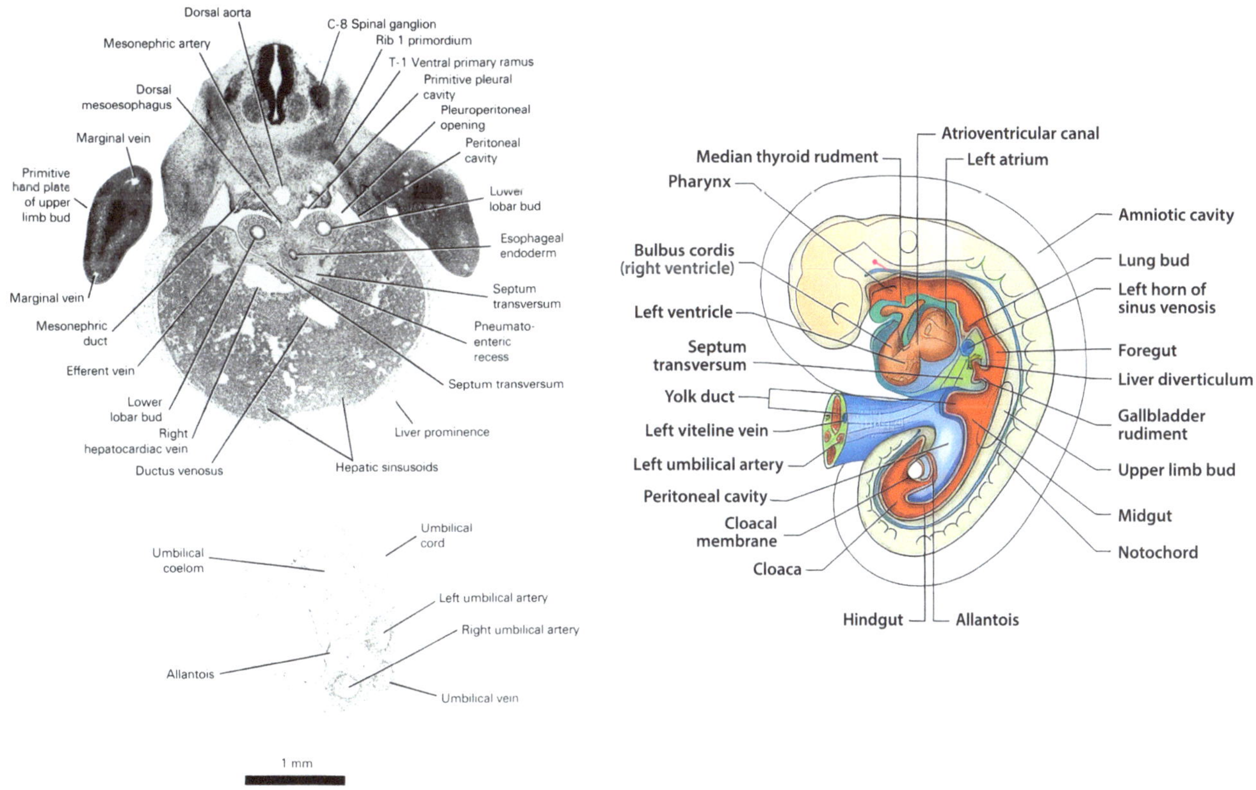


**Figure 2.13 – Lung Development in Early Gestation.** Transverse section of an embryo at 5 weeks (right) and illustration of development at 4 weeks (left). Reprinted from Standring[22] and Gasser.[23]

It is possible to consider everything growing off the endodermal tube to just be a gland. The stomach is a gland growing off that endodermal tube; the trachea branches off from that endodermal tube; then two little lung buds develop early in the third month.

The liver in an embryo grows as a semi-solid jelly; it widens and descends relative to the brain and completely traverses the width of the embryo, so it is directly related to the diaphragm. The liver is bigger on the right, as it is predominantly a right-sided organ, and it grows like an expanding piston. With every little bit of growth the embryo goes through, the liver gets a little bit wider, a little bit larger and a little bit heavier, and it drags on the adjacent tissues. As the neural tube expands and lifts, the diaphragm drops, resulting in **the growth dynamic of a suction field** for the lungs to develop into. There is a hunger for nutrients and the need for venous evacuation. In "The Biodynamic Model of Osteopathy in the Cranial Field," John McPartland summarised Blechschmidt's discussion on metabolic fields:

> "Blechschmidt elaborated six different mechanisms by which fluids "behave internally," creating function out of which emerges structure: contusion, distusion, dilatation, retension, detraction,

> and densation. Later he added corrosion, loosening, and suction mechanisms. These mechanisms are driven by the metabolism of cellular tissues. Cell metabolism potentizes or depletes various fluids."[24]

Shea suggested that Blechschmidt originally said that when the newly fertilised zygote starts moving, there is a reciprocal movement in its fluids. Blechschmidt called this a *suction field* and said that this was the pre-exercising of the respiratory function.[25] However, Blechschmidt himself said that "zones adjacent to limiting tissues, in which suction arises during growth, are known as **suction fields**....For example, they can arise when the more rapidly growing epithelium tends to lift away from the more slowly growing stroma."[26]

The suction field has more force on one side than the other side, so there is more drag on the right lung, which thus forms three lobes. In contrast, the left lung forms two lobes to accommodate the developing heart. Thus, these growth movements explain the growth functions.

Considering the vectors of the growth of the lungs, there is the space expanding posteriorly with the straightening of the spine; there is the space expanding superiorly with the growth of the brain; and then there is the space expanding inferiorly with the liver and anteriorly with the heart.

These are all the vectors for lung growth laterally, superiorly, medially, and inferiorly, and they all relate to the anatomy and functions. Figure 2.14 A and B illustrate the development of these lung buds in relation to surrounding tissue. The first lung cell buds from the sides of the endodermal tube. This occurs in the upper cervical somites and, as the lungs grow, they carry this innervation, which becomes the phrenic nerve. Observe the future mouth, the pharyngeal pouches and the first two lung buds, which are asymmetrical. Observe two little cells, one slightly bigger than the other because the suction forces underneath and around it are a little bit stronger.

In Figure 2.15, note how the space is expanding, allowing the wedge-shaped cells to grow and expand into a watery cavity (intraembryonic coelom). The

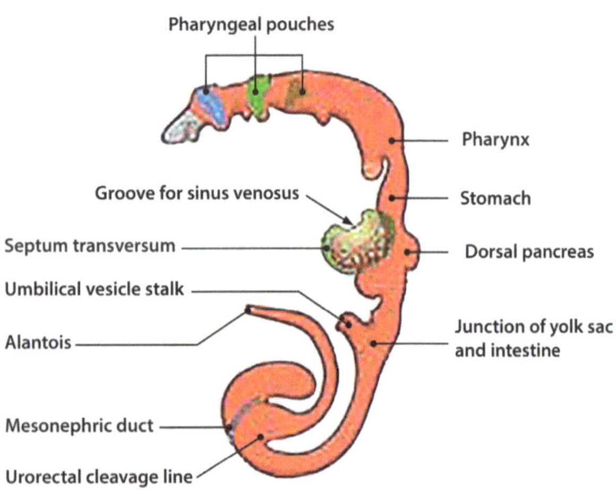


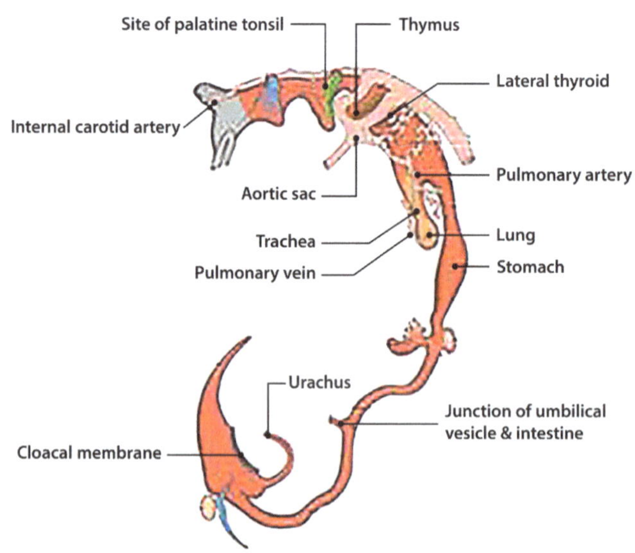


**Figure 2.14 A and B – Development of Lung Buds.** Illustrations of a cross-section of developing lung buds in a human embryo at stage 12 (left) and stage 13 (right). Reprinted from Standring's *Gray's Anatomy*.[27]

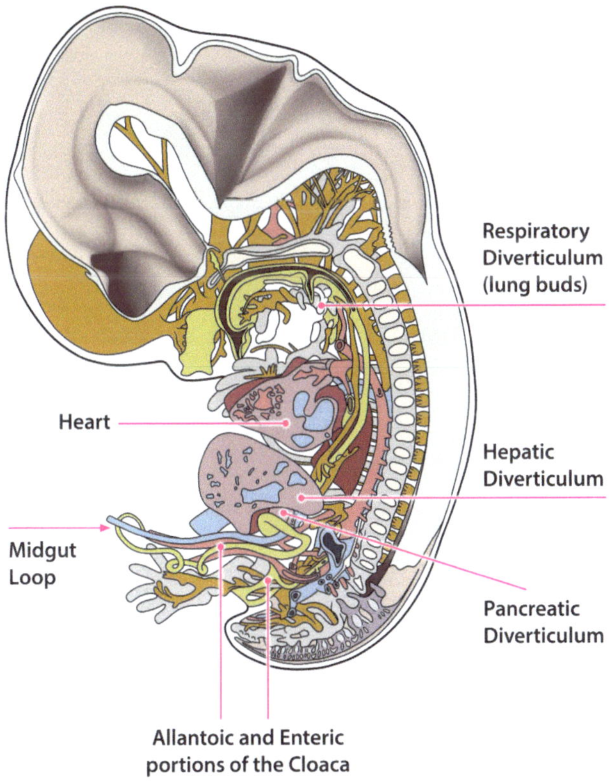


**Figure 2.14 B – Lung Development in Embryo.** An illustration of developing lung buds within surrounding tissues. Note the separation of the respiratory diverticulum, the elongation of the foregut and expansion of the stomach, the formation of the hepatic and pancreatic diverticula, the lengthening of the midgut loop which protrudes into the umbilical cord, and the separation of the cloaca into enteric and allantoic portions. Illustration by Hugh France.

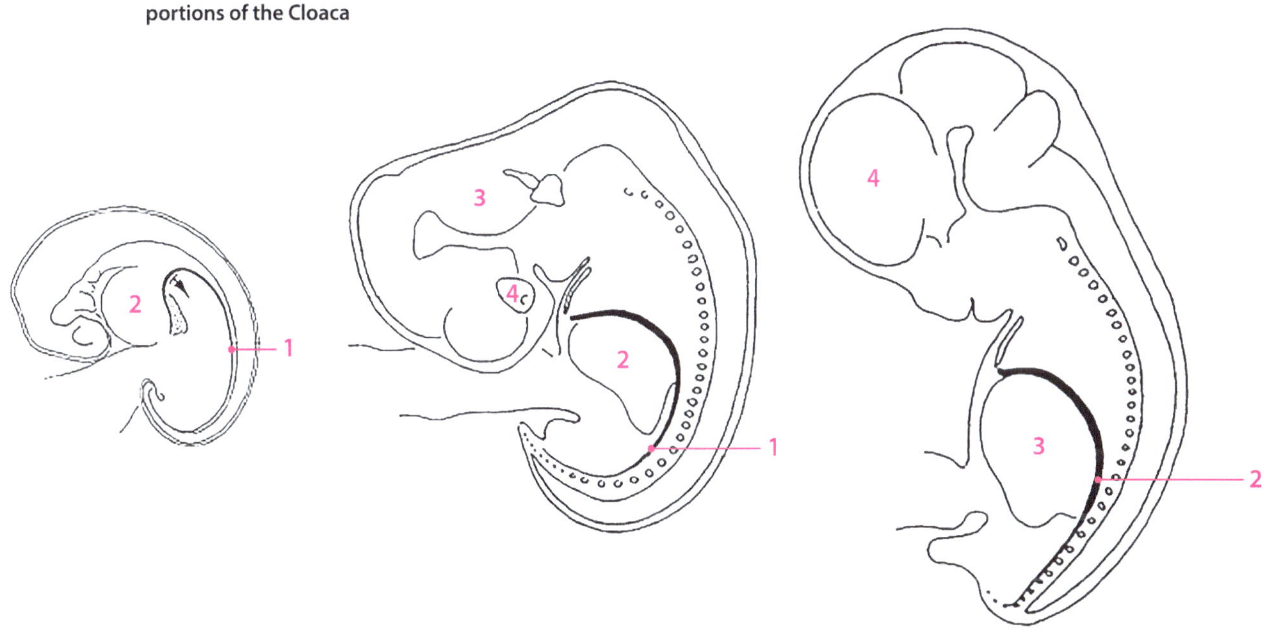


**Figure 2.15 – Developing Mediastinum.**
**Left:** Human embryo 4.2 mm long (Carnegie stage 13). 1 = inferiorly attached part of diaphragm, 2 = heart bulge.
**Middle:** Human embryo 10 mm long (Carnegie stage 17). The diaphragm has descended relative to the cranial end of the vertebral column. 1 = diaphragm in lumbar region, 2 = liver, 3 = hindbrain with otic vesicle, 4 = eye.
**Right:** Human embryo 29 mm long (Carnegie stage 23). The embryo has become relatively narrow in the neck region during extension of the trunk and descent of the heart, liver, and diaphragm. 1 = vertebral column, 2 = angle between vertebral column and diaphragm (vertebral diaphragmatic recess), 3 = inferior part of diaphragm, 4 = right cerebral hemisphere. Reprinted from Blechschmidt.[28]

diaphragm is at the superior margin of the liver and the mesenchyme is compressed into the central tendon between the liver, heart and lungs. The liver is larger on the right, as is the lung, because of stored elastic energy. This stored elastic energy is very important.

What is seen in Figure 2.15 is that early on in the embryo, there is a small liver, a heart bulge and the future diaphragm, which is connected to all of the tissues. Then, with another growth movement (middle drawing), the space for the lungs and the function of the mediastinum expands with the growth of the whole. In the third image, it is getting closer to looking like the future child. The lungs develop in the expanding suction cavity, which draws the lungs into that space.

The lung field is larger on the right-hand side because the drag and the pull of the liver was more powerful on that side. This is what Blechschmidt described as the elastic recoil or the stored elastic energy in the liver.[29] So, there is an expanding piston (liver) dragging on the related fascia and then recoiling. All of the lung tissue, the lung parenchyma, is exposed to the suction-compression, expansion-contraction and growth torsions, and that condenses elastic fibres in the intercellular spaces. It is those growth movements that are kneaded into the tissues so as to have a contractile quality (Figure 2.16).

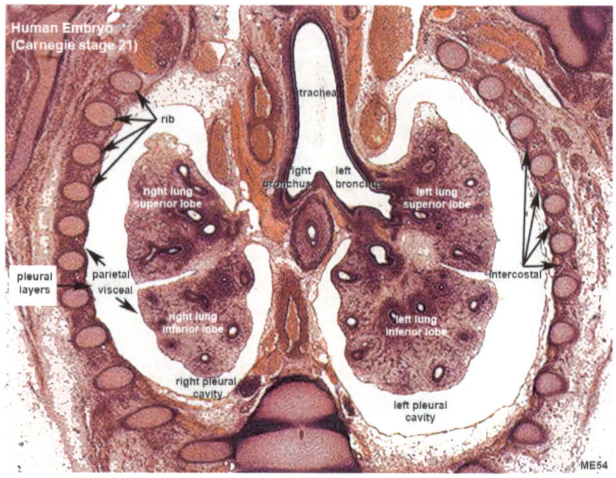


**Figure 2.16 A – Human Embryo Stage 21: Growth Inspiration**. As the embryo grows into extension, there is an inspiratory movement of fluids, which are paving the way for adult breathing. The fluids are byproducts of metabolism, which ebb into the spaces between the cells and are drawn in through the stomodeum. Each movement gradually dissolves the oropharyngeal membrane. Reprinted from Hill.[30]

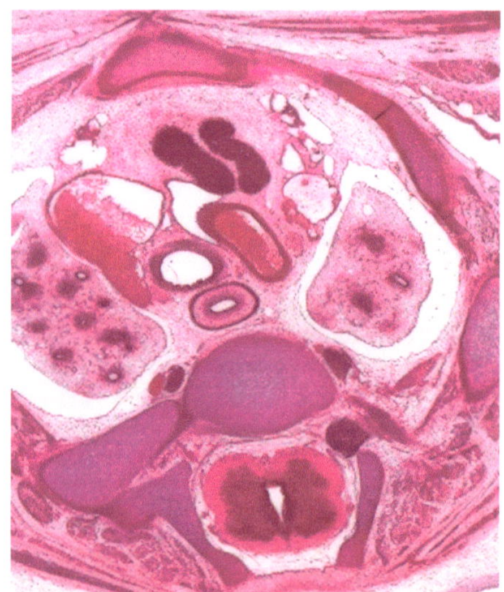

**Figure 2.16 B – Human Embryo Stage 21: Growth Expiration**. As the embryo grows into flexion, the fluids ebb out of the embryo and into the surrounding amnion. The movement of amniotic fluid ebbs in and out with the growth movements, at first taking days to complete a cycle but gradually developing into adult patterns. Reprinted from Hill.[31]

In his lectures, Freeman described the lungs as the elastic engines of the thorax. The lungs expand in relation to atmospheric pressure, but this expansion is not solely because of muscular action. The atmosphere is pushing on us at approximately 10 $kg/cm^2$ (14.7 $lbs/inch^2$). So, atmospheric pressure pushes into the lungs, expands them, and then the elastic recoil allows the lungs to expire. They grew that way and so they function that way. Easy, normal breathing should be effortless due to atmospheric pressure and the elastic recoil of the lungs.

Figure 2.17 illustrates "growth breathing", and the red colouring represents the developing lung field. There is a small suction field where the lung grows. As the growth occurs, the lungs develop into that field, and all of the organs and the functions around them relate to the anatomy of the lungs.

This rhythmic growth can be seen in the serial sections of an embryo seen in Figure 2.17. Growth inspiration and expiration are seen as the embryo grows into extension. There is an inspiratory movement of fluids, which paves the way for future breathing. The fluids are byproducts of metabolism that ebb into the spaces between the cells and are drawn in through the stomodeum. Each movement gradually dissolves the oropharyngeal membrane.

In Figure 2.17, you can also see flexion/inspiration on the above right and extension/expiration just below on the right. If this were live, coiling and uncoiling would also be seen. If it were possible to show three dimensions, the growth torsions that are occurring simultaneously would be observable. The top half rotates forward (anteriorly) and the bottom half rotates backward (posteriorly). The liver acts as an expanding piston. The principle that applies to this process is that the mediastinum and the functions of the lungs will develop in this area in relation to the context of the whole.

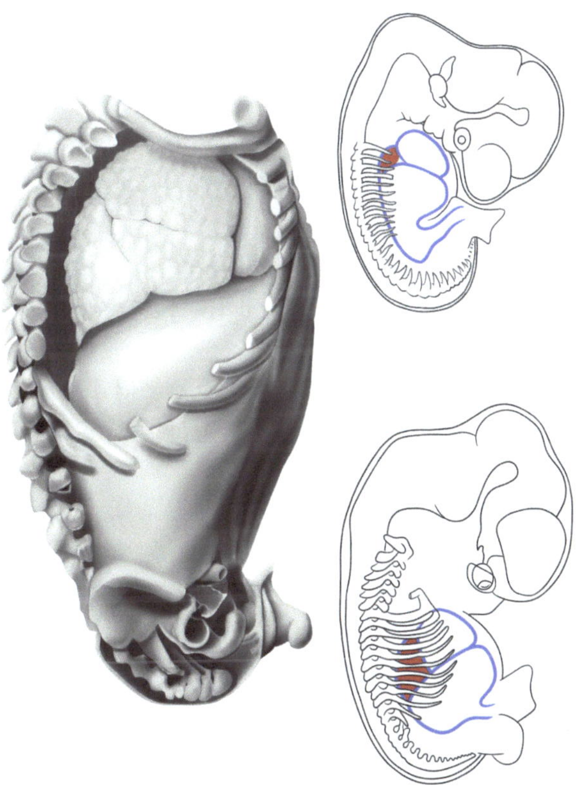

**Figure 2.17 – Development of the Organs of Respiration.** The lung field (depicted in red) develops before the lungs. Illustrations by Hugh France.

Freeman brought our attention to the fact that breathing is not only an outcome of muscular action. It is important to recognise that, as elastic engines, the lungs respond to atmospheric pressure. All anatomy is a condensation of function. The liver, the heart and the head respond to thoracic respiration in the same way that they contributed embryologically to the growth movements of the lungs.

A video posted online by Emmanuel Roche provides an excellent view of respiration. Please take a moment to watch the YouTube video, which you can access by visiting https://www.youtube.com/shorts/K1gZ2DrPRrE or by scanning this QR code:

The video shows a lateral view, highlighting the dome of the liver. Notice how every cell is responding to thoracic respiration. The lung field, the kidney, the viscera, and the response of **every** cell to thoracic respiration and therefore primary respiration, which gave birth to thoracic respiration, is visible. Observe the spiralling movements of blood in the abdominal aorta, the coiling and uncoiling of the heart and the response of the liver to the breathing movements. It grew that way; it functions that way. Every single cell is connected: reciprocal biomechanical cohesion via metabolism. It happens between two cells, it happens between two **trillion** cells.

In the video, the superior mediastinum, which contains some musculature that runs from the sternum up into the neck, can also be observed. The thymus can be found in the superior mediastinum along with lymph nodes, the thoracic duct, the brachiocephalic vein and brachiocephalic trunk, the subclavian arteries and veins, the left common carotid artery, the aortic arch, the trachea, the esophagus, the vagus, the phrenic and recurrent laryngeal nerves and more.

Observe, too, the anterior, middle and posterior divisions of the inferior mediastinum. The middle mediastinum is broad and contains the heart and the pericardium, the ascending aorta, superior vena cava, tracheal bifurcation, both main bronchi, pulmonary trunk, right and left pulmonary arteries and veins and the phrenic nerve.

The diagram in Figure 2.18 shows the connection between the hyoid bone, the pharyngeal fascias, the thyroid fascias and the trachea coming down into the pericardial tissue and then connected to the diaphragm. The septum transversum and the heart and the brain are all directly connected.

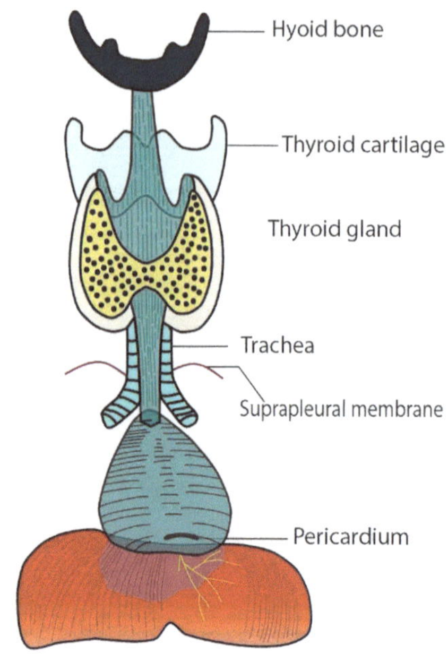


**Figure 2.18 – Connection of the Pretracheal Fascia From the Hyoid to Diaphragm.** Reprinted with permission from Prue Eddie.

## Applications to Osteopathic Practice

The development of the lungs, the mediastinum, and thoracic respiration occurs in a suction field, which precedes and prepares the embryo for future functions. This suction field develops in a region where the early lungs will grow into an expanding space, and the ebb and flow of fluids in and out of the lungs precedes expiration and inspiration of air.

The examination of breathing becomes an experience of whole body biomechanics to identify organs or soma that may be restricting the quality and quantity of the breath.

The elastic recoil of the lungs, which optimises the efficiency of breathing, is palpated in the context of the lungs responding to atmospheric pressure. The lungs, as the elastic engines of the thorax, are perceived as primary in the biomechanics of breathing.

The response of the ribs, muscles and diaphragm is understood to augment thoracic respiration.

Patients describe ailments and symptoms that often appear unrelated. When these clues are viewed through a biodynamic lens and the living connections with which they grew, the symptoms often make sense. A unique anatomical pattern emerges in every encounter with a patient, and this pattern of compensatory distortions helps explain the source of the symptoms and provides clues as to the cause of the problem. An understanding of the living connections between cells, organs, and tissues can be of great benefit to our patients.

## Chapter 2 Endnotes

1. A.T. Still, *Autobiography of Andrew Taylor Still* (Kirksville, MO: A.T. Still, 1908), 149.

2. Brian Freeman, "The Heart Arises at the Transverse Confluence of Two Tubes, not From Their Lengthwise Fusion," Powerpoint Presentation, *Drawing on Anatomy: Art and Science of the Human Body*, http://www.drawingonanatomy.com.au/newsD/index.html.

3. Erich Blechschmidt, *The Ontogenetic Basis of Human Anatomy: A Biodynamic Approach to Development From Conception to Birth* (Berkeley: North Atlantic Books, 2004).

4. Erich Blechschmidt and Raymond F. Gasser, *Biokinetics and Biodynamics of Human Differentiation: Principles and Applications* (Springfield, IL: Charles Thomas Publishing, 1978).

5. Guy Dudley Hulett, *A Text Book of the Principles of Osteopathy* (Kirksville, MO: Journal Printing Company, 1906).

6. Nan Cheney, *Hemisection of Head*, 1951, Clinical Anatomy, University of British Columbia, accessed April 13, 2023, http://www.clinicalanatomy.ca/illustrationsCheney.html#chenBrain.

7. Blechschmidt, *The Ontogenetic Basis of Human Anatomy.*

8. Georg-August-Universität Göttingen,"Provenance research 'The Blechschmidt Collection,'" The University of Göttingen Centre of Anatomy, accessed April 5, 2023, https://www.uni-goettingen.de/en/575416.html

9. Mark A. Hill, "Carnegie Stage 6," in *Embryology,* The University of New South Wales, last modified October 5, 2018, https://embryology.med.unsw.edu.au/embryology/index.php/Carnegie_stage_6.

10. Henry Gray, "Ovum Embedded in Uterine," in *Anatomy of the Human Body* (Philadelphia: Lea & Febiger, 1918), accessed September 26, 2023, https://commons.wikimedia.org/wiki/File:Gray32.png.

11. Blechschmidt, *The Ontogenetic Basis of Human Anatomy*, figure 5-9, p 128.

12. Blechschmidt, *The Ontogenetic Basis of Human Anatomy*, figure 10-5, p 131.

13. Lara Planas-Paz et al, "Mechanoinduction of lymph vessel expansion," *The EMBO Journal* 31, no. 4 (February 2012): 788-804, https://10.1038/emboj.2011.456.

14. Blechschmidt and Gasser, *Biokinetics and Biodynamics of Human Differentiation.*

15. Blechschmidt, *The Ontogenetic Basis of Human Anatomy*, figure 4.11, p 104.

16. Blechschmidt, *The Ontogenetic Basis of Human Anatomy*, 102.

17. *Flight: The Genius of Birds,* directed by Lad Allen (Illustria Media), originally released May 14, 2013, accessed October 12, 2023, https://www.youtube.com/watch?v=-Ah-gT0hTto.

18. George L. Streeter, "The Developmental Alterations in the Vascular System of the Brain in the Human Embryo," *Contributions to Embryology* 8 (1918): 5–38.

19. Miguel Marín-Padilla, "The Human Brain Intracerebral Microvascular System: Development and Structure," *Frontiers in Neuroanatomy* 6 (September 2012): 38, https://doi.org/10.3389/fnana.2012.00038.

20. Timothy J. Kinsella, Jason Sohn, and Barry Wessels, "Principles of Radiation Oncology," in *Oncology: An Evidence-Based Approach*, eds. Alfred Change et al (New York: Springer, 2006), 594, https://doi.org/ 10.1007/0-387-31056-8_3.

21. A.T. Still, *Autobiography of Andrew T. Still With a History of the Discovery and Development of the Science of Osteopathy* (Kirksville, MO: published by the author, 1897): 219.

22. "Chapter 73: Development of the Peritoneal Cavity, Gastrointestinal Tract and Its Adnexae," in *Gray's Anatomy: The Anatomical Basis for Clinical Practice*, ed. Susan Standring (UK: Elsevier, 2020), accessed October 28, 2020, https://clinicalgate.com/development-of-the-peritoneal-cavitygastrointestinal-tract-and-its-adnexae/

23. Raymond F. Gasser, "Chapter VI: The Sixth Week of Life: Late Bronchial Arch and Limb Bud Period," *Atlas of Human Embryos*, figure 6-17, accessed April 13, 2023 https://www.ehd.org/classics/gasser_ch6.php.

24. John M. McPartland and Evelyn Skinner, "The Biodynamic Model of Osteopathy in the Cranial Field," *EXPLORE* 1, no. 1 (January 2005): 21-32.

25. Michael Shea, "What does 'Biodynamic' Mean? Implications for Manual Therapists"(Michael Shea, PhD, 2006), https://bti.edu/pdfs/Shea_The-Meaning-of-Biodynamic.pdf.

26. Blechschmidt, *The Ontogenetic Basis of Human Anatomy*, 74.

27. "Chapter 73: Development of the Peritoneal Cavity, Gastrointestinal Tract and Its Adnexae."

28. Blechschmidt, *The Ontogenetic Basis of Human Anatomy*, 176.

29. Blechschmidt, *The Ontogenetic Basis of Human Anatomy*.

30. Mark A. Hill, "Respiratory System Development," in *Embryology*, accessed July 27, 2023, https://embryology.med.unsw.edu.au/embryology/index.php/Respiratory_System_Development.

31. Hill, "Respiratory System Development."

Chapter Three

# Water, Flow and Function

*"Comprehend and copy nature."*
- Viktor Schauberger

*"Life is water dancing to the tune of solids."*
- Gerald H. Pollack

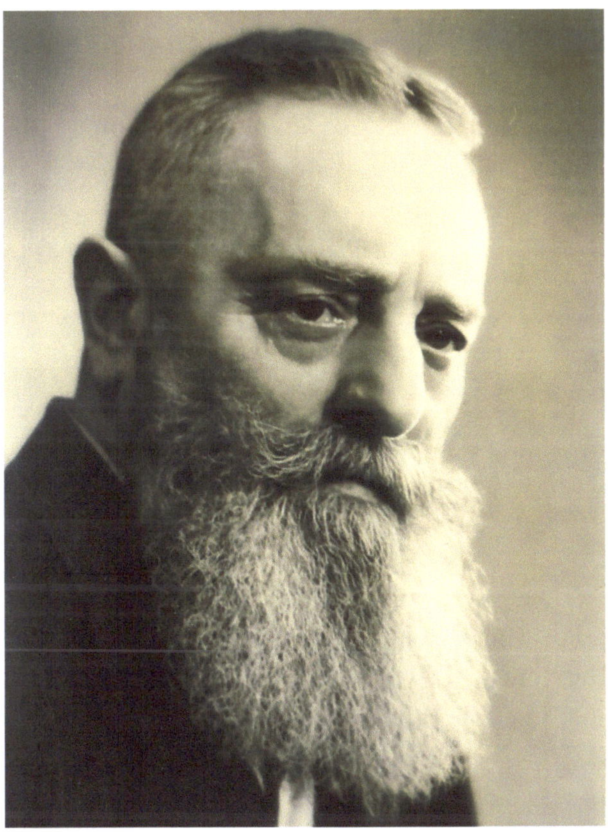

**Figure 3.1 – Viktor Schauberger, February 28, 1938.** Viktor Schauberger, Forest Scientist (June 1885–September 1958). © Schauberger Archive.

The insights provided by naturalist and inventor Viktor Schauberger on the combination of charge and spiralling of water was the genesis of the Rule of the Artery programs that we have taught in Australia, New Zealand, Europe and the United States. So, we begin this chapter on water with a brief description of his work.

Schauberger (pictured in Figure 3.1) came from a long line of foresters. At age 18, with the support of his mother, he refused to follow in the footsteps of his two elder brothers and attend university. He did not want to have his natural way of thinking moulded by people he considered to have lost contact with nature. Instead, he became a warden in a remote forest in Austria. It was here that Schauberger gained his inspiration from studying the water of fast-flowing streams in pristine forested areas.

From his intense and astute observation of nature he developed an understanding of implosion, the phenomena of spirals or vortexes that occur in liquids and gases throughout the natural world. These phenomena have "a concentrating, ordering effect and decrease the temperature of the medium, in opposition to the dictates of 'modern' thermodynamics".[1] According to his Implosion theory, the process results in no destruction or pollution.

In 1937, Schauberger applied his theory in designing an implosion motor, which produced a thrust of 1,290 m/sec, considerably out-performing other motors of the era.[2] According to electrical engineer, Swedish conservationist and author of *Living Waters* Olof Alexandersson, Schauberger "...developed his Trout Turbine, named after his observations of trout moving upstream. Later renamed the *Implosion Machine*, it could generate power without fuel. The implosion motor is centripetally operated. It produces its own driving source through the diamagnetic use of water and air. It does not require any other fuel such as coal, oil, uranium or energy derived from atom splitting, since it can produce its own energy (atomic power) by biological means in unlimited amounts—almost without cost."[3]

Schauberger developed what he called his "natural way of thinking" on which he relied for the rest of his life. He described his thought process succinctly:

> "The majority believes that everything hard to comprehend must be very profound. This is incorrect. What is hard to understand is what is immature, unclear and often false. The highest wisdom is simple and passes through the brain directly into the heart."[4]

The following description illustrates Schauberger's "natural way of thinking" in his observations of the behaviour of trout in the alpine streams that he frequented.

> "It was spawning time one early spring moonlit night. I was sitting beside a waterfall waiting to catch a dangerous fish poacher. Something then happened so quickly; I was hardly able to grasp it. The moonlight falling onto the crystal clear water picked up every movement of a large shoal of fish gathered in the pool. Suddenly they dispersed as a big fish swam into the pool from below, preparing to confront the waterfall. It seemed as though it wanted to scatter the other trout as it quickly darted to and fro in great twisting movements.
>
> "Then, just as suddenly, the large trout disappeared into the huge jet of falling water that shone like molten metal. I could see it fleetingly, under a conically shaped stream of water, dancing in a wild, spinning movement, which at that moment didn't make sense to me. When it stopped spinning it seemed then to float motionlessly upward. On reaching the lower curve of the waterfall it tumbled over and with a strong push reached behind the upper curve of the fall. There, in the fast-flowing water, and with a strong movement of the tail, it disappeared.
>
> "Often subsequently, I witnessed the same sequence of behaviour of a trout leaping up a high waterfall. After decades of similar observations that manifested like rows of pearls on a chain, I should be able to come to some conclusion. But no scientist has been able to explain the phenomenon to me.
>
> With the right lighting, it is possible to see the path of levitational currents as an empty tube within the veil of a waterfall. It is similar to the tunnel in the middle of a circulating vortex of water plunging down a drain, which brings up a gurgling sound. This downwardly-directed whirlpool drags everything with increasing suction with it into the depths. If you can imagine this whirlpool or watercyclone operating vertically, you get the picture of how the levitational current works and you can see how the trout appears to be floating upward in the axis of fall."[5]

There were many questions that Schauberger asked himself following this observation. How did the trout actually manage to find just the right spot that was cut off by a 16-meter waterfall? How was it able to flee upstream in the waterfall, like a streak of lightning, against the laws of gravity? How was it possible for this fish to stand motionlessly, steering itself with the slightest of movements of its tail fins, in the wildly torrential flow of water?

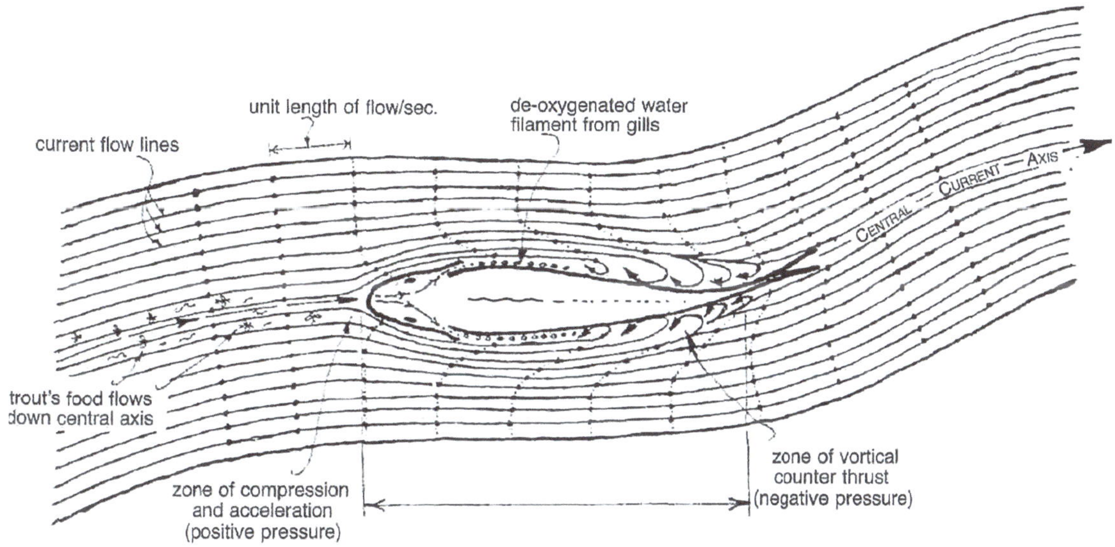


**Figure 3.2 – Diagram of a Trout Swimming Upstream.** Image courtesy of Callum Coats.[8]
The following QR code will lead you to a more detailed explanation from Coats:

Schauberger's observations and a gradual and growing understanding of the fundamentals of the flow of water led him towards his many groundbreaking inventions.

From his observations, Schauberger concluded that the trout was best able to hold its position where the water was coldest, densest and had the most potential energy. Schauberger thought that the gills of the fish acted like guide vanes, which could direct the water flow into a powerful backward vortex, and that the scales, whilst minimising friction with the water, also created scores more of tiny vortices with the effect of amplifying the upstream counter-current.

The trout swimming upstream (depicted in Figure 3.2) became the basis for Schauberger's implosion "flying saucer", which would utilise a vortex engine that "used friction between vortices and the surrounding air to force the air downwards, thus creating an overall lifting effect".[6] Modern researchers are currently attempting to develop a "flying saucer" utilising science very similar to Schauberger's principles and designs.[7]

Another illuminating experience occurred one winter night when Schauberger was hunting and his quarry (a large elk buck) had fallen into a deep ravine. As he tried to retrieve it, he lost his footing and slid and tumbled to the bottom of a snow chute, landing near a stream. As he stood to survey his exit strategy, he noticed something strange happening in the stream at his feet. Because of ice dams and other obstructions, there wasn't much current, but he watched several green logs sink to the bottom, and then rise back to the surface. More curious still, he watched as a large stone "began to gyrate on the bottom, and then came to the surface, where it was immediately surrounded by a halo of ice".[9] He saw this happen with several other stones and after further observation concluded that water could carry heavier loads when below a certain temperature. This observation also demonstrated the principle of levitation that Schauberger applied in his later work.

Experts considered Schauberger completely mad and said so often and publicly. All of that changed in 1922, when a chance meeting with Princess Schaumburg-Lipp led to a meeting with Prince Adolf zu Schaumburg-Lippe. Princess Schaumburg-Lipp was a big fan of the gambling establishments of Monte Carlo and had brought the family to the brink of bankruptcy. The Prince hoped to avoid such humiliation by selling off timber in his forests where Schauberger was a warden, but because of the trees' location, he feared most of the timber would be destroyed in the conventional methods of log transport by oxen. Hoping there were some better ideas out there, he offered a prize for the engineer who could get most of the timber down the mountain intact.

Schauberger said that he could design a system to float the logs down the creeks, which would reduce overall costs by 90 percent. Other engineers called his plan ridiculous arguing that oak and beech were too heavy to float.

Schauberger submitted his plans, which utilised the lessons he had learned from his observations and conclusions about water's movement in nature. His plan would require the work be completed on very cold nights in troughs with slats of larchwood angled to "implode" the flowing water. The Prince gave him a chance on the condition that he footed the bill for construction costs until his plans proved true. When it came time to implement his plan, "The heavy logs went forward like bullets shooting out of a rifle. They twisted about their own axis without ever bumping against the walls of the trough, even at full capacity."[10] Schauberger's plan was so successful experts came from all over Europe to study the flume.[11,12]

To watch the original 1930 film on Schauberger's project *Tragendes Wasser*, visit https://m.youtube.com/watch?v=QWsUGpKfP8A or scan the following URL code:

More than once, Schauberger challenged professional hydrologists to disprove the principles that he championed. For instance, in 1952 he asked the Stuttgart Technical University to assess an experiment, which he offered to fund, if they would observe the test. He approached Franz Popel, the director of the Institute of Hygiene at that time, who initially refused. However, after Popel was encouraged by the German government to participate (in the hope that Schauberger would be discredited), he agreed to do so.

The test compared the movement of water through eight distinct types of pipe, differentiated by various forms of friction in each pipe. Surprisingly, the straight pipes constructed of glass and copper produced the most friction, while the pipes made with more flexible material had less. Schauberger's creation of the spiral helicoid copper pipe (which had an effect similar to that of the scales on a trout described above) had almost zero friction. It "directed the water flow in an involuting flow movement away from the walls, giving the greatest reduction in friction, to zero or perhaps even below (negative friction or acceleration) at specific velocities."[13]

Sadly, Popel's report omits any mention of the fact that the measured frictional values went below the line of frictional values (negative friction), which is a paradox in physics and which Popel was unable or unwilling to contemplate/comprehend.

Fluid **motion** and **temperature** became the two cornerstones of Schauberger's theories and discoveries. Based on his prolonged and careful studies of water, Schauberger published a paper on "Temperature and the Movement of Water".[14] Central to these was the influence of **minute** differences in **temperature**, which are presently ignored by modern hydraulics and hydrology. Schauberger showed that in natural, living water (conventionally regarded as a homogeneous substance), electrical discharges can be observed. He saw that water was composed of many strata, or layers, with subtle variations in temperature and electric charge that influence the water's motion, its form of flow and its physical properties, inside the vortex. It was Schauberger's recognition of layered water carrying charge that formed the basis for understanding our perception of electrical charge and magnetic field in blood flow.

In paying attention to temperature, Schauberger recognised that, in particular, coolness optimised fluid flow and argued that "small variations in temperature are as crucial to the healthy movement of water and the sap of a tree, as they are to human blood."[15] He paid particular attention to water's variations around the temperature of +4°C (39°F), which is the physical and chemical "anomaly point" of water when it is at its densest and expresses its greatest vitality, health and energy content.

To demonstrate the importance of temperature, Schauberger conducted an experiment with Philipp Forchheimer (an internationally recognised hydrologist). Schauberger arranged for his foresters to build a fire under a large cauldron to heat up the 100 litres of water it contained. This was done about 150 metres upstream from the stationary trout that Viktor was observing. When satisfied that the water was hot enough, Schauberger gave the signal to release the water into the stream. Whilst this had only a minute effect on the temperature of the water in the creek, the trout downstream at Schauberger's observation point were no longer able to hold their stationary position but were swept downstream in the fast flowing water. Forchheimer was astonished because the science of the day did not recognise the importance of very small variations in temperature.

Schauberger had discovered that temperature changes in response to varying patterns/cycles that activate life or trigger the decline of health. He found that "Temperature controls the innate energies that produce the pulsations that punctuate and control all life's processes. These energy pulsations, which at one moment dissociate or disconnect, and at another recombine both energy and matter, are the mechanism for creating the countless individualities and qualities that make up life as we know it."[16]

He realised that cool running water increases its directional, and hence ordered, energy. That ordered energy is much easier to convert into work. He also understood that the dramatic response to a minute change in the temperature of the creek that he was observing was evidence of this.

Schauberger believed that, just as the earth behaves like an organism—with the conditions for life being maintained within very narrow limits, in spite of the enormous variation in the sun's radiation and the effect of harmful cosmic rays—that the human body works in a similar way: as a self-regulating system that maintains the blood temperature in the narrow range essential for health (around 37°C/98.4°F). He also felt that in the right conditions, water creates dynamic structures, mainly vortices where the phenomenon of "implosion" occurs. He observed that suction forces act in the direction from the periphery or edge of the vortex towards its centre and on the other side moves in the opposite direction to the movement of water, thus creating a funnel. This funnel is just like the one described in relation to the trout's ability to appear to effortlessly float upwards in the waterfall whilst spinning.

In pondering the human body's ability to maintain blood temperature at approximately 37°C, we recall that in Chapter 1, we saw that the heart produces a magnetic field that is 5000 times more powerful than that produced by the brain.[17] The magnetic field generated by the muscular activity of the heart varies from moment to moment. This variation of the magnetic field may induce an electromotive force that drives the electric current in the blood, thereby making **minute** changes in the temperature of the blood. It is noteworthy that the formation of a vortex in liquid water occurs at a critical temperature (4°C), the exact measurement at which water has maximum density. Alick Bartholemew in *Hidden Nature* observed that "[t]his seems to work in a similar way to the self-regulating system in the human body that maintains the blood temperature in the narrow range essential for health (around +37°C/98.4°F). A mechanistic scientist would insist that this is just a computer function, but computers don't operate with purpose and meaning."[18]

The second cornerstone of Schauberger's thinking about water was motion. Like Still, Schauberger knew that life is motion and that spirals are basic to many of nature's forms. In water, those spirals become complex vortices that develop order from chaos.

Schauberger saw spirals as a universal expression of nature, from the structure of galaxies down to the atom. In the blood, spirals can be very complex with a central spiralling core and helicoid forms sprouting out from the core. Other examples of spirals are found in tissues such as ligaments and the connective tissue matrix where the triple helix of collagen can be found (Figure 3.3). Spiral fractures can occur within long bones because of the lines of the Haversian canals lying within the bone. The fingerprint is a spiral, as is DNA at the micro level.

Spirals are found in muscles, and Torrent-Guasp showed,[20] by blunt dissection, how the spiraling of the ventricular myocardial band can be understood. He demonstrated how a continuous ventricular myocardial band extends between the points of origin of the right ventricle at the pulmonary artery root to termination at the aortic root in the left ventricle. These components include a spiral, horizontal basal loop that surrounds the right and left ventricular cavities and changes direction to cause a second spiral, produced by almost vertically oriented fibres, giving rise to the helical configuration of the ventricular myocardial band.

In a documentary clip titled *The Helical Heart*, the narrator highlights Torrent-Guasp's findings during the dissection of a heart. To view the full video, visit https://www.youtube.com/watch?v=NHl4DUu1bEI (dissection starts at 6:12). Alternatively, scan the following QR code to be taken to the dissection segment of the video:

Schauberger saw that there is little internal friction between molecules forming a vortex where the water molecules are rotating at similar speeds and

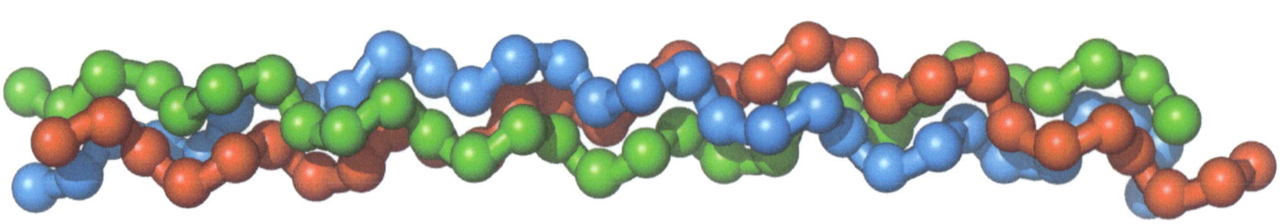

**Figure 3.3 – Triple Helix of Collagen.**[19]

frequencies, such that they behave coherently. The qualities associated with coherence are connectivity and integrity, which result in an ability to maintain that coherence over considerable distance. Spirals facilitate information transfer. Like Still,

> "Schauberger observed that all life is motion. Natural movement is not in straight lines, but in spirals, or in spiraling vortices. Spirals are the actual shape of fluid energy evolving order from chaos. Viktor Schauberger saw them as the natural movement of life, from the structure of galaxies down to the atom. The spiral is the most common vehicle for 'correspondences'— as above, so below.
>
> The spiral can develop in a number of different ways: as a vortex, moving upwards or downwards, round in a circle, or doubling back on itself. Whenever there is movement, spirals form visibly with water; but gases, and even electrical fields, express themselves in spirals or doughnuts. Sinews, tissues, blood and bones and so many formations in organic life are spiral in form.
>
> The vortex is a window between different qualities or levels of energy. The vortex and spiral became hallmarks for Viktor Schauberger. For him they were the key to all creative movement. Creative energy moves spirally in the form of a vortex. The creative process takes place as the energy containing the blueprint of what is being created moves in whatever way it needs to in order to create the system it wishes. It draws down matter as a mirror image of the idea or blueprint. This is why the physical is said to be the shell of the organic reality."[21]

Schauberger would often insist, in a similar vein, that a bird "is flown" and a fish "is swum". On many occasions he said that the heart is not a pump but that it "is pumped". He saw the heart as a regulator of blood flow, the real function of which is to stimulate pulsation in blood flow.[22]

For us, as osteopaths, this last observation of Schauberger's was central to Still's statement that the heart imparts knowledge (information) to the blood.

As described in Chapter 1, when reviewing the literature, we found that the spiralling is intrinsic to the movement of blood. Bremer[23] performed a remarkable series of observations of blood circulation in the 1930s in very early chick embryos—**before** the formation of the heart valves. Bremer filmed the beating embryonic heart in which the already spiralling blood is boosted by the pulsating heart without creating turbulence in the blood.

The Stuttgart experiment, described earlier, revealed that when the water flow was in resonance with the configuration of the pipe, there was no friction. Likewise, resonance between the blood and the capillaries and arteries enhances flow. In addition, blood vessels pulsate naturally in a peristaltic action, the Traube-Hering wave, continuing the influence of the heart into the periphery. The Traube-Hering wave (discussed more fully in Chapter 5) provides an ebb and flow, a tidal motion that provides a tidal wave to which the fractaline helical waves relate.

Around 1927, some years before Bremer, Prof Kurt Bergel of Berlin University recorded this automatic pulsation in small warm blood vessels around the egg sac of a bird's egg a few days after incubation, although no heart had yet been formed. Bergel also rejected the popular theory of the heart as a pump, insisting that this function was carried out by "the millions of highly active capillaries permeating the body" and that "health or disease are primarily dependent on the faultless or disturbed activity of the capillaries".[24]

Bergel thought that the pulsation of the capillaries initiate the circulation of the blood, augmented by the configuration of the blood vessels themselves. As part of this function there was a provision that the viscosity of the blood would be reduced in the finer blood vessels, so that its ability to flow freely would not be compromised!

The total length of blood vessels in the average human adult is estimated to be about 96,500 km (60,000 miles)! On the basis of conventional hydraulic calculation, "it is inconceivable that the actual power output of the heart, about 1.5 watts, would be sufficient for this huge task".[25]

## Gerald Pollack and the Fourth Phase of Water

We now turn to the pioneering and groundbreaking insights of Gerald Pollack, professor of bioengineering at the University of Washington in the USA. Pollack built on the work of predecessors like Szent-Gyorgi, Ling, Gurwitz, Nasonov and Lepeshkin, who questioned the conventional view that even if there was a zone that was organised in bulk water, it would not exceed more than a very few layers—a few nanometres at most. However, Pollack revealed that in the vicinity of hydrophilic surfaces, a very thick layer of charged water (that he termed the *exclusion zone,* or *EZ*) exists and from which solutes are completely excluded.

In 1972, Szent-Gyorgi had shown by experimentation that this layering effect of water could extend outwards for about 500 nm, implying hundreds of adherent layers of water. Prof Pollack was able to show that under certain conditions, the thickness of the EZ reached **hundreds** of **microns.**

The water in this zone was neither solid (ice) nor liquid nor gas (steam). Hydrogen bonding between water molecules (positively charged hydrogen atom on one molecule attracted to negatively charged oxygen atom on another molecule) becomes important. Ice has relatively fixed hydrogen bonds, whereas steam has essentially none. Liquid water is characterised by bonds that distort and break as molecules pass over each other. But EZ water was ice-like, having a hexagonal ring from which one hydrogen molecule had been cleaved off. As can be seen in Figure 3.4, it has a crystalline lattice structure, which Pollack described as $H_3O_2$, or a hydronium ion.

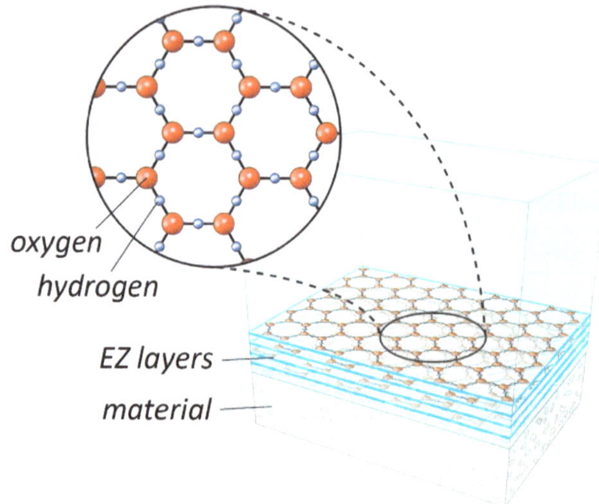


**Figure 3.4 – A Hydronium Ion Honeycomb.** This illustration shows the honeycomb structure of ice-like water in the exclusion zone. Reprinted from Pollack.[26]

In *The Fourth Phase of Water*, Pollack proposed a model for structured water that was essentially a stacking of water molecules (Figure 3.5).

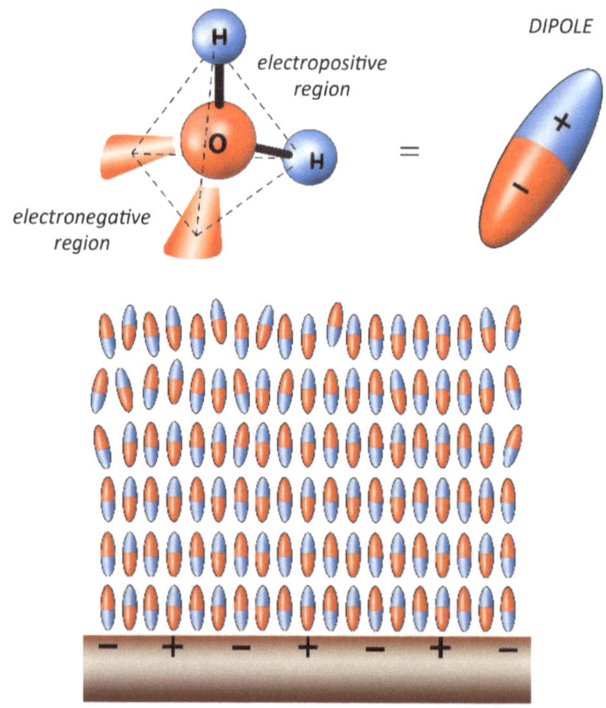


**Figure 3.5 – Structured Water.** In this earlier model, the structure of water is charge driven. Reprinted from Pollack.[27]

Pollack described how he developed a different model (Figure 3.6) based on a hexagonal ring, where one hexagram is slightly offset against the other so that the opposite charges could be linked, thereby maintaining the structure as a whole.[28] Pollack found that the same model had been proposed in 1969 in an article published by Ellis Lippincott in *Science*. Lippincott called it *polywater*.[29]

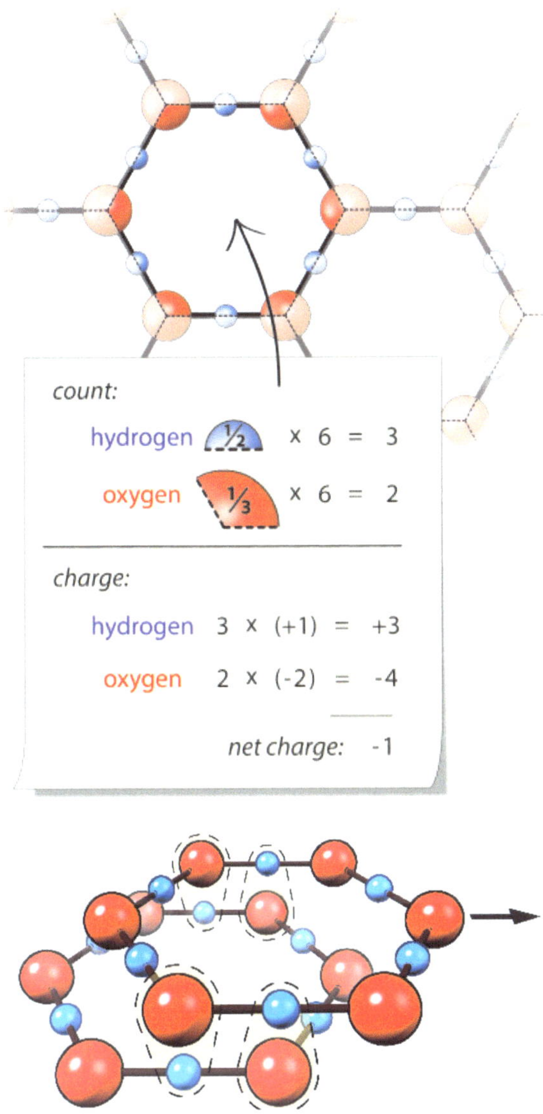


**Figure 3.6 – Hexagonal Ring Model and Shifting Planes.** Structure and charge of the hexagonal ring model (left) and linking allowing shifting planes. Reprinted from Pollack.[30,31]

Pollack was able to show that there is a measurable flow of charge between the EZ and the adjacent water into which the hydronium ions had been moved. Pollack named this "The EZ Battery". However, a pressing question arose: How could such a battery be sustained over time without running down?

It was one of Pollack's postdoctoral fellows, Jim Zheng, who discovered part of the answer. He noticed that when he placed a sheet of nafion (a hydrophilic experimental substance) between it and the EZ zone that was immediately adjacent and switched the microscope lamp on, there was a progressive doubling of the size of the EZ zone. Further enquiry showed that infrared light at 3000 nm was most effective at maintaining an optimal EZ zone (Figure 3.7).

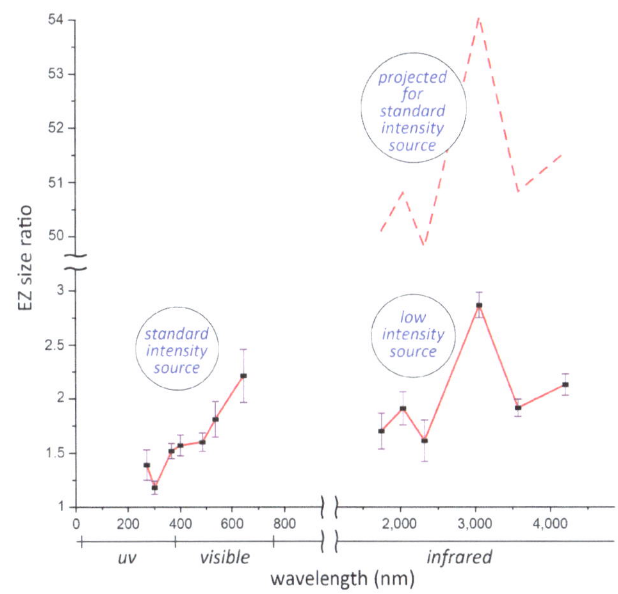


**Figure 3.7 – Effect of Incident Light on Exclusion Zone (EZ) Growth.** Infrared light at 3000 nm has the greatest effect on biowater.[32] Reprinted from Pollack.[33]

Infrared light is ubiquitously present night and day, demonstrating how the EZ zone of structured water could maintain itself indefinitely over time.

Renowned physicist Richard Feynman coined the phrase "like-likes-like through an intermediate of unlikes",[34] and Pollack showed how this could be applied to his model, where positive charges concentrated between the two negatively charged spheres allowed a powerful and electrodynamic attraction between spheres to develop (Figure 3.8).

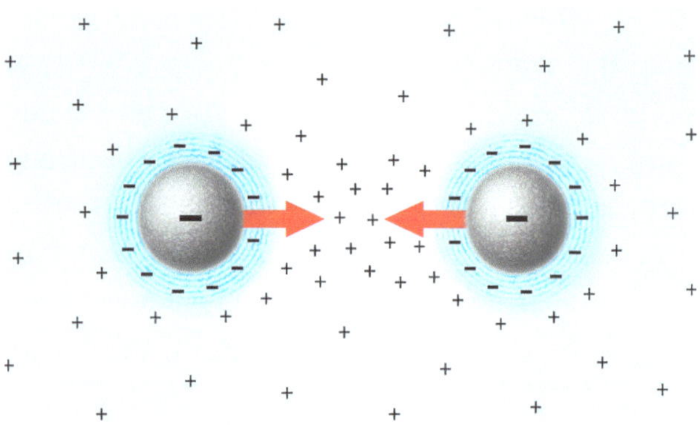

**Figure 3.8 – Attraction Between Spheres.** The space between spheres has opposite polarity, which allows attraction.

This helps to explain the organisation of cellular ensembles in the flow of red blood cells in the vasculature. The red blood cell has a layer of negative charge surrounding it but is able to remain discreetly separate from adjacent red blood cells by virtue of the very thin zone of a positive charge that exists between them (Figure 3.9).

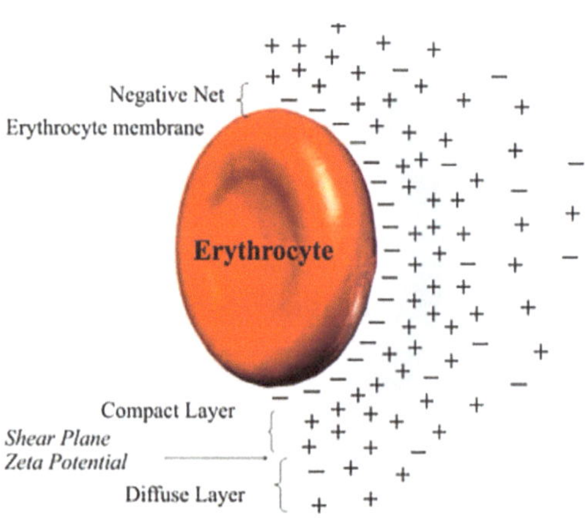


**Figure 3.9 – Red Blood Cell Charge-Based Motion**[35]

This like-likes-like layering of charge has been described as the sheer plane of Zeta potential. Fernandez et al determined that "intermolecular forces may be involved in agglutination with cell clumping occurring when the aggregation force is greater than the force of repulsion. Repulsive force is generated by negative charges on the red blood cell surface that occur due to the presence of the carboxyl group of sialic acids in the cell membrane; these negative charges create a repulsive positive zeta potential between cells."[36]

In the EZ, water is 10 times more viscous than normal water,[37] and so it excludes not only colloidal particles but also high and low molecular solutes. The EZ water is also evenly oriented.

Pollack found that, unlike bulk water that is transparent for UV light right down to 200 nm, the EZ water exhibits a profound peak light absorption at 270 nm and fluoresces when excited at this wavelength, as seen in Figure 3.10.

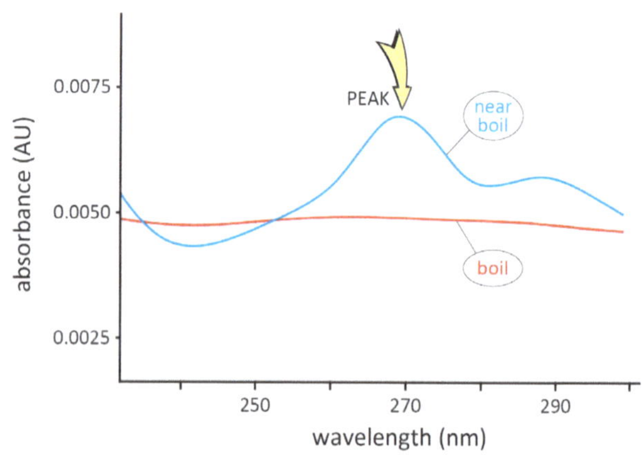


**Figure 3.10 – Exclusion Zone Water at Peak Light Absorption.** Reprinted from Pollack.[38]

Pollack was also able to show how it was possible to have continuous flow occurring through a Nafion tube. Figures 3.11 and 3.12 provide a model for how this might work. The key element is the hydronium ion build-up in the tube core depicted in Figure 3.12.

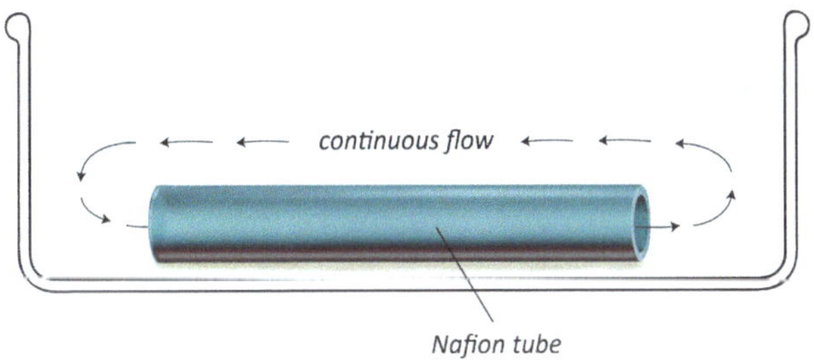


**Figure 3.11 – Continuous Flow Through Nafion Tube.** Reprinted from Pollack.[39]

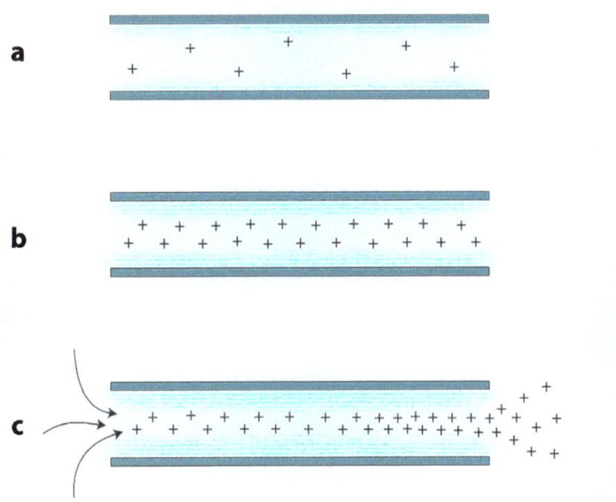


**Figure 3.12 – Hydronium Ion Build-up.** Prof Pollack's description and illustration of his experiment, which demonstrates continuous flow, is shown above: "An exclusion zone (EZ) demonstrably builds just inside the tube (a); we can see it. The EZ generates a buildup of hydronium ions in the core of the tube (b); we can measure it. When the hydronium ion concentration builds sufficiently, those positively charged water molecules must begin escaping at one end of the tube or the other, to the fluid outside. That escape initiates the flow (c). The escape draws fresh water into the other end of the tube. The incoming water gets protonated, which perpetuates the flow." Reprinted from Pollack.[40]

Schauberger envisaged the spiraling of the collagen in the multi-layered arterial wall, the spiraling of the endothelial cells and the moment-to-moment rifling of the endothelial wall of the arteries providing reinforcement to the spiraling once the heart has gone through its spiraling motion at systole as the basis for the development of charge and its related motion. Pollack reported, "All water-containing (hydro)gels produced exclusion zones, including gels made of biological molecules and artificial polymers. We also saw exclusion zones next to natural biological surfaces; they included endothelial cells lining the insides of blood vessels."[41]

Nafion's Teflon-like backbone contains many negatively charged sulfonic acid groups, which make this polymer one of the more potent "excluders". Its negatively charged sulfonic acid groups are similar to blood vessel walls.

Pollack sees the negative charge of the vessel wall producing a similar effect to the Nafion tube, producing a negatively charged exclusion zone and a positively charged central core with red blood cells being "squirted" along by this ambient charge. Pollack's model is supported by Seneff[42] and Ling.[43] Whilst the models developed independently by Schauberger and Pollack differ substantially, both envisage the possibility of continuous flow of water or blood without the need for a pump or motor. The complex and beautiful structure of blood vessel walls provides a hydrophilic tube that would enable blood to flow continuously through the vast distances of the vascular tree (Figure 3.13).[44]

## Behaviour of Water in the Fascia

This chapter has been devoted to blood flow. However, as the fascia is ubiquitous within the body, a brief discussion of the behaviour of water in the fascia, or extracellular matrix, will be included here.

So, we turn now to the work of Prof Emilio Del

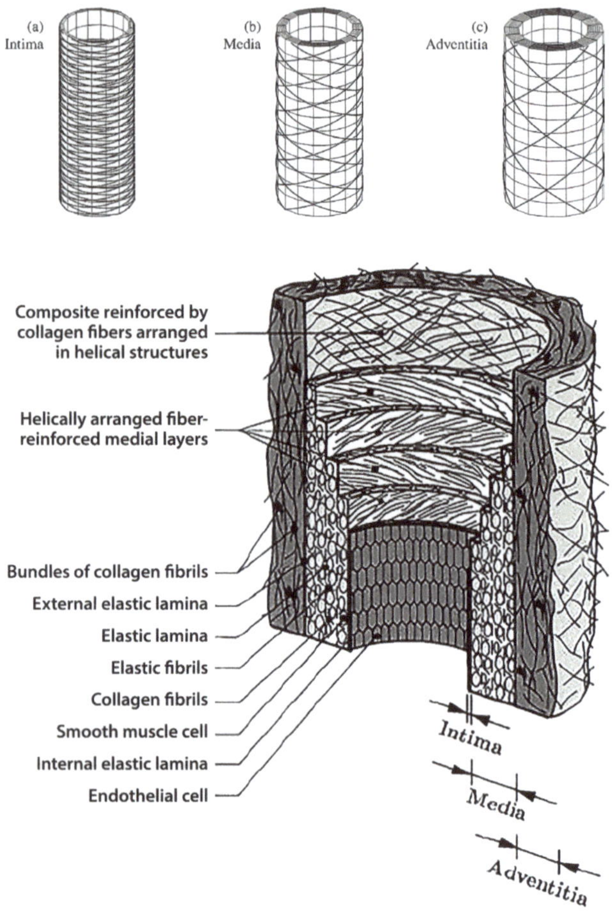


**Figure 3.13 – Structure of Blood Vessel Walls.** Reprinted from Holzapfel.[45]

Guidice, a high-energy physicist who worked at the Niels Bohr Institute in Copenhagen and collaborated with Giuliano Preparata and Nobel Prize winner Luc Montagnier.

These researchers showed that the interaction between the electromagnetic field of a physical vacuum and a liquid such as water could lead to the appearance of areas in which water molecules begin to congregate in unison so that they become "phased" or enter a coherent state. These special areas in liquid were described by Del Guidice and his team as "coherent domains".[46]

Del Guidice and colleagues presented a detailed mathematical model of quantum electrodynamics (QED) as it applies to living systems. They observed that collagen can, by virtue of its structure, orient water molecules. Water is strongly attracted to glycose-aminoglycans (GAGs) of the ECM, which associates with large volumes of water in hydrogen-bonded chains.

The water molecules linked to GAGs can form a channel without walls for electromagnetic signals while collagen shields the channel from outside influences. Collagen is a structural protein, is less interactive with water and behaves as an insulator, but GAGs bind large volumes of water through their sulfate moieties and act as electric conductors. More organised signals transit channels that display more organised molecular arrangements of GAGs and collagen.

Recall the paravasal mantle, or perivascular space, described by Hauk in Figure 1.9 in Chapter 1. The line drawing shows gel and sol islands, the explanation for which may be provided by the work of Del Giudice and colleagues. The fluid pathways, which are without walls, shown in Figure 3.14, may be the channel for information transfer. The gel islands would be the region where water rotations are less correlated.

Del Giudice envisaged a wave of energy (information) oriented with the GAGs and resulting in coherently spinning water molecules that are the

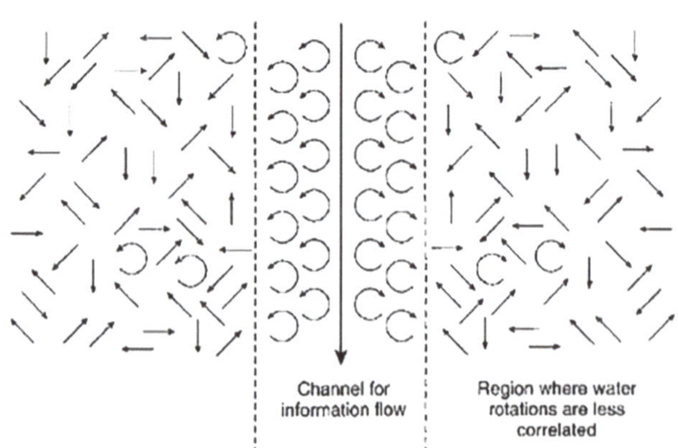


**Figure 3.14 – Channel for Information Flow.** Reprinted from Del Giudice et al.[47]

carriers for information. The dotted lines show the interface between the ordered (sol) and the disordered (gel) water phases that lie on either side of the information channel.

The composition of the extracellular matrix enables incoming waves of energy to convert coherent domains of water into vortices that are coherent. So, if for instance, water is stirred or shaken (eg, by contraction of the blood vessel wall), then vortices are produced belonging to the coherent domains. This rotation is motion without friction. It equates to the suction and implosion of fluid described by Schauberger.

The ability of water to become structured is central to the heart being able to impart **knowledge** or information to the blood so that it can proceed correctly with all its work. Using nuclear magnetic resonance spectroscopy, Pollack showed two water–proton resonances, one representing intimate water layers next to the polymer surface, the other corresponding to water lying beyond.[48] Pollack has shown that EZ water is more constrained,[49] more stable,[50,51] viscous and aligned,[52] all of which emphasises the ability of water to be the medium for information transfer. Chai[53] suggested that the EZ that may exist adjacent to hydrophilic surfaces has unexpected absorption of specific wavelengths and then emission at a longer wavelength, which are qualities that imply the water has a different structure to "bulk water". Messori refers to Chai's work and suggests that "Quantum Electrodynamic (QED) field theory has led to a concept of water in a liquid state, which, because it can be configured as described by Pollack, del Guidace and Chai, may provide the means for long-range communications."[54]

Finally, in discussing his hypothesis of information transfer, Pollack noted that oxygen has five states (dependant upon whether it has gained or given up one or two electrons), which gives it immense power in terms of the complexity of information storage or transfer. The images in Figure 3.15, from Pollack, show how information transfer may occur, including the contribution of oxygen.

Brini et al reviewed how the properties of water may be encoded within water's molecular structure and energies.[56] Water is an oscillating dipole and as a molecule is nearly spherical; however its hydrogen bonding results in a pyramid shape with a flat polygon base. The team discussed how small molecules and ions diffuse through liquids:

> "Small molecules and ions diffuse through liquids. Their diffusion rates typically depend on the radius of the diffusant and the viscosity of the solvent. However, when the liquid is water, there is a remarkable exception. Water's own component breakdown products — its protons and hydroxide ions — diffuse much faster than other ions do in water...This implies that there is a distinctive transport mechanism for $H^+$ and $OH^-$ compared to other ions in water. Ionic diffusion in water plays crucial roles in processes in biology (e.g., proton transfer in enzymes and biological channels)...The protons in water forms a hydronium ion, $H^+(H_2O)$ or $H_3O^+$, which is itself short-lived.[57] The hydronium ion can donate three hydrogen bonds. Hydronium makes strong hydrogen bonds,[58] which can influence more than 100 surrounding waters,[59] and can form hydronium chains. Manfred Eigen suggested that the proton is localized on an individual water molecule, and that the $H_3O^+$ gets further solvated by three water molecules, i.e. $H_3O^+(H_2O)_3$ or $H_9O_4^+$; this is called the Eigen cation."[60]

## Applications to Osteopathic Practice

For years we had been perceiving charge in the tissues but not understanding its source or its nature. It came in a sudden realisation when seeing Schauberger's diagram of water flowing in a pipe and carrying charge. So, our first efforts were directed at trying to link what we were perceiving with earlier efforts at understanding the nature of water in biological

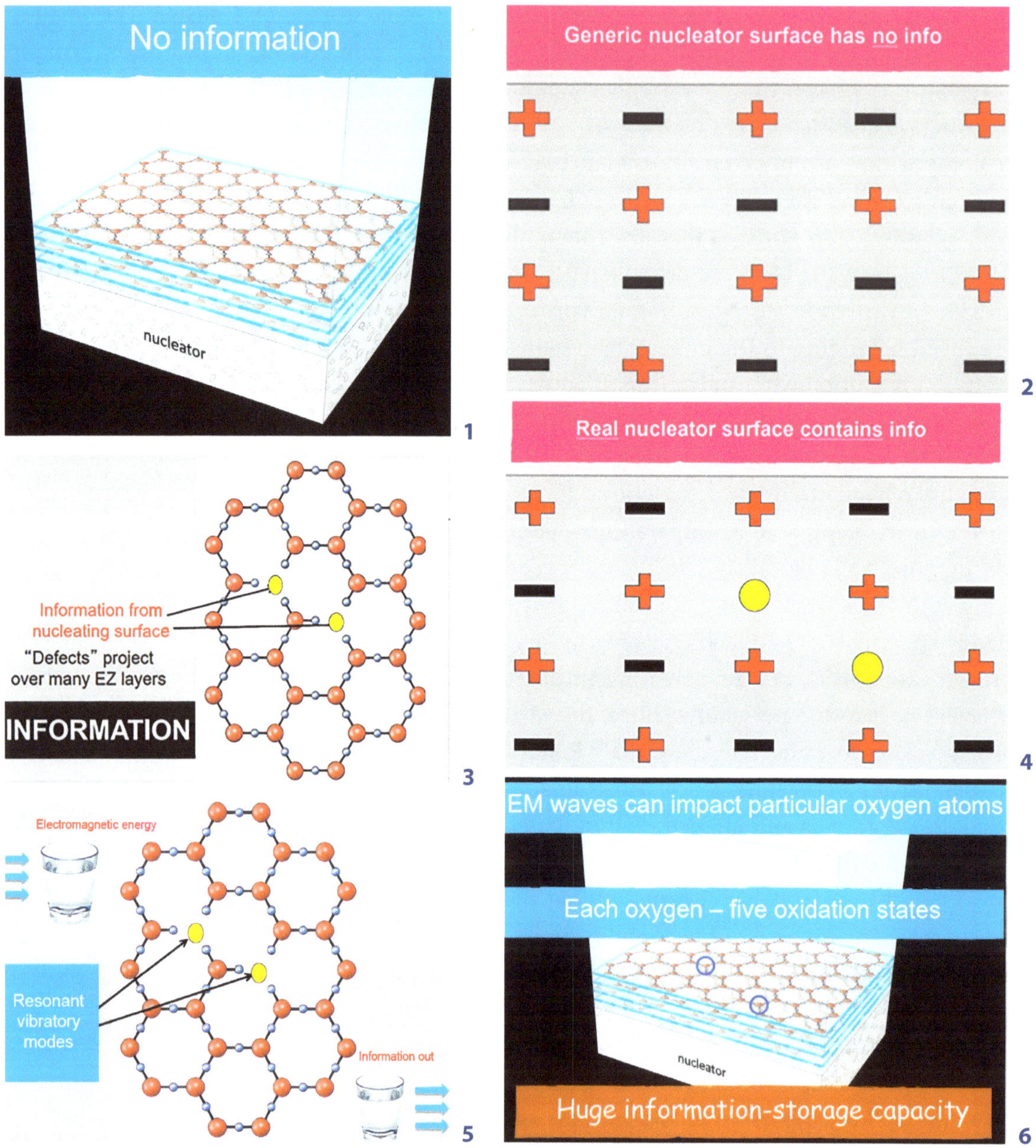


**Figure 3.15 – Information Transfer.**[55] From a lecture by Gerald H. Pollack, PhD, titled *The Fourth Phase of Water: A Central Role in Health* presented in Kobe Japan in November 2016. In image 1, the liquid crystal is arranged in a characteristically symmetrical pattern with the symmetrical charge pattern shown in 2. Where there is an irregularity or "defect" in the crystalline pattern, this allows for transmission of information from the nucleating surface; a deviation from the pattern both static and dynamic communicates information about the molecule in the water, which changes the three-dimensional shape of the hexagonal structure seen in image 3 and its charge state shown in 4. Regions of resonant vibration can occur as in image 5 where the nucleator is exposed to electromagnetic (EM) waves that match the natural vibrational frequencies of the nucleator molecular bonds. Resonant EM waves can impact particular oxygen atoms by resonant absorption. Oxidation states referred to in 6 will change the vibrational frequency. Each oxygen atom can have five oxidation states, which contributes to its potential for storing information: the oxidation states represent a distinct bonding pattern for the oxygen atom, allowing it to encode information through variations in the oxidation state.

systems. We came to understand that the natural movement or flow of water was expressed in a spiral with a related charge. The charge was maintained by a combination of the orientation of the endothelial cells lining the blood vessel walls and the charge of those cells' connective tissues that help to organise adjacent water.

The relationship between temperature and flow of water is still not well understood. In a personal communication with Rob Gourlay (the inventor of the Phion water-structuring device), he referred to his conversations with a student of Schauberger who understood from Schauberger that it was the magnetic field developed by the heart that managed temperature within the blood. As mentioned earlier, the magnetic field of the heart is 5000 times stronger than that of the brain.[61] So, the heart is constantly involved in maintaining a temperature with a small variance on either side of 39°F. This concept is further discussed in Chapter 7: The Heart as a Generator.

Pollack was able to show continuous flow in a tube without any pumping required. Bremer was able to demonstrate that there was an intrinsic nature of blood with spiralling occurring before the heart started to pump. Neither Schauberger nor Steiner believed that the heart was capable of pumping blood through all the vessels of the human body which, in an adult, is estimated to be about 96,500 km. They thought it was inconceivable that the power output of the heart (about 1.5 watts) would be sufficient for this huge task.

Still said, "A disturbed artery marks the period to an hour and minute, when disease begins to sow its seeds of destruction in the human body".[62] However, the opposite is also true. When feeling turbulence in a vessel and treating osteopathically to achieve the restoration of normal charge and vortical flow, we can sense a moment when the shift in the viscosity and flow of fluid indicates the restoration of normal charge and flow.

When the "ionars" described by Nordenström (collections of positively charged ions, such as calcium ions near the capillary bed in the ECM) express normal physiological patterns, the ionic fluctuation occurs seamlessly and there is nothing that stands out. This is just as Irwin Korr and his colleagues described[63] when using the metaphor of soldiers marching as a group. When they march in perfect order nothing stands out, but when one is out of step, then that becomes immediately apparent. In just the same way, when there is a stretch, compression or strain within the connective tissue matrix, the charge within this liquid crystalline system is perceived to function differently. This relationship is what Still meant when he said, "As an electrician controls electric currents, so an Osteopath controls life currents and revives suspended forces."[64]

There are many times when we, as osteopaths, have felt thickening in connective tissues. During treatment we seek to achieve balanced tension in the membrane, ligaments, joint capsules and the fascia or extracellular matrix. As a result, we may experience a phase shift, from gel to sol, with a resultant softening, warming and a greater sense of fluidity in the tissue. Coincident with these changes is a change in the function within the sol and gel islands and the ability of water to move through these functional conduits within the fascia.

As mentioned, Dr Still emphasised that health, or the lack of it, starts with the fascia: "By its action we live and by its failure we wither and die."[65] As a single, continuous, interconnected system that links the circulatory system, nervous system, digestive tract and musculoskeletal system together, it must be borne in mind continuously during treatment that, as a liquid crystalline material, fascia also has semiconductor properties.

One of these semiconductor properties is piezoelectricity, meaning "pressure electricity". This means that when you squeeze, twist or stretch the fascia, there is a momentary burst of electrical activity. So, in every movement of the body, in every pressure and every tension, an analog wave of bioelectric signals or microcurrents is produced. The signals form a pattern or symphony that is recognisable to the body and that spreads throughout the body as a result of the continuity of the connective tissue matrix.

However, when the stretch, twist or compression is beyond the modulus of the tissue, there is a resulting distortion in the bioelectric pattern that results. This distortion then produces a shift from sol to gel, which is what osteopaths are trained to perceive as tissue congestion, the hallmark of dysfunction and focus for treatment.

It was mentioned earlier that the hunger of the tissues sucks the blood towards the cells of the body. As mentioned in the first chapter, 20% of the blood is arterial whereas 80% is in the venous system. This is because there are smaller numbers of cells drawing the blood back to the heart. There are roughly 8 trillion cells in the lungs compared to the 35 trillion cells in the body as a whole. This distribution of cells is why patterned breathing can have such a powerful effect on the venous return. Such an effect is particularly noticeable in cases of venous congestion within the lumbar spinal canal, as the veins in this area are avalvular.

## Chapter 3 Endnotes


1. James Odel, "History - Viktor Schauberger," Bioregulatory Medicine Institute, accessed October 20, 2022, https://www.biologicalmedicineinstitute.com/viktor-schauberger.

2. Alick Bartholomew, *Hidden Nature: The Startling Insights of Viktor Schauberger* (Edinburgh: Floris Books, 2003).

3. Alison Davidson, review of *Living Water - Viktor Schauberger and the Secrets of Natural Energy* by Olof Alexandersson, in Tom Brown, ed., *Implosion Instead of Explosion. Part II: More Implosion than Explosion* (BSRF, 1986), 4.

4. Ernst O. Attinger, "Hydrodynamics of Blood Flow" (unpublished), as quoted in Callum Coats, *Living Energies: An Exposition of the Concepts Related to the Theories of Viktor Schauberger* (Dublin, Ireland: MH Gill & Co., 2001), 190, 192.

5. Alick Bartholomew, *Hidden Nature: The Startling Insights of Viktor Schauberger* (Edinburgh: Floris Books, 2003), p. 10. Taken from The Schauberger Archives, Linz, January 1952.

6. Michael West, "Investigation of Viktor Schauberger's Vortex Engine" (B.Sc. Thesis, The University of Queensland School of Engineering, 2005), https://doi.org/10.14264/300139.

7. Larry Greenemeier, "The World's First Flying Saucer: Made Right Here on Earth," *Scientific American*, July 7, 2008, https://www.scientificamerican.com/article/worlds-first-flying-saucer/.

8. Callum Coats, *Living Energies: An Exposition of the Concepts Related to the Theories of Viktor Schauberger* (Dublin, Ireland: MH Gill & Co., 2001), 142.

9. Bartholomew, *Hidden Nature.*

10. Albert Zock, "Viktor Schauberger and His Work," *Journal of Borderland Research* (May-June 1979), reprinted in Riley Hansard Crabb and Thomas Maxwell Thompson, eds., *Implosion Instead of Explosion. Part I: Implosion – Viktor Schauberger and the Path of Natural Energy*, rev. ed. (1985), 41, accessed November 13, 2023, https://alkimist.net/wp-content/uploads/2015/11/Implosion-Viktor-Schauberger-and-the-Path-of-Natural-Energy-1985.pdf.

11. Viktor Schauberger, "Nature Was My Teacher," trans. Albert Zock, reprinted in Riley Hansard Crabb and Thomas Maxwell Thompson, *Implosion Instead of Explosion. Part I: Implosion – Viktor Schauberger and the Path of Natural Energy*, rev. ed., (1985), 49–50, accessed November 13, 2023, https://alkimist.net/wp-content/uploads/2015/11/Implosion-Viktor-Schauberger-and-the-Path-of-Natural-Energy-1985.pdf.

12. Bartholomew, *Hidden Nature.*

13. "The Popel Report" (Stuttgart: Institute of Hygiene at the Stuttgart University of Technology, February to March 1952).

14. Viktor Schauberger, "Temperature and the Movement of Water," *Die Wasserwirtschaft: The Austrian Journal of Hydrology*, vol. 20 (1990).

15. Bartholomew, *Hidden Nature.*

16. Bartholomew, *Hidden Nature.*

17. Ali M. Alshami, "Pain: Is It All in the Brain or the Heart?" *Current Pain and Headache Reports* 23, no. 88 (November 2019), https://doi.org/10.1007/s11916-019-0827-4.

18. Bartholomew, *Hidden Nature.*

19. Triple Helix Collagen, CC BY-SA 3.0, https://commons.wikimedia.org/wiki/File:Collagentriplehelix.png.

20. Francisco Torrent-Guasp et al., "The Structure and Function of the Helical Heart and Its Buttress Wrapping. I. The Normal Macroscopic Structure of the Heart," *Seminars in Thoracic and Cardiovascular Surgery* 13, no. 4 (October 2001): 301–19.

21. Bartholomew, *Hidden Nature*, 54.

22. Coats, *Living Energies*, 188.

23. J. Bremer, "Presence and Influence of Spiral Streams in the Heart of the Chick Embryo," *American Journal of Anatomy* 49 (1932): 409–40.

24. Viktor Schauberger, *Our Senseless Toil* (Vienna: Krystall Verlag, 1933), 34.

25. Ernst O. Attinger, "Hydrodynamics of Blood Flow" (unpublished), as quoted in Callum Coats, *Living Energies: An Exposition of the Concepts Related to the Theories of Viktor Schauberger* (Dublin, Ireland: MH Gill & Co., 2001), 190, 192.

26. Gerald H. Pollack, *The Fourth Phase of Water: Beyond Solid, Liquid, and Vapor* (Seattle, WA: Ebner and Sons Publishing, 2012),

27. Pollack, *The Fourth Phase of Water,* 50.

28. Pollack, *The Fourth Phase of Water,* 89.

29. Ellis R. Lippincott,et al., "Polywater: Vibrational Spectra Indicate Unique Stable Polymeric Structure, *Science* 164, no. 3887 (June 1969): 1482–7, https://doi.org/10.1126/science.164.3887.1482.

30. Pollack, *The Fourth Phase of Water,* 56.

31. Pollack, *The Fourth Phase of Water,* 59.

32. Pollack, *The Fourth Phase of Water,* 87.

33. Pollack, *The Fourth Phase of Water,* 87.

34. Norio Ise, "Like Likes Like: Counterion-Mediated Attraction in Macroionic and Colloidal Interaction," *Physical Chemistry Chemical Physics* 12, no. 35 (2010): 10279–87.

35. Heloise Fernandez, Carlos Lenz Cesar, and Maria de Lourdes Barjas-Castro, "Electrical properties of the red blood cell membrane and immunohematological investigation," *Revista Brasileira de Hemoterapia e Hematologia* 33, no. 4 (2011): 297–301.

36. Ferandez et al., "Electrical properties of the red blood cell membrane and immunohematological investigation."

37. Pollack, *The Fourth Phase of Water.*

38. Pollack, *The Fourth Phase of Water,* 228.

39. Pollack. *The Fourth Phase of Water,* 112.

40. Pollack. *The Fourth Phase of Water,* 113.

41. Pollack. *The Fourth Phase of Water,* 32.

42. Stephanie Seneff et al., "A Novel Hypothesis for Atherosclerosis as a Cholesterol Sulfate Deficiency Syndrome," *Theoretical Biology and Medical Modelling* 12 (2015): 9.

43. Gilbert N. Ling, "Life at the Cell and Below-Cell Level: The Hidden History of a Fundamental Revolution in Biology" (New York: Pacific Press, 2001).

44. G.A. Holzapfel, "Collagen in Arterial Walls: Biomechanical Aspects," in *Collagen: Structure and Mechanics*, ed. Peter Fratzl (New York: Springer, 2008), 285–324.

45. Holzapfel, "Collagen in Arterial Walls: Biomechanical Aspects."

46. Emilio Del Giudice, Giuliano Preparata, and Giuseppe Vitiello, "Water as a Free Electric Dipole Laser," *Physical Review Letters* 61 (August 1988): 1085.

47. Del Giudice et al., "Water as a Free Electric Dipole Laser."

48. Hyok Yoo, Rajan Paranji, and Gerald H. Pollack, "Impact of Hydrophilic Surfaces on Interfacial Water Dynamics Probed With NMR Spectroscopy," *The Journal of Physical Chemistry Letters* 2, no. 6 (February 2011): 532–6.

49. P.P. Olodovskii and I.L. Berestova, "On Changes in the Structure of Water Due to Its Contact With a Solid Phase. I. NMR-Spectroscopy Studies," *Journal of Engineering Physics and Thermophysics* 62 (1992): 622–7.

50. Yoo et al., "Impact of Hydrophilic Surfaces on Interfacial Water Dynamics."

51. Jian-Ming Zheng et al., "Surfaces and Interfacial Water: Evidence That Hydrophilic Surfaces Have Long-Range Impact," *Advances in Colloid and Interface Science* 127, no. 1 (November 2006): 19–27. https://doi.org/10.1016/j.cis.2006.07.002.

52. Mae-Wan Ho, *The Rainbow and the Worm: The Physics of Living Organisms,* 3rd ed. (World Scientific Publishing Co., 2008).

53. Bing-hua Chai et al., "Spectroscopic Studies of Solutes in Aqueous Solution," *The Journal of Physical Chemistry* A 112, no. 11 (March 2008): 2242-7.

54. Claudio Messori, "Deep Into the Water: Exploring the Hydro-Electromagnetic and Quantum-Electrodynamic Properties of Interfacial Water in Living Systems," *Open Access Library Journal* 6, no. 5 (May 2019): 1-62.

55. Pollack, *The Fourth Phase of Water.*

56. Emiliano Brini et al., "How Water's Properties Are Encoded in Its Molecular Structure and Energies," *Chemical Reviews* 117, no. 19 (September 2017): 12385–414, https://doi.org/10.1021/acs.chemrev.7b00259.

57. Christopher A. Reed, "Myths About the Proton. The Nature of H+ in Condensed Media," *Accounts of Chemical Research* 46, no. 11 (July 2013): 2567–75, https://doi.org/10.1021/ar400064q.

58. Omer Markovitch and Noam Agmon, "Structure and Energetics of the Hydronium Hydration Shells," *The Journal of Physical Chemistry A* 111, no. 12 (March 2007): 2253–6, https://doi.org/10.1021/jp068960g.

59. Kenta Mizuse, Asuka Fujii, and NaohikoMikami, "Long Range Influence of an Excess Proton on the Architecture of the Hydrogen Bond Network in Large-Sized Water Clusters," *The Journal of Chemical Physics*, 126 (June 2007): 231101, https://doi.org/10.1063/1.2750669.

60. Manfred Eigen and L. De Maeyer. "Self-Dissociation and Protonic Charge Transport in Water and Ice," *Proceedings of the Royal Society of London, Series A* 247, no. 1251 (October 1958): 505–33, https://doi.org/10.1098/rspa.1958.0208.

61. Alshami, "Pain: Is It All in the Brain or the Heart?"

62. A.T. Still, *Journal of Osteopathy* VII, no. 9 (February 1874): 33.

63. Irvin Korr, *The Physiological Basis of Osteopathic Medicine* (San Rafael, CA: Insight Publishing Company, 1982).

64. A.T. Still, *Autobiography of Andrew Taylor Still* (Kirksville, MO: A.T. Still, 1908): 224.

65. A.T. Still, *Philosophy and Mechanical Principles of Osteopathy* (Kansas City, MO: Hudson-Kimberly Publishing Co., 1902), 63.

# Chapter Four

# The Embryology of the Heart

*"Turn the eye of reason to the heart; and observe the blood start on its journey."*[1]

—Andrew Taylor Still

Vascular function is the earliest to develop in the embryo. Emerging from a cardiogenic field, it meets the rising needs for nutrients and oxygen, outstripping the capability of diffusion alone to supply the need of the tissues.[2,3,4] Aristotle was the first to record this discovery based on his study of chick embryos in the fourth century B.C., when he proclaimed the heart the most important of all organs and the seat of intelligence.[5] Throughout history, the heart has been heralded not only as the seat of intelligence, but as the source of passion, emotion and the soul.

In the *Philosophy and Mechanical Principles of Osteopathy*, Still agreed, at least in part, when he waxed poetically, "First is formed the material heart, in which the spiritual establishes an office in which to dwell and enforce the requirements of the specifications for constructing the human body or that of any animal, fish, reptile, or bird."[6] Still knew that we must have a way to organise, facilitate and augment the complex materials transportation, construction and waste removal processes necessary to create life and that this need is met by the development of the heart.

## Early Embryonic Development

Before we explore embryogenesis of the heart and how and why this is intrinsically related to the whole, we must first understand early oocyte development: preconception, fertilisation and implantation.

The immature eggs within the mother's ovaries, otherwise known as primordial follicles, begin to mature approximately 10 months prior to ovulation in a process known as folliculogenesis. Numerous primary follicles may be stimulated to grow in any month, and some—but not all—will grow to the vesicular follicle stage.

There is an associated shape change and fluid accumulates centrally with metabolic activity. This is important, and while students may focus on what's happening to the developing cells, the fluids have important morphokinetic and morphogenetic influences at every stage. *Morpho* comes from morphology, referring to the development of structure, while *kinetic* refers to movement, therefore *morphokinetic* refers to structural movement. *Morphogenetic*, on the other hand, refers to the development of structure in relation to genetics.

Therefore, the fluid influences movement, structural organisation and genetic expression.

As shown in Figure 4.1, as the granulosa cells develop, the fluid forms centrally and is encapsulated by the zona pellucida surrounding the oocyte still contained within the ovary. The zona pellucida and surrounding antrum provides a source of sugars and nutrients for the oocyte, with the antrum present 2 months before ovulation. In each menstrual cycle, one vesicular follicle will grow to become the dominant follicle in any single cycle.

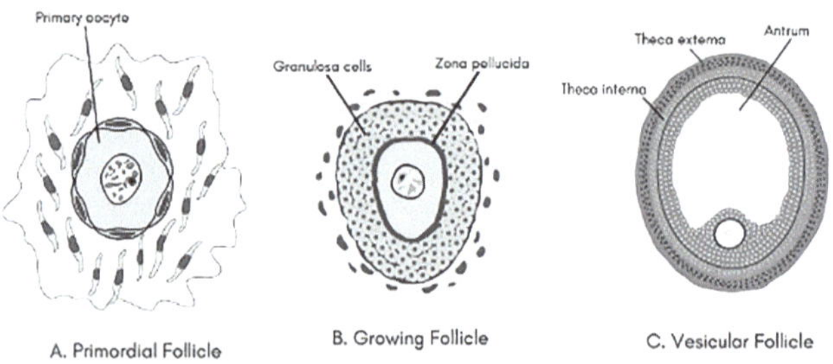


**Figure 4.1 – Development of an Ovarian Follicle.**

The development of the fluid-filled antrum continues until it gets so big that it bursts out of the ovary. The liberated oocyte is captured by the fluid movements of the fimbriae of the fallopian tube and it gets drawn towards the maternal nutrition of the uterine lining, with potential fertilisation occurring 12–24 hours after ovulation.

## First Week of Development

When a sperm successfully penetrates an oocyte, the spark of life transforms the fertilised egg, now referred to as the conceptus. The conceptus is visible in the image on the left in Figure 4.2. The image on the right shows two important phenomena, the first being *reciprocal biomechanical cohesion by metabolism,* which we will discuss in more depth in Chapter 6.

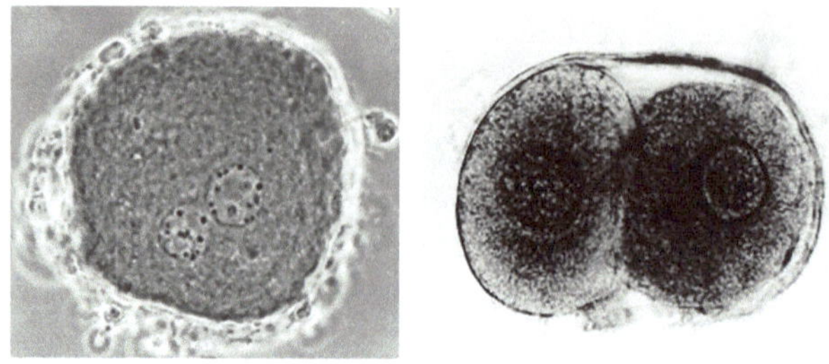

**Figure 4.2 – Fertilised Conceptus and First Cellular Multiplication.** Reprinted with permission from The Endowment for Human Development: Raymond Gasser's Atlas of Human Embryos.[7]

What this phenomenon means is that even from the first cellular division, the two cells are completely reliant on each other and function as a single cohesive unit. They are bound together by their metabolic and growth needs, with fluid flowing around them.

There is a constant flow of information, biomechanically as well as nutritionally, between the two. If the cells are separated, they are unable to survive. They work as a team: when one releases waste products, the other absorbs what it can from the surrounding environment in order to continue growing to survive. They communicate, pressing and shearing on one another, their cell membranes receptively coordinating the information from outside in and then back to the outside and with one another. There is a movement, backwards and forwards, with synthesis and turnover of biochemical signals, hormones and other metabolites. This is the beginning of local intra-, inter- and extracellular communication.

The second observable phenomenon is what occurs after the first cell multiplication. While the multiplication results in two genetically identical cells, it is important to note they are not the same, that a structural *asymmetry* is observed. The cells are not identical in shape, size or biochemistry or in context with the environment. With each division, there is increasing complexity, but essentially

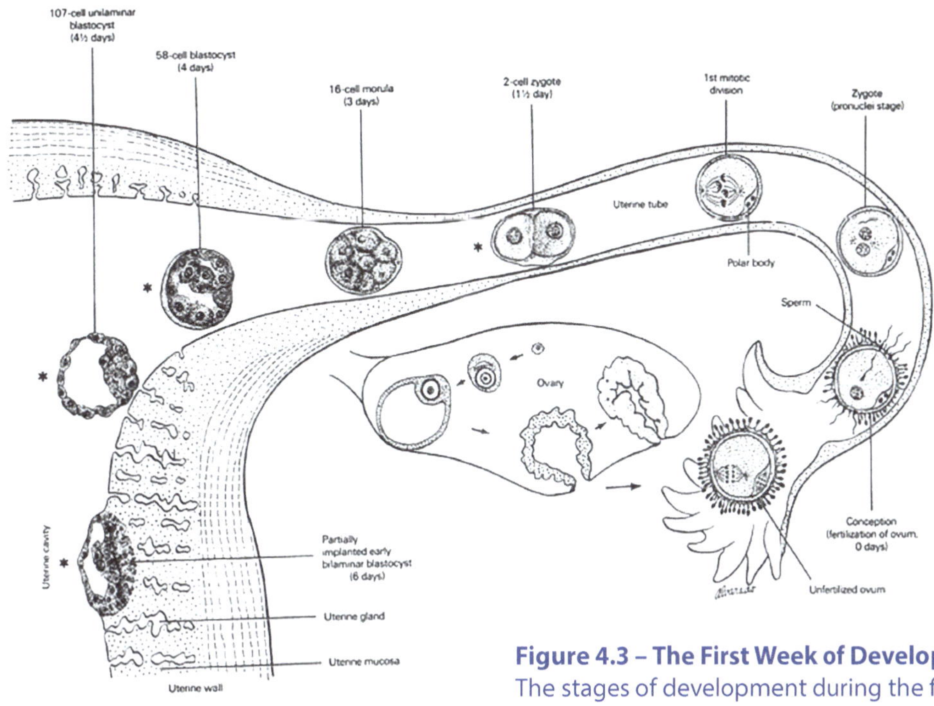


**Figure 4.3 – The First Week of Development.** The stages of development during the first week and the general location of each in the uterine tube or uterus. Reprinted with permission from Gasser.[8]

the needs remain the same. The cells work together as a single unit of function, dependent and reliant on each other for life to continue, but evolving and differentiating according to their unique environmental conditions, hence the asymmetry.

With progressive increased complexity, space restriction, growth forces, and local differences in access to nutrition, some cells grow faster than others. Some cells swell and expand faster while others are flattened, stretched and relatively starved. Fluids are produced and flow, sculpt and influence shape and structure. The living, breathing functional requirements of a cell to sustain life, in conjunction with each cell's position and access to nutrients, have the strongest influence on structural development. The movements of the cell, or group of cells, and the fluctuation of fluids sculps the tissues into form.

By day 3, there are approximately 6–10 cells. At this stage, cells begin to multiply more rapidly and they're becoming smaller and smaller. By around day 5, there are approximately 70–100 cells, which remain firmly adhered to and dependent on one another. With this new growth, the conceptus is now referred to as a blastocyst.

As the single fluid antrum pools centrally, the cells are moved towards the outside, creating a ring around the edge, with a pocket of more densely developing cells. This is referred to as the *inner cell mass*. The living blastocyst pulsates while growth and increasing pressure lead to thinning, precipitating the rupture of the zona pellucida, ultimately leading to hatching of the blastocyst. The rapidly developing and hungry inner cell mass (from which the future embryo will form) orientates itself towards the nutrient-rich uterine wall (Figure 4.3).

The embryo starts to digest the maternal tissues and embed itself into the endometrium of the uterus, forming the syncytiotrophoblast. It is an important name that refers to a syncytium of cells forming an interface between the mother's blood and that of the fetus, and that interface facilitates and regulates the exchange of nutrients and gases.[9] They share a cytoplasm and a nucleus over a large number of cells.

During the second week, a second fluid chamber and embryonic tissue layer are formed. Once again, the fast-growing cells are producing a lot of fluid, leading to the development of a cavity and surrounding membrane: the future yolk sac (Figure 4.4).

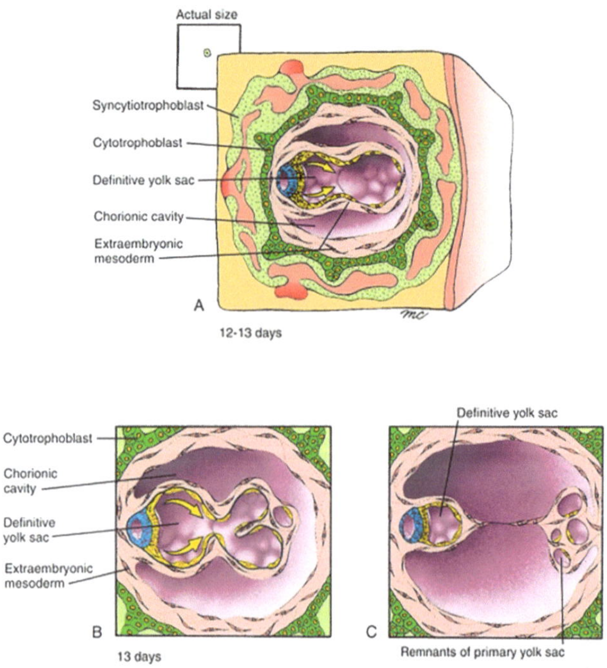


**Figure 4.4 – Formation of the Secondary (Definitive) Yolk Sac and Degeneration of the Primary Yolk Sac.** A: On days 12 and 13, a second wave of migration of hypoblast cells produces a new membrane that migrates out over the inside of the extraembryonic mesoderm, pushing the primary yolk sac in front of it. This new layer becomes the endodermal lining of the secondary (definitive) yolk sac. B and C: As the definitive yolk sac develops on day 13, the primary yolk sac breaks up and is reduced to a collection of vesicles at the abembryonic end of the chorionic cavity. Reprinted from Schoenwolf et al.[10]

The future amniotic cavity forms because these cells are metabolising so rapidly that fluid accumulates in between them. This facilitates division of the embryo into its two layers: *ectoderm* and *endoderm* (Figure 4.5). The importance of a fluid space, in terms of sculpting cells, is considerable—it bathes the fast-growing cells, which will later form the brain. This future brain tissue is considered to be an external tissue with an open communication with the external environment, but through growth it is encapsulated as an internal tissue. Through this process, some amniotic fluid from the external environment is enveloped into the internal body to become part of the function of the cerebrospinal fluid (CSF) postnatally. The yolk sac is important for stimulation and development of the digestive system.

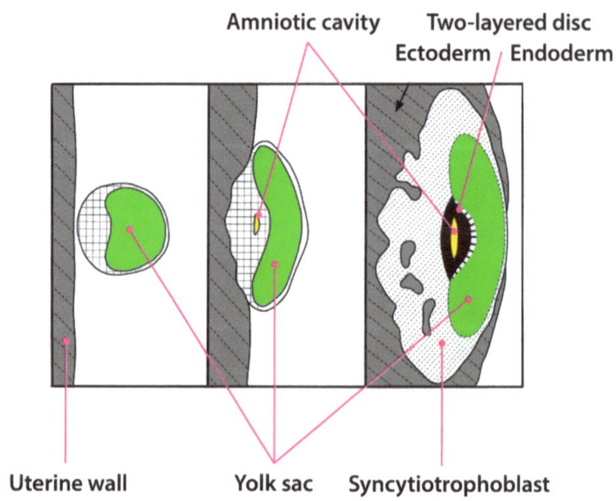


**Figure 4.5 – Third Week of Development: Three Chambers, Three layers.** Adapted from Blechschmidt.[11] Illustration by Hugh France.

As growth continues, in the third week, a third fluid chamber forms called the chorionic cavity (also referred to as the extraembryonic coelom), which expands rapidly.

## Permeation and Parmeation

Adjacent to the chorionic cavity, blood islands appear and become sources of nutrients that will flow directly perpendicular, at close to a 90° angle, to the embryo. This is referred to as *permeation*, which is important because the flow direction makes for efficient and effective uptake of nutrients from the fluid. As the blood islands are closer to the maternal tissues, the hungry cells support a trajectory of flow towards them. There is also a flow of nutrients parallel to the tissues, described as *parmeation* of nutrients. It is worth noting that nutrients are coming from every direction and that this will affect how effectively nutrient uptake will be achieved by the developing cells, as seen in Figure 4.6.

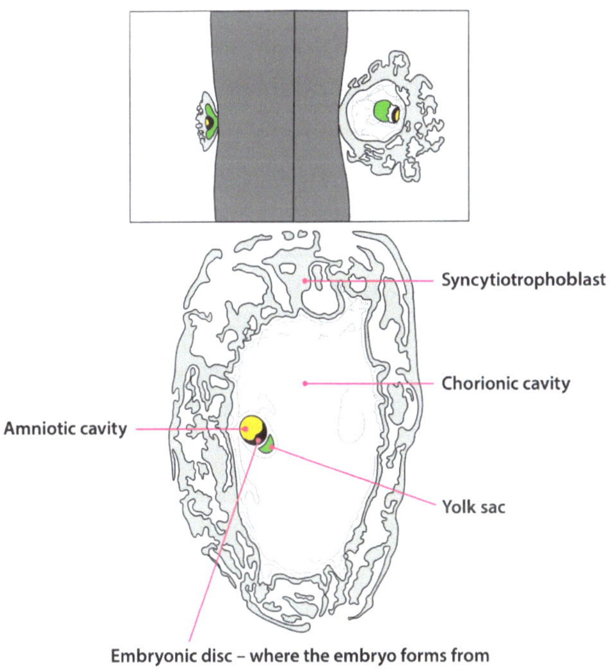


**Figure 4.6 – Permeation and Parmeation.** Illustrations by Hugh France. Adapted from Blechschmidt.[12]

The embryonic disc, made of up two layers, endoderm and ectoderm, can be seen in Figure 4.7 along with the developing chorionic cavity, the future amniotic cavity, and yolk sac. As it grows, the embryo lengthens. The ectoderm is a layer of embryonic tissue, which acts as a precursor to the development of the nervous system, including the brain, spinal cord and peripheral nerves as well as the skin, pineal and pituitary gland, hair, nails, kidney marrow, cornea, teeth and sweat glands. The endoderm stimulates formation of the inner lining of the respiratory and gastrointestinal tracts.

## Development of Brain and Notochord

In Figure 4.7, the ectodermal layer, which forms the future neural tube, is shown in the left image. The cut edge of the amniotic sac is visible, as is the future brain bulge from the front in the right image.

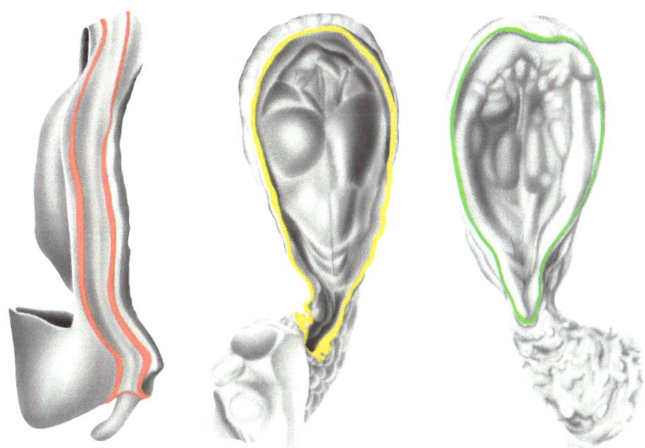

**Figure 4.7 – The Forming of the Future Neural Tube.** The ectodermal layer forms the future neural tube (left). Cut edge of the amniotic sac shows the future brain bulge. Illustrations by Hugh France. Adapted from Blechschmidt.[13]

In Figure 4.8, the centre illustration of the right image is bulging out of the page while the image to the right is the *impansion pit*,[14] a term used by Erich Blechschmidt to describe the dorsally concave part of the endocyst disc, which develops as a consequence of the rapid growth of the cranial end of the disc with the "retarded" growth of the caudal region atop a non-expanding basement membrane. At this point the start of the formation of the notochord occurs. What is important about this is that it is curving outwards—out of the page towards you, the reader. The future brain bulge is just one bulge initially.

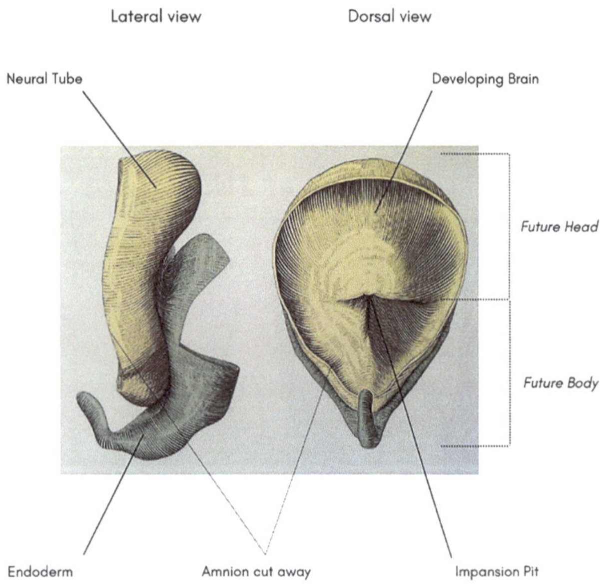


**Figure 4.8 – The Impansion Pit.** Adapted from Blechschmidt and Gasser.[15]

Following many dissections, Blechschmidt concluded that, as the conceptus is growing, it is creating an area of tension below that creates the impansion pit. As growth is occurring in a restricted space and some tissue is growing a little faster, it creates a fulcrum, folding over (at the rolling rim) and initiating formation of the axial process, the precursor of the notochord.

As shown in Figure 4.9, everything is organised around the null point. It is a dynamic point that is constantly changing. The point stays neutral and, as growth occurs, the growth comes from below and then moves up towards the neutral or null point.

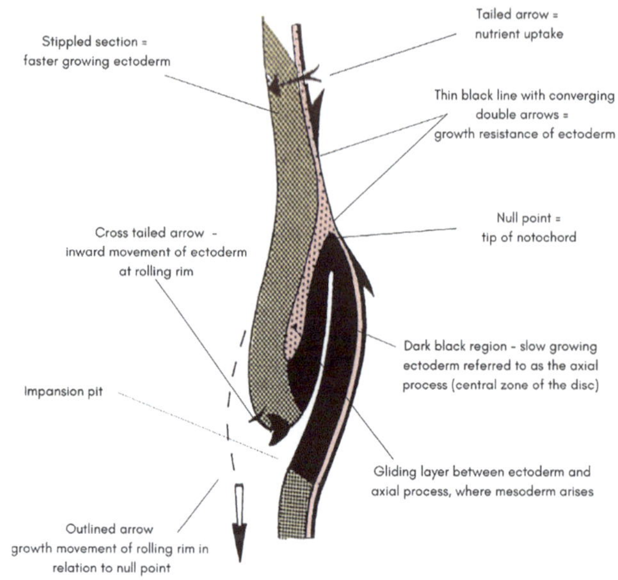


**Figure 4.9 – The Null Point.** Adapted from Blechschmidt and Gasser.[16]

The starting point of the notochord is a reference point for the whole multidimensional function of the embryo. It is constantly a null point because no matter where it is, it is at the centre of all function, with all subsequent biomechanical movements and biodynamic forces referenced in relation to it.

In one of his lectures, Brian Freeman theorised that the reason that the notochord develops from this point has to do with the whole. It is only in the context of the whole that we can understand the notochord and its functions.

In osteopathic philosophy, this null point is **function** creating **structure**; when observing or perceiving function, the practitioner has an opportunity to witness this esoteric process in action. Function comes from beyond the physical product in the realm of Still's celestial world, whereas the outcome of the process, the notochord, is within Still's terrestrial world. (Refer to *The Philosophy and Mechanical Principles of Osteopathy* for more information about these concepts.[17]) The study of embryology is replete with this basic osteopathic concept of function creating structure.

## Development of the Mesoderm

In Figure 4.10, on the left is a dorsal aspect of an embryo at the end of the third week of development, showing the developing brain with the neural groove centrally and the tail end below. Observe the asymmetry in those brain bulges. The right brain bulge, which is the future right hemisphere, is slightly bigger and a slightly different shape than the left.

The right image in Figure 4.10 is a transverse section, showing the neural groove and the notochord centrally, with the ectoderm in black and endoderm beneath it. The ectoderm, which takes up nutrition predominantly via permeation, grows faster and away from the slower growing endoderm and starts to lift. As it pulls away, it leaves behind cells. These cells become stretched and spindle-like, and they are under mechanical strain, aligning themselves radially between the ectoderm and endoderm.

As a result, a loose layer of intermediate tissue forms between them—the *mesoderm*—from which all of the future connective tissues develop. This includes the formation of blood and lymphatic vessels, muscle, fascia, tendon, cartilage and bone and contributes to the formation of many viscera. The stretched cells that are underneath lose and release some of their intracellular fluid, which collects in the spaces between the cells.

The intercellular spaces communicate with each other and fluid starts to trickle through them. So, the mesoderm is spongy and rich in fluid and permits extensive transport of metabolites as well as nutrients, parallel with and perpendicular to the surface ectoderm.

With further growth, ongoing rupturing of cells continues, increasing the fluid of the chorion, taking some cells with it, lining the cavity and extending to cover the endoblast, with a transitional region called

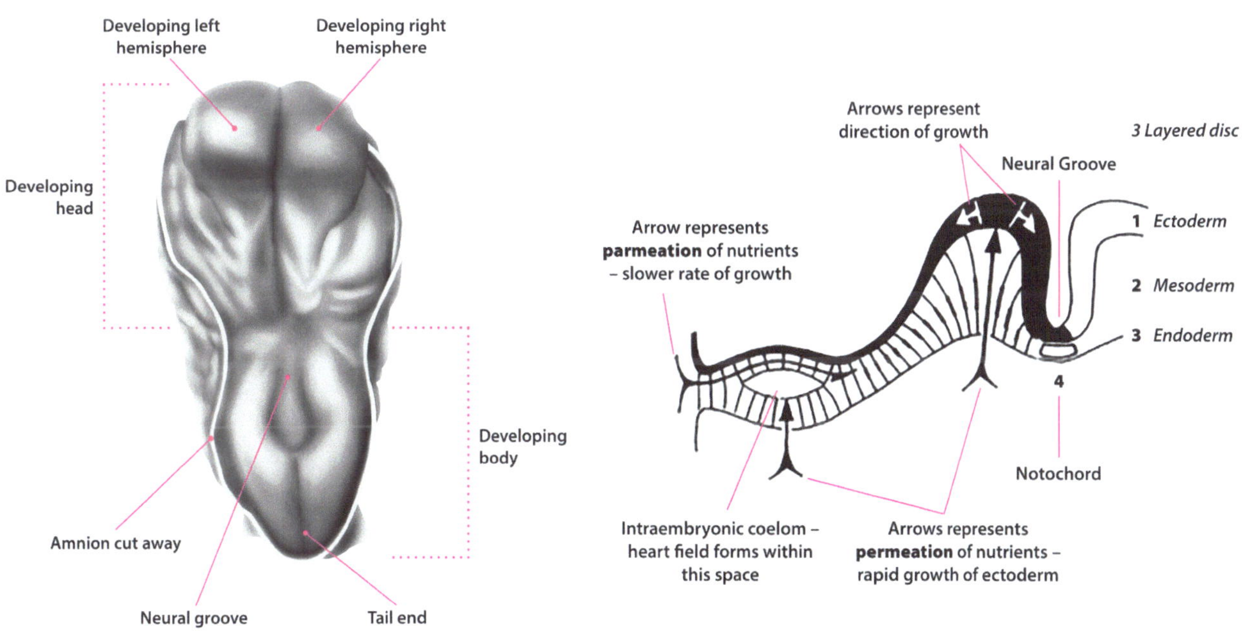


**Figure 4.10 – Third Week of Development: Development of the Mesoderm.** Reprinted from Blechschmidt.[18]

the connecting stalk. Substances from the yolk sac, chorion (outer membrane of the chorionic sac) and between the layers of the embryonic disc flow and create the precursor for the pathway for the umbilical cord. Small volumes of fluid trickle within and over the surface of the conceptus, the precursor to the development of blood vessels.

## Development of the Intraembryonic Coelom

A cavity starts to form within the layer of the mesoderm, and as other cells are growing away in different directions, this forms the intraembryonic coelom.

Function always fills a vacuum. As this space (the coelom) opens up, interstitial fluid collects, allowing more space between the cells for nutrients to flow into that space. Through the combination of flexion and growth of the embryo, the precursor heart tissue will soon be enveloped by the coelom. This forms the future mediastinum, and within the cardiac jelly, the heart chambers start to form. Meanwhile, the septum transversum, in conjunction with growth and folding in the transverse plane, will allow the development of the diaphragm to separate the cavity from the peritoneum.

## Feeding the Hungry Embryo

Figure 4.11 is an illustration of the vascular syncytiotrophoblast. The hungry embryo will access nutrition from wherever it can source it, including the yolk sac. In time it forms blood islands (accumulations of extraembryonic mesoderm from the amniotic membrane), along with the chorion, which is marked with a red C in Figure 4.12.

The blood islands eventually canalise as the flow inside and around them increases. The pericardial

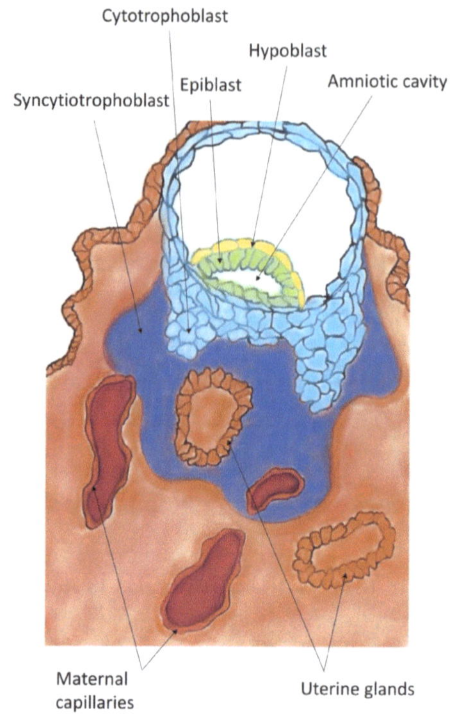


**Figure 4.11 – Illustration of an Implanted Embryo.** Reprinted from Wikipedia.[19]

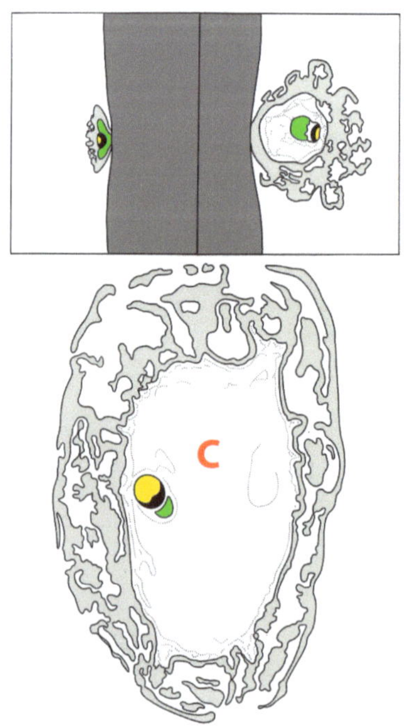


**Figure 4.12 – Chorion.** The chorion is marked with a red C. Illustration by Hugh France. Adapted from Blechschmidt.[20]

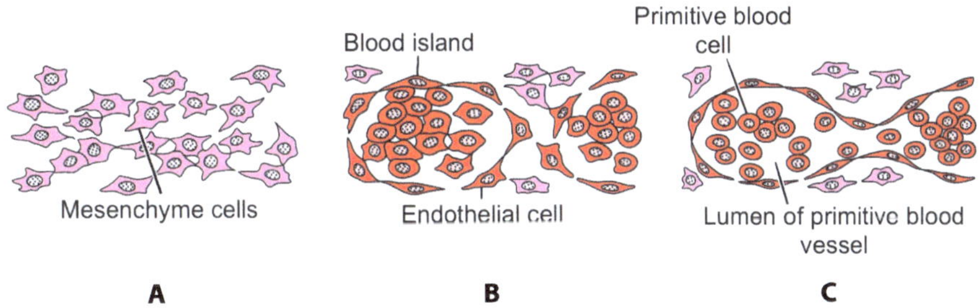


**Figure 4.13 – Successive Stages of Blood Vessel Formation.** (A) Undifferentiated mesenchyme cells. (B) Blood island formation. (C) Primitive capillary. Note the differentiation of mesenchymal cells into primitive blood cells and endothelial cells. Illustration by Hugh France.

cavity can be thought of as mesenchyme dense with early immature vessels and red blood cells. The ectoderm, endoderm and all of these blood islands are sources of nutrients. As the syncytiotrophoblast starts to become more involved in the maternal tissues, these blood islands start to become less important (Figure 4.13).

At 18 days, the blood islands concentrate and coalesce around the head region and the yolk sac and can be observed surrounding the developing embryo. These represent sources of nutrients, and the embryo draws nutrients from wherever it can.

A thick ectoderm forms where the epithelial cells form in relation to the amnion and due to its proximity to the nutrients (Figure 4.14).

The way these blood islands form as a result of the development of corrosion fields. A corrosion field is a type of metabolic field forming between two vessels in which fluid is traveling in the same direction. Corrosion occurs between those two walls, creating a unified single pathway and hence forming one vessel. When flow occurs in opposite directions, the movement creates a distusion field flow in the opposite direction, resulting in the formation of a venous and an arterial vessel. At the bottom of the lower image in Figure 4.14, there is a tiny capillary bed that results in blood trickling through the mesenchyme.

With growth, the flow becomes stronger and the vessels coalesce to form distinct vessels. This takes place between the syncytiotrophoblast and chorion to initiate formation of the placenta.

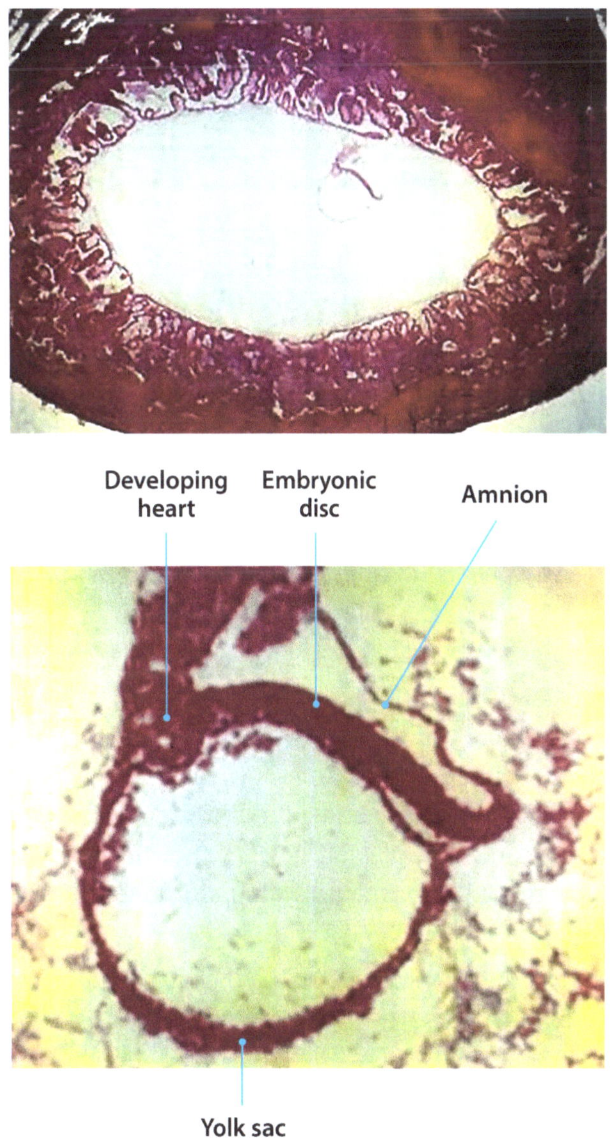


**Figure 4.14 –** Detail of embryonic disc showing extra-embryonic cavities (amnion and yolk sac), developing heart and blood islands. Reprinted from Fujimoto[21] and Schoenwolf et al.[22]

## Growth Relationship of the Heart and Brain

The horse-shaped future heart (cardiogenic area) can be seen in Figure 4.15. The cardiogenic area develops where a mesh of fine vessels coalesce to meet the metabolic needs of the neural tube. There is a dense accumulation of these vessels above, lateral and ventral to the neural folds.

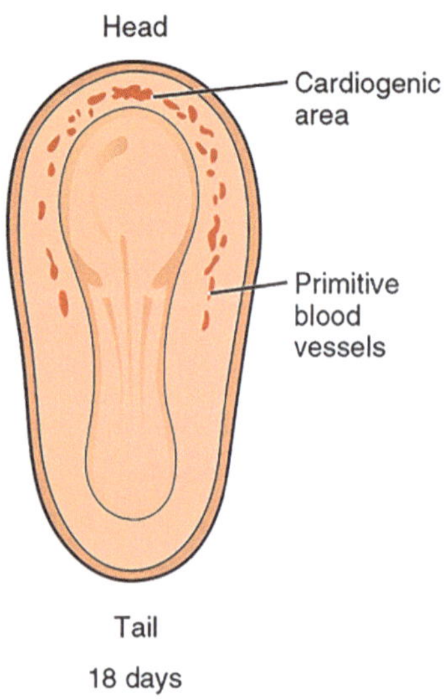


**Figure 4.15 – Embryonic Development of the Heart.** At day 18, the paired endothelial cords canalise into tubes like trickling water in sand that fuse in the midline to form a single heart. Reprinted with permission from Schoenwolf.[23]

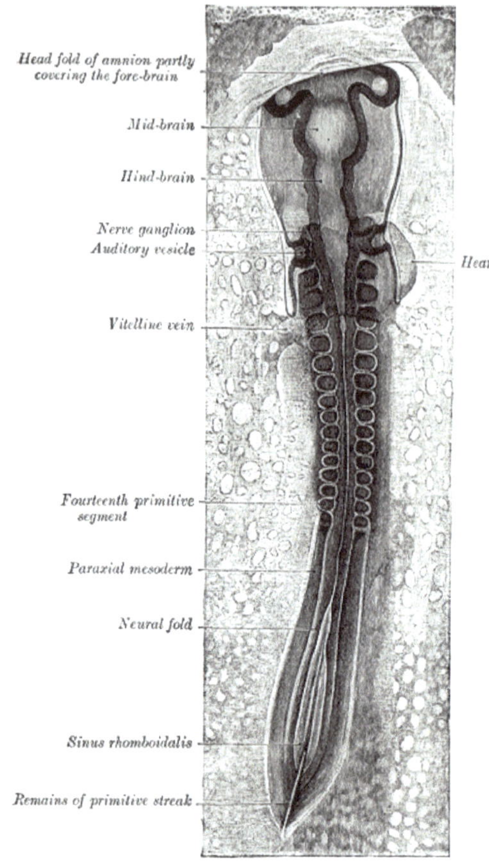


**Figure 4.16 – Neural Tube Development.** Reprinted from Gray.[24]

As the neural groove matures, the walls fuse like a zip. The nutrients in the undifferentiated mesenchyme and early plexiform vessels flow in the same direction towards the neural tube. The neural tube continues to grow and is impacted by 2 factors: nutritive and mechanical.

At this stage, there is equal access to nutrition along the neural plate. The mechanical presence of the yolk stalk (connecting between the yolk sac and the midgut) creates a relative compression on the caudal end compared to cephalad, and it tends to retard the growth of a tail. In Figure 4.16, the neural tube proliferates longitudinally and laterally.

The lateral development is greatest at the cephalad end primarily because there is the space to develop. This rapid proliferation of neural cells/ectoderm soon approaches the potential to access nutrients by diffusion from the amniotic fluid, and so the demand—the hunger—for another nutritional source is created. Through this need, structures develop to support this growth, namely the developing cardiogenic area.

With the rapidly enlarging brain growing away from the nutritional source of the yolk sac, the mesenchymal layer vessels become restrained. In order to continue to grow, the embryo folds forwards, towards the nutritional source, and slightly rotates towards the left, leading to the septum transversum, coelom, cardiogenic area (future heart) and bilateral aortic arches, relatively descending anteriorly and inferiorly (Figure 4.17). This is the first flexion and rotation motion of the embryo, a pattern of growth movement the embryo will repeat many times over.

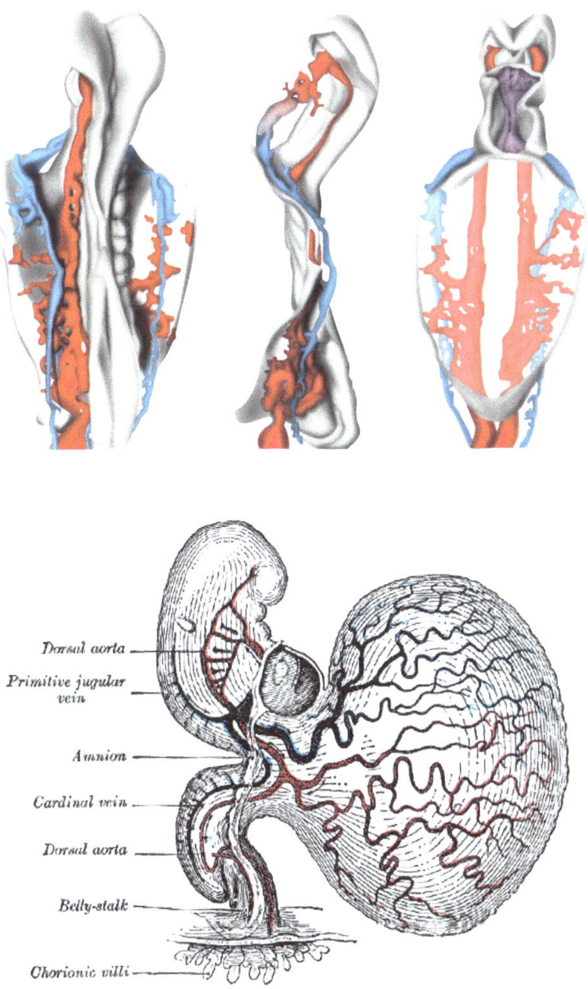


**Figure 4.17 – Developing Brain and Neural Tissue.** Neural development of a 7-somite embryo (top) and human embryo of about 14 days, with yolk-sac (bottom). Reprinted from Payne[25] and Gray.[26]

Between days 18–22, the neural tube closes and a single heart tube and aorta forms in the midline.

With growth of the whole embryo, the heart tube (with the cardiac jelly) initiates formation of the heart chambers and grows into the pericardial cavity, forming the future mediastinum (Figure 4.18). This is broad transversely and rests on the septum transversum, the future diaphragm, which, with growth, will partition the cavity from the peritoneum. All of this is happening in just a couple of days, at the end of that third week or start of the fourth week.

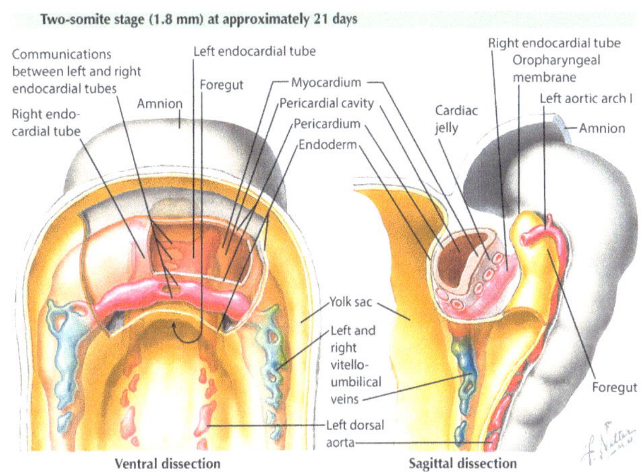


**Figure 4.18 – Two-Somite Stage at Approximately 21 Days.** Reprinted from Netter.[27]

## Development of the Heart

The primitive heart is 1.5–1.8 mm around days 18 to 20. The heart tube can be seen in the midline, and the septum transversum appears around day 22, dividing the area where the heart and lungs develop from the gut.

In relation to growth movements and twisting of the whole embryo, the heart follows; it folds to the left, which is the initiation of changes in shape that result in the heart being positioned to the left of the midline.

The folding of the embryo is directly related to the folding of the heart. This tube, which has rich, oxygenated blood pouring into it, grows more quickly than the other tissues around it. As a result, it buckles in on itself.

This is a key moment. As the tube folds, the curvature of the tube provides more resistance to blood flow. Because of the spiralling blood flow pouring into this area under significant pressure, the area of that original tube starts to dilate apart. From that single tube the left and right ventricles develop.

In Figure 4.18, we see the future atria, which are part of the inflow tract (which initially appear in the area below the heart), the future ventricle, the bulbus cordis and the future arch of the aorta.

The blood flowing in expands the single chamber, and with the inflow tract, two chambers start to form when dense connective tissue forms the *endocardial cushions* that will later form the septum that separates the chambers of the heart. The endocardial cushions coincide with where the fold of the tube is and create some resistance to blood flow; in response, further folding develops.

In every image of the embryo you see the growth torsions that represent normal growth movements. As the upper half of the embryo is growing and twisting to the left, the lower half is growing and twisting to the right. The patterns of blood flow match these movements because they are responding to the demands of whatever region is more metabolically active.

Figure 4.19 is a photograph titled "A Child is Born" by Lennart Nillson. In this image, you can observe the closing neuropore, the first fold of the heart tube and the first two pharyngeal arches. Equally importantly, you can observe the growth torsion in the early embryo.

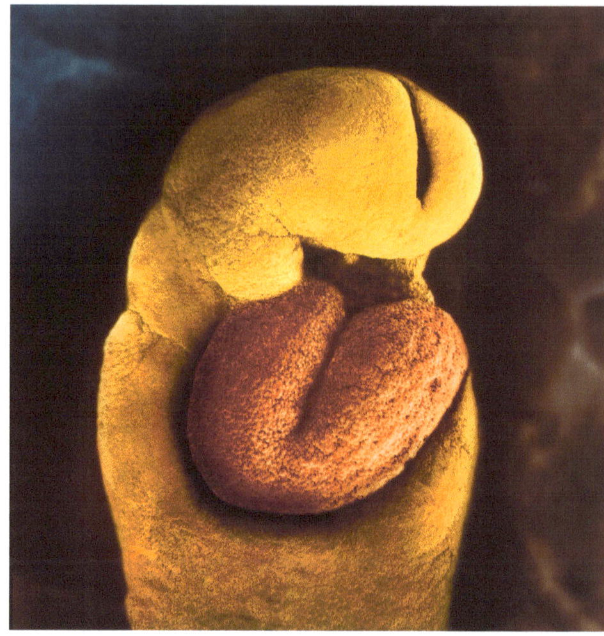

**Figure 4.19 – Embryo at 24 Days.** Reprinted from Lennart Nilsson, TT/Science Photo Library.[28]

An important point about the foramen ovale and its related atrioventricular septum[29] is that it actually stays relatively the same size throughout the process. The expansion and dilation of the tissues around it makes this orifice become relatively much smaller until it finally coalesces and closes. It is the growth of the whole heart that eventually closes the septum.

In Figure 4.20, observe how much more the heart is twisted upon itself. More of the coelom breaks down with the increasing development of the pericardium with a separation from the dorsal wall.

The heart originally is just a tube, but as the flow dilates the chamber, the heart tube starts to fold. That fold becomes the edge of where the endocardial cushions form. And then further maturation of the chambers and the continued folding of the tube occurs, so that the ventricular portion of the heart lies below the atria.

To summarise, there is the neural tube and the future heart field. There is a linear heart tube that buckles to the left, expanding the left ventricle, then the two ventricles coalesce to form one chamber, then the fold in between these areas becomes the area where the endocardial cushions form. That endocardial cushion eventually closes off to form two separate ventricular chambers.

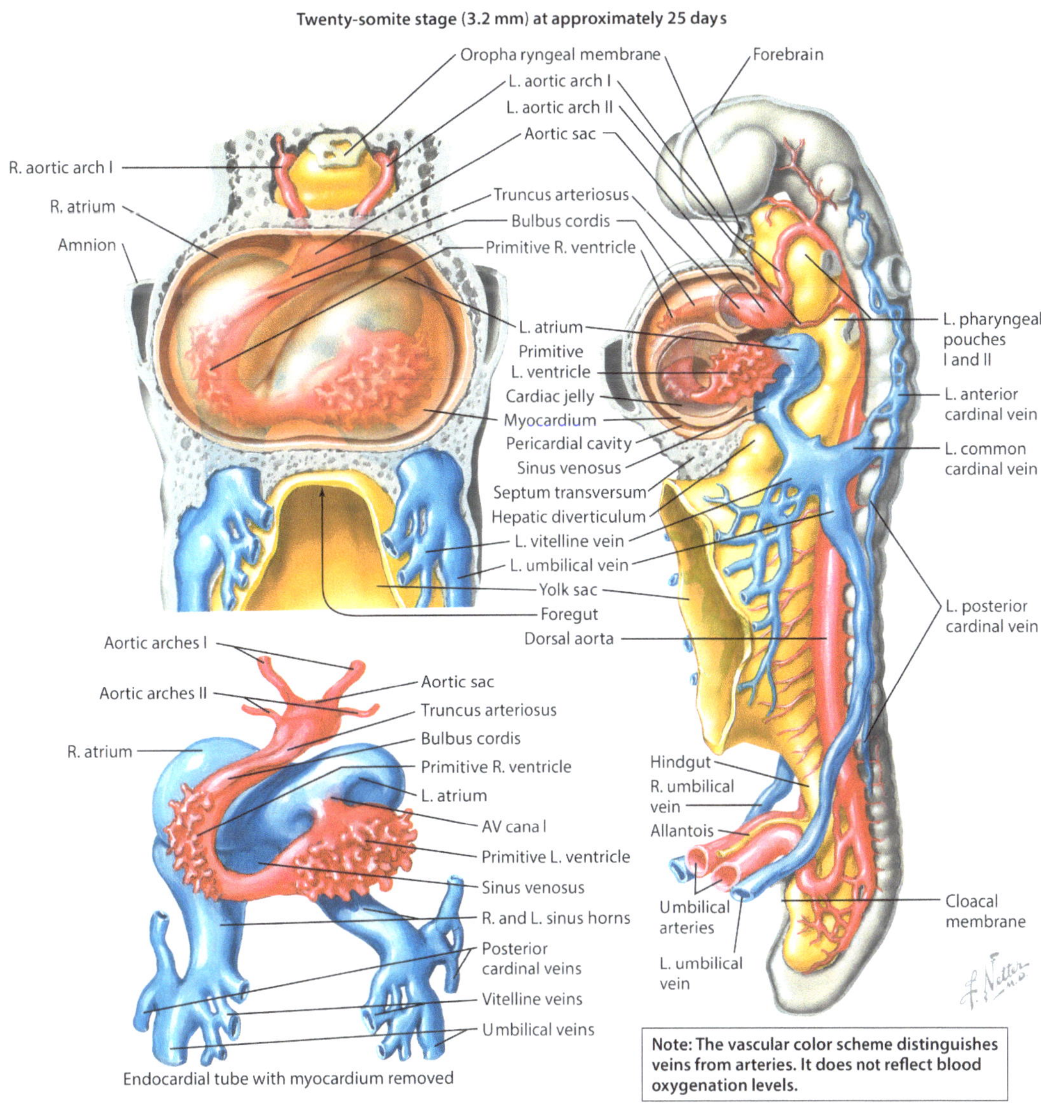


**Figure 4.20 – Twenty-Somite Stage at Approximately 25 Days.** Reprinted from Netter.[30]

## Vortical Flow Sculpts Tissue Into Form

Let us briefly review the importance of vortical flow from Chapter 3 and integrate it with the information from this chapter. The blood does not flow in the same way that water flows out of a tap. Blood has an innate spiral quality to it. Blood comes into the ventricle as a spiral and then gets ejected as a spiral. The endocardial cushions form and separate the chambers. There is only one outflow tract, but that spiralling creates another two little chambers that coalesce to separate the pulmonary arteries.

The formation of these two little chambers relates to that spiral flow. There is an outflow tract to the body and to the lungs, and the division of that outflow tract comes from that spiraling flow. Some

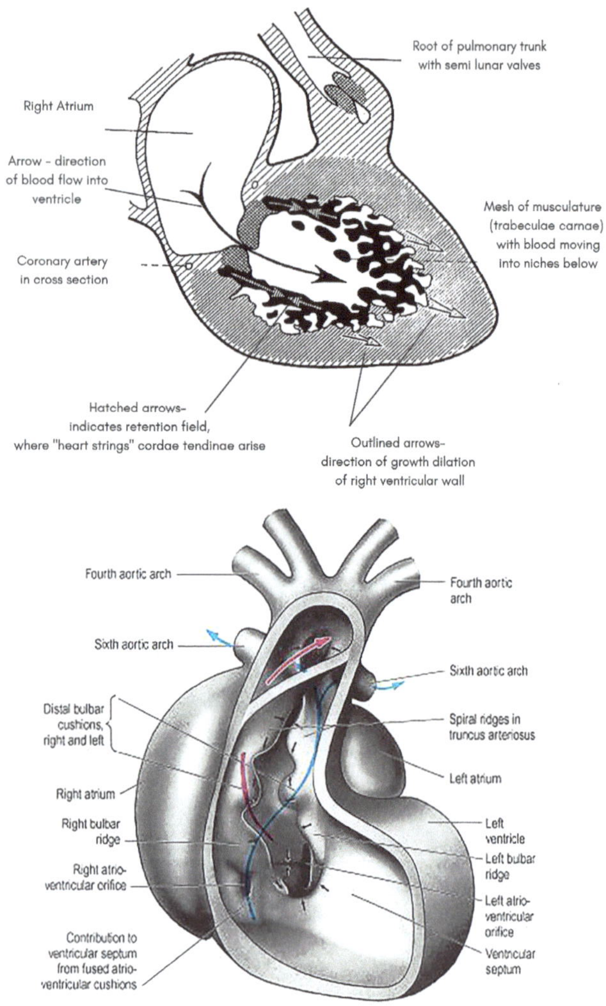


**Figure 4.21 – Fluid Flow Sculpts Tissue.** Reprinted from Blechschmidt[31] and Standring.[32]

of the cells in that flow come up against a tiny little ridge, and that ridge develops more and more into a separation of the whole outflow tract.

In Figure 4.21, the tailed arrow shows the main direction of blood flow spiralling into the right ventricle and sculpting and stretching the cardiac jelly, which under the associated forces will develop into cardiac muscle. The ventricle expands and then recoils, spiraling the blood out through the outflow tracts. The jelly-like consistency allows for niches to develop in the wall of the ventricle.

Fluid flow carves small pathways between the niches, leading to the development of a reticulated or mesh-like network of cells to form the chordae tendinae. The local forces on these cells involve pulling the tissue taut, which is described as a retention field and is in response to the spiralling flow. The spiralling flow in the outflow tract sculpts the mesenchymal tissue and divides the single outflow tube into the future aortic arch and pulmonary arteries.

The bottom image in Figure 4.21 depicts how vortical flow and folding sculpts and moulds the shape of the adult heart. This is where the formation of the septa occurs that separates the aortic and pulmonary channels in the embryonic heart. The red arrow indicates the aortic channel and the blue arrow the pulmonary channel. Where the red and blue lines cross, the ridge indicates the separation between the two ventricles. This is where the chambers expand on each side of the developing ventricular septum and flow precedes form in the division of the chambers and outflow tracts.

The blood flowing into the heart acts like a "commutator," a switch. It changes the direction of the flow. It also facilitates the vortical flow going into it and the vortical flow going out of it.

## Applications to Osteopathic Practice

Studying and understanding embryological motion and development can extend beyond the academic interest of the practitioner. Understanding the sculpting of form by the biokinetics of flow leads to an understanding of function.

Movement is not only an essential expression or consequence of life, but rather it is integral to the whole process of embryological development and ongoing homeostatic processes beyond the womb into the outside world. Essentially, what is being proposed is that the movements expressed through formation are the same movements associated with the maintenance and expression of health throughout life. The osteopath works with these inherent motions with their patients at all stages of their life, from the newborn through old age.

Understanding these movement patterns not only assists the osteopath in facilitating and supporting the patient's tissues towards health, but it can also help explain some of the observations or otherwise unexplained experiences shared in the therapeutic dynamic.

While the structure of anatomy and key physiological processes can be learnt from a textbook, the normal variance of the individual cannot. One must understand the application of principles and how to apply scientific knowledge in conjunction with listening to the patient's tissues. For example, the unobstructed flow of blood supports the body's ability to self-repair while impeded or altered flow may act as a precursor to the development of dysfunction.

Working with newborn babies often provides the practitioner with the opportunity to feel the function of flow sculpting the tissues, particularly in the closing of the foramen ovale or ductus arteriosus. The anatomy changes according to the changes in the whole environment, particularly the need to breathe on one's own. However, it is also important to recognise that this is in relation to changes in the internal environment, the wringing out like motion patterns of the expanding lungs twisting on the patent ductus arteriosus and effectively shutting it off. When this process is interrupted or impeded, the function of flow continues, leading to a lack of stimulus driving structural change.

Furthermore, the work of Torrent-Guasp helps us understand how the embryological spiraling of the ventricular muscle ends up.

> "The exhaustive and painstaking anatomical dissection studies of Francisco Torrent-Guasp in over a thousand hearts of diverse species, carefully prepared in order to dissolve the collagen scaffolding without distorting the preferential linear or laminar pathways, have shown that the heart can be unraveled into a continuous myocardial band that extends from the pulmonary artery to the aorta. This band forms a basal loop in continuity with an apical loop consisting of a descending and an ascending segment, the sequential contraction of which determines the isovolumetric contraction (basal loop), ejection (descending) and 'isovolumetric relaxation' (ascending) phases [*Figure 4.22*] of the cardiac cycle."[33]

The orientation of all of the ventricular fibres relate to function. In the lengthening and suction in the chambers and in the widening and uncoiling of the chambers, the ventricular myocardial band is oriented to emphasise and support function: the lengthening during suction and the widening and narrowing during ejection.

When the heart beats, there is a single impulse that spreads throughout the whole of the myocardial band, and it is the contraction of that single myocardial band that is involved in both phases of the heartbeat: diastole and systole. As one part of the band begins to contract, it spirals down towards the apex. As it contracts, the fibres shorten,

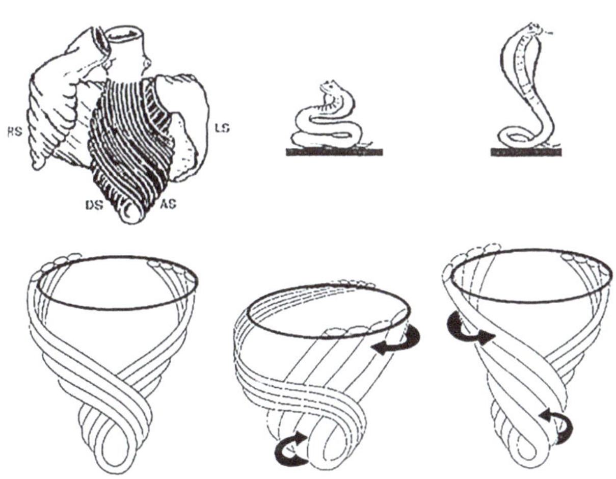


**Figure 4.22 – Twisting of the Heart Segments.**
Reprinted from Buckberg.[34]

the heart rotates around and these fibres become more vertical.

Next, the electrical impulse passes through the myocardial band and turns the corner at the apex. The fibres on the ascending part again shorten and rotate the heart back around the other way. So, each beat of the heart is generated by a single electrical impulse that runs through the whole of that myocardial band. It functions in the same way as a coiled cobra. It elevates itself into a standing position; the heart starts in this long and thin shape, becoming coiled and then lengthening again using the same muscular agents.

Notice the heart ascending and descending through the orientation of the myocardial fibres and the fibres formed secondarily to support the function of that coiling and uncoiling.

Take a moment to watch "The Helical Heart" video by visiting https://www.youtube.com/watch?v=v75tpamodY4 or scanning the following QR code:

In this video, Torrent-Guasp describes his method of blunt dissection of the heart. The serial images at the end of the video are an excellent overview of the orientation of the fibres of the left and right ventricles.

To understand the interventricular septum, it needs to be seen in the context of a single band of muscle with a wrap-around circumferential band at the base and septum composed of helical fibres that are oblique and cross each other at 60° angles. When the helical band contracts, the base is drawn downward towards the apex in a spiraling motion. The ventricular septum forms a wall between the left and right ventricle and is a midline structure that we can use to observe the charge in the left and right chamber. The helical band, with its cyclic shortening and lengthening, produces 80% of the ejection fraction or output of the heart.

Figure 4.23 illustrates Torrent-Guasp's summary of the process of cardiac contraction, which is as follows:

- The spiral formation of the helical loop produces a twisting effect that causes a counterclockwise rotation of the heart, including the apex, which remains in a fixed position.
- The shortening and twisting of the apical loop squeezes the ventricular cavity to raise pressure and opens the aortic valve to eject blood to the body.

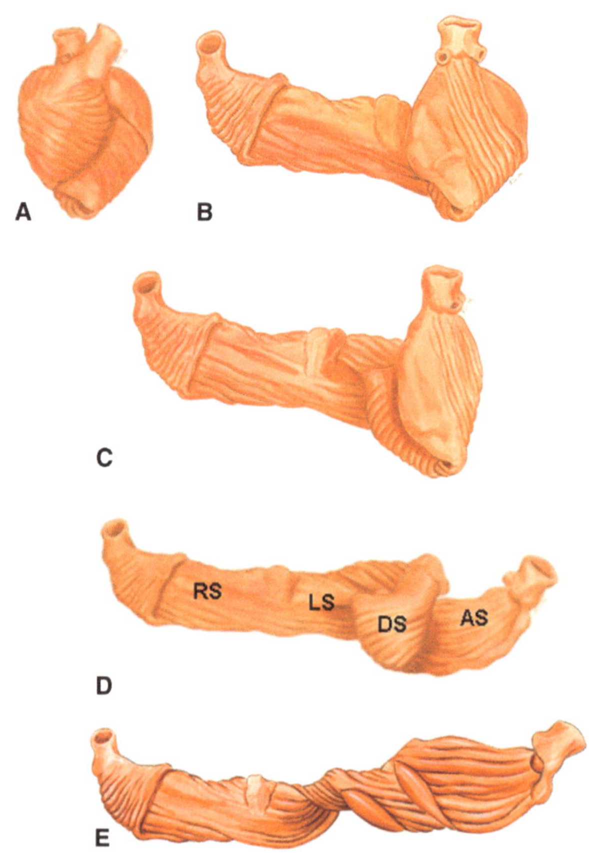


**Figure 4.23 – Torrent-Guasp's Unscrolling Myocardial Band.** Reprinted from Buckberg et al.[35]

- From the osteopathic perspective: The fulcrum within the interventricular septum is dynamic and shifting, is suspended between the two ventricles and has a nodal point at the apex.
- The contraction of the descending loop shortens the ventricle.
- The adherence of the apical loop to the rigid basal loop pulls the stiff outer shell down towards the apex.
- The fibrous connection of the great vessels descends with the basal loop.
- When the basal loop contracts, it constricts or narrows the ventricles to compress the underlying muscle.
- The sequence starts with the right ventricle and then goes to the left segment to cause a clockwise cocking before beginning ventricular shortening.

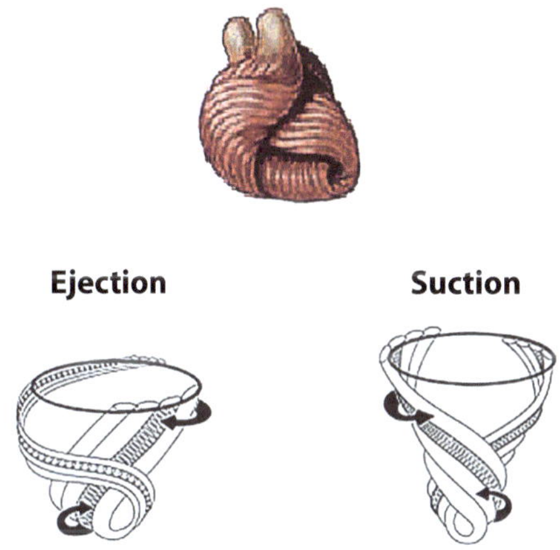


**Figure 4.24 –** Cardiac Suction and Ejection.

The delivery of electrical impulses through the heart's specialised conduction system results in a wave contraction that follows the path of the ventricular band from the pulmonary arteries to the aorta. Active contraction moves along the band as the wave progresses.

Figure 4.24 illustrates cardiac suction and ejection. The clockwise twist at the apical loop produces a potential vacuum and begins to lengthen the ventricle, pushing the basal loop back up. The untwisting opens the atrioventricular valve so that atrial blood is actively sucked into the ventricle; this causes widening of the cavity as 50%–60% of effective filling occurs as the ascending atrial segment rises.

The helical course of the contraction continues with a vortex or figure eight around the apex. Contraction of the ascending segment twists its fibres, resulting in a clockwise rotation of the heart.

The object of the osteopath is to use this knowledge of flow, function and form from embryo to the postnatal period to become aware of the charge differential between the left and right ventricle and to feel the quality of the two ventricles; for example, you may feel that the right ventricle feels denser and less vital.*

*For a discussion of the palpatory qualities of paramagnetic (venous) and diamagnetic (arterial) blood, see Chapter 8, p. 133.

## Chapter 4 Endnotes

1. A.T. Still, *Philosophy and Mechanical Principles of Osteopathy* (Kansas City, MO: Hudson-Kimberly Publishing Co., 1902), 58.

2. Philip Mathew and Bruno Bordoni, "Embryology, Heart," In *StatPearls* (Treasure Island, FL: StatPearls Publishing, 2022), last modified August 8, 2022, https://www.ncbi.nlm.nih.gov/books/NBK537313/.

3. Mary F. Donovan and Marco Cascella, "Embryology, Weeks 6-8," In *StatPearls* (Treasure Island, FL: StatPearls Publishing, 2022), last modified October 10, 2022, https://www.ncbi.nlm.nih.gov/books/NBK563181/.

4. Richard C.V. Tyser, "Formation of the Heart: Defining Cardiomyocyte Progenitors at Single-Cell Resolution," *Current Cardiology Reports* 25 (2023): 495–503, https://doi.org/10.1007/s11886-023-01880-z .

5. "The History of the Heart," Early Science Lab, Stanford University, accessed June 30, 2023, https://web.stanford.edu/class/history13/earlysciencelab/body/heartpages/heart.html.

6. Still, *Philosophy and Mechanical Principles of Osteopathy*, 48.

7. Raymond F. Gasser, "The First Week of Life: Conception to Implantation Period," *Atlas of Human Embryos* (R.F. Gasser, 1975), Fig. 1-1, reprinted in The Endowment for Human Development, https://www.ehd.org/classics/gasser_ch1.php.

8. Gasser, "The First Week of Life."

9. Winifrida B. Kidima, "Syncytiotrophoblast Functions and Fetal Growth Restriction during Placental Malaria: Updates and Implication for Future Interventions," *BioMed Research International* 2015 (2015): 451735, https://doi.org/10.1155/2015/451735.

10. Gary C. Schoenwolf, et al., *Larsen's Human Embryology* (Philadelphia, PA: Churchill Livingstone, 2015).

11. Erich Blechschmidt, *The Beginnings of Human Life* (Springer, 1977).

12. Blechschmidt, *The Beginnings of Human Life.*

13. Blechschmidt, *The Beginnings of Human Life.*

14. Erich Blechschmidt and R.F. Gasser, *Biokinetics and Biodynamics of Human Differentiation: Principles and Applications* (Berkely, CA: North Atlantic Books, 1978).

15. Blechschmidt and Gasser, *Biokinetics and Biodynamics.*

16. Blechschmidt and Gasser, *Biokinetics and Biodynamics,* 36.

17. Still, *The Philosophy and Mechanical Principles of Osteopathy.*

18. Erich Blechschmidt, *The Ontogenetic Basis of Human Anatomy: A Biodynamic Approach to Development from Conception to Birth,* (Berkely, CA: North Atlantic Books, 2004).

19. "Implantation (Embryology)," Wikipedia Foundation, last modified January 21, 2024, https://en.wikipedia.org/wiki/Implantation_%28embryology%29

20. Blechschmidt, *The Beginnings of Human Life.*

21. Toyoaki Fujimoto. "Nishimura's Collection of Human Embryos and Related Collections," *Congenital Anomalies* 41, no. 1 (March 2001): 67–71, https://doi.org/10.1111/j.1741-4520.2001.tb00875.x.

22. Schoenwolf et al., *Larsen's Human Embryology.*

23. Schoenwolf et al., *Larsen's Human Embryology*, Figure 7.1.

24. Henry Gray, *Anatomy of the Human Body* (Philadelphia, PA: Lea & Febiger, 1918), accessed August 4, 2023, https://commons.wikimedia.org/wiki/File:Gray18.png.

25. F. Payne, "General Description of a 7-Somite Human Embryo," *Contributions to Embryology* 16 (1925): 115–23.

26. Gray, *Anatomy of the Human Body*, accessed January 3, 2024, https://commons.m.wikimedia.org/wiki/File:Gray459.png#mw-jump-to-license.

27. Frank Netter, *Two-somite stage 21 days*. Used with permission of Elsevier. All rights reserved. Netterimages.com, https://www.netterimages.com/

28. Lennart Nilsson et al., *The Everyday Miracle: A Child Is Born* (Allen Lane, The Penguin Press, 1967).

29. Michelle R. Annabi, Connor C. Kerndt, and Amgad N. Makaryus, "Embryology, Atrioventricular Septum," in StatPearls (StatPearls Publishing, 2023), last updated May 1, 2023, https://www.ncbi.nlm.nih.gov/books/NBK482372/.

30. Frank Netter, *Twenty-somite stage 25 days*, Used with permission of Elsevier. All rights reserved. Netterimages.com, https://www.netterimages.com/

31. Blechschmidt. *The Ontogenetic Basis of Human Anatomy*.

32. Susan Standring, ed., *Gray's Anatomy: The Anatomical Basis of Clinical Practice*, 40th ed. (London, UK: Churchhill Livingston, 2008).

33. H. Cecil Coghlan et al., "'The Electrical Spiral of the Heart': Its Role in the Helical Continuum: The Hypothesis of the Anisotropic Conducting Matrix," *European Journal of Cardio-Thoracic Surgery* 29, supplement 1 (April 2006): S178–87, https://doi.org/10.1016/j.ejcts.2006.02.046.

34. Gerald Buckberg, "The Helix and the Heart," *The Journal of Thoracic and Cardiovascular Surgery* 124, no. 5 (November 2002): 863–883, https://doi.org/10.1067/mtc.2002.122439.

35. Gerald Buckberg et al., "Structure and function relationships of the helical ventricular myocardial band," *The Journal of Thoracic and Cardiovascular Surgery* 136, no. 3 (September 2008): 578–89.e11, https://doi.org/10.1016/j.jtcvs.2007.10.088.

# Chapter Five

# The Fascia and the Code

*"The secret of life and of nature is the fundamentality of waves waving within one another."*[1]

– Irving Dardik

In *Philosophy and Mechanical Principles of Osteopathy*, Dr Still wrote:

> "I know of no part of the body that equals the fascia as hunting ground. I believe that more rich golden thoughts will appear to the mind's eye as the study of the fascia is pursued than of any other division of the body…In every view we take of the fascia a wonder appears. The part the fascia takes in life and death gives us one of the greatest problems to solve. It surrounds each muscle, vein, nerve, and all organs of the body. It has a network of nerves, cells, and tubes running to, from, and through it; it is filled with millions of nerve centres and fibers which carry on the work of secreting and excreting fluids vital and destructive."

In the words of Still, "By its action we live and by its failure we wither and die."[2]

Without doubt, the connective tissue is "the most abundant, widely distributed" tissue of animal matter.[3] It forms the bulk of the animal body, consisting of "extracellular matrices, integrins, cytoskeletons, nuclear matrices"[4] and all aspects of materials that create and maintain it. Keep that in mind a moment.

Still also said that the heart "imparts the attributes of life and **knowledge** to the blood so that it can proceed correctly with all its work".[5] We have called this "The Heart's Code", the phrase being an echo of the book written by psychologist Paul Pearsall[6] that carries that title, in which he presents research on cellular memory and energy cardiology. Indeed, the shape and orientation of red blood cells affect the sound energy (introduced in Chapter 1) in the blood they flow through, with certain shapes and orientations leading to a loss of sound energy and an effect on health.[7]

These two great insights of Still's—the heart imparting knowledge to the blood and that we live and die by the **action** of the fascia—are the focus of this chapter.

The heart's code is delivered to the arterial tree, which is estimated to be 161,000 km (100,000 miles) long. From there, nutrients and oxygen pass across the capillary beds into the bloodstream and extracellular matrix or fascia.

Now, recall from Chapter 1 that the helical-vortical flow of blood and the charge existing within the blood facilitates flow. Additionally, recall that the blood from the heart flows in an oscillatory wave that has been named the *Traube-Hering wave*. Ludwig Traube and Karl Ewald Hering independently discovered a slow oscillation in pressure underlying standard blood pressure recordings from carotid arteries of dogs in the mid-1800s. This oscillation has become known as the Traube-Hering wave. Its rate coincides with the rate of the fluctuation of fluid that osteopaths call *primary respiration* or *The Tide*.[8]

James Oschman discusses this phenomenon in terms of charge, also indicating that an oscillating direct current can be measured in arteries and nerves.[9,10] The flow of blood in arteries is vortical and helical. The helical impulse, we assert, is the representation of this oscillating, direct current and fluctuant pressure that is measurable and palpable in the bloodstream and known to science as the Traube-Hering wave.[11]

This oscillatory wave is a whole body phenomenon that exhibits a rate that is typically slightly less than, and independent of, respiration: about 7–10 times per minute. This is similar to one of the rates described for the primary respiratory mechanism.[12,13]

In addition to blood flow being a consequence of the suction of the 35 trillion cells expressing a metabolic need (also introduced in Chapter 1), and to nitric oxide production and sulphate charge, the Traube-Hering oscillation effects a cyclic delivery of more, and then less, electrolytes at the capillary bed with a resultant oscillatory concentration of ions in the extracellular matrix.

Recall that in Chapter 1 we referred to the paravasal plasma mantle (PVM), or perivascular space, as a way in which the heart's code is entrained with the fluid in the extracellular matrix adjacent to the PVM.[14–16] In addition to the PVM, Hauk[17] showed that there are islands within the extracellular matrix that are relatively more, and then less, gelatinous. This gel/sol oscillation occurs continuously within the matrix and is also referred to in Chapter 3.

Still mentions electricity **170 times** in the four books he published, and so we will briefly review how the electrical properties of the blood link to the electrical qualities of the extracellular matrix.[18,19,20,21] These electrical qualities derive from the crystalline form of the fascia or extracellular matrix, its piezoelectric and colloidal properties and the presence of *ionars*, or groups of ions, and their effects. Together these form the basis for information (**knowledge**) transfer via an atomic and subatomic messenger or communication system.[22]

## Ionic Fluctuations

The Traube-Hering pressure oscillation affects a cyclic delivery of more, and then less, electrolytes at the capillary bed with a resultant oscillatory concentration of ions in the extracellular matrix. Dr Björn Nordenström, professor emeritus of radiology at the Karolinska Institute and former chairman of the Nobel Assembly in Sweden, identified these ionic concentrations as ionars.[23] Nordenström developed the principle of Biologically Closed Electric Circuits (BCEC) as a result of decades of research and described the structural and functional effects in his book *Biologically Closed Electric Circuits*. In his writing, Nordenström emphasised the electrical nature of our world and how close the relationship is between electricity, particles and wavelengths. We witness this in the technology that has become an integral part of our lives. Similarly, though frequently more complex and therefore less immediately apparent, electrical circuits and functions exist in biology.[24] According to Nordenström:

> "Matter derived from electromagnetic energy, supplied with the electrically powered BCEC systems, inherits prerequisites to become biological matter. This is possible because mechanisms of BCEC systems contain the capacity to initiate structur-

> ing and functioning of matter…BCEC systems… may provide the important primary steps that are necessary for the transfer of non-biological into biological matter. Secondly, other factors are evidently contributing to biological differentiation, including for instance the principle of differential selection of species. Due to their basic role, the BCEC systems can nevertheless be recognized to be involved in the majority of structural and functional expressions in biology. This rests on the fact that our physical world once developed from energy and specifically its representation of electric energy."[25]

The Vascular-Interstitial Closed Circuit (VICC) is one specific BCEC system that uses mechanical circulation and functions as a charge-based system. Because its efficiency partly depends on its capacity to provide bidirectional transport of ions, the VICC is an "in vivo electrophoretic-dielectrophoretic system that is powered by metabolic energy or injury currents".[26]

In his book *Interface: Mechanisms of Spirit in Osteopathy,* Dr R. Paul Lee devotes a section of his book to the extracellular matrix. Lee draws attention to Pischinger's observation that "the most suitable energy form through which open biological systems create and maintain structure and organisation is information input and processing.[27] *Such information is in the form of electrostatic charge and electric current* [emphasis added]."[28] According to Becker,[29] these charges exist in the water and fibres of the connective tissue. Lee states that "these charges and currents transmit information in the form of molecules, ions, protons and electrons as well as via hydrophobic forces, hydrogen bonds, electrostatic forces and van der Waals forces."[30] The phase transition that occurs in the ECM is an important part of the process of information transfer within the matrix. Pollack describes the sol-to-gel and gel-to-sol phase transition as happening in an instant when there is a shift in pH, temperature, ion content, biophoton output, electrical field and mechanical stress.[31]

Nordenström determined that the VICC activation leads to transports of metabolites, new structuring and healing of an injured tissue. There are groups of ions that collect in the extracellular fluid because of the electrophoretic-dielectrophoretic system's metabolic activities and local differences in capillary bed circulation, matrix properties and ionic size and mobility.

According to Nordenström, groups of ions represent an electromotive force and participate in the fluctuation of charge. They are responsible for actual structural modifications and are associated with movement of water. Fluctuation of polarity is created when an injury potential or physiological polarisation is accompanied by an opposite reaction to balance the polarity. As these actions increase in this process, fluctuation is established.

Nordenström found that healing results from the ebb and flow of ions and that fluctuations occur in different degrees in injured and normal tissue and in morphogenesis. Oxidation/reduction reactions were found to occur in the fluids next to fibrous membranes.

Nordenström explored the electrical activity in the extracellular matrix. He found that there were 5 mV and 1 mV alterations of potential in the tissues that he was recording with microelectrodes. He established a whole new technology using microelectrodes to record cellular activity. The electrical potentials recorded are for a 1-minute duration. So Nordenström was recording electrical activity, a potential change in the tissue, that was at the rate of 7 times per minute, the same rate as the vascular Traube-Hering oscillation and consistent with primary respiration. Osteopaths are familiar with this rate, as they have shown it is possible to perceive it by somatic palpation on a blinded basis.[32,33] Importantly, not only did Sergueef et al show that it is possible to palpate the Traube-Hering wave, but they also demonstrated that cranial manipulation favourably affects the Traube-Hering wave.[34]

## Crystalline Form of the Fascia or Extracellular Matrix

When crystals are mentioned, we usually think of solids such as diamonds. However, crystals in living tissue are liquid and pliable structures consisting of long and thin molecules that are soft and flexible.[35] These crystalline forms are the rule rather than the exception in biological forms. They can be found in collagen arrays that are ubiquitously found in fascia, phospholipids that form part of cell membranes and the myelin sheaths of nerves, contractile arrays in muscles, microfilaments and other fibrous components of the cytoskeleton.

As long ago as 1941, Nobel laureate Prof Szent-Györgyi suggested that a large number of molecules may join to form energy continua, along which energy may travel some distance as excited electrons. He wrote that:

> "If a number of atoms be arranged in close proximity, as for example in a crystal lattice, single valency atoms cease to belong to one or two atoms only, and belong instead to the whole system."[36]

In 1988, Herbert Fröhlich suggested that crystalline molecular arrays would vibrate strongly and coherently.[37] James Oschman found that "In crystals, a great number of atoms or molecules are packed closely together in a lattice arrangement. The bonding electrons that hold the crystal together, which are called *valence electrons*, are actually mobile. They are not fixed in place and do not belong to any particular atom, molecule or bond but instead belong to the whole system."[38] As a result, many atoms or molecules can join together to form an energetic continuum, composed of excited electrons, moving about within the crystalline lattice.

Pienta and Coffey[39] combined the concepts of the living matrix, vibratory and resonant interactions, cellular and tissue continuity, coherence and solid state biochemistry. They envisioned a continuous interaction between the capillary bed, the matrix and the cellular cytoplasm and cytoskeleton whereby dynamic vibration with complex harmonics can be transferred bidirectionally. Fröhlich[40] predicted that biological systems must produce coherent oscillations. Lee hypothesizes that a calcium flux, with its resultant phasic increase and decrease of ions, ultimately leads to a cyclic sol and gel phase within the extracellular matrix (see Appendix).

Pischinger[41] proposed that, in addition to the cellular oscillations predicted by Fröhlich, the extracellular matrix also has an oscillatory pattern. This oscillation is due to the constantly changing pH, ion concentration, viscosity, hydrostatic pressure and electrostatic charge in the matrix.

As seen in Figure 5.1, hyaluronan, with its heavily sulphated moieties that carry a negative charge, can load calcium and release water,[42] triggered by fluctuations in ionic concentrations, pH and electrostatic charge. The result is that there is a phasic loading and unloading of water. This release of water in turn causes a shift from gel to sol in the surrounding tissue. The oscillation from gel to sol occurs at a rate of 7 cycles per minute, or what osteopaths describe as primary inhalation and exhalation or flexion and extension and which is also a similar oscillation rate to the Traube-Hering wave.

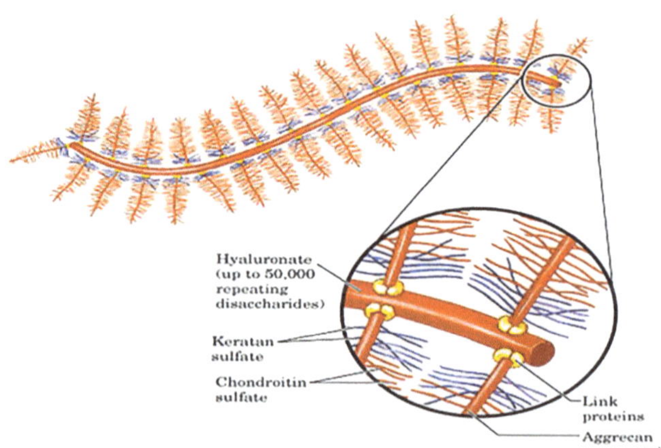


**Figure 5.1– Aggregates of Proteoglycan.** The extracellular matrix of cartilage is mainly composed of proteoglycan aggregates, collagen and glycoproteins such as integrins and fibronectin. Reprinted from Oschman.[43]

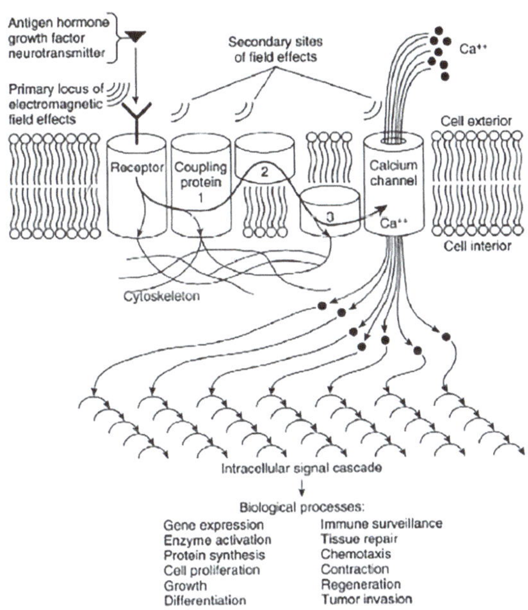


**Figure 5.2 – Wide-Ranging Intracellular Action of Calcium.** Reprinted with permission from Oschman.[45]

In addition to the oscillation occurring in the fascia (matrix), there is also a cellular oscillation. The calcium flux influences the cell in many ways, as illustrated in Figure 5.2.[44]

The oscillation includes the cell's swelling and receding in a cyclical fashion, as flexion and extension occur from the moment of conception onwards.[46–48]

There is also a slower rate occurring intracellularly within the cytoplasm occurring at a rate of seven cycles in 10 minutes, which is similar to that found by Prof Seifriz[49] in his extensive work on the inherent motion of protoplasm in slime mould (shown and discussed more fully in Chapter 6).

The pattern of motion from the capillary bed into the fascia (matrix) is described by Jacobson as follows:

> "The inward stream of signals into cells is the result of a complex sequence, beginning with binding of humoral molecules that provide stimulation at their specialized binding sites. A rippling effect is elicited extending along the membrane's outer layer. Altered calcium binding to glycoproteins affects membrane related proteins serving receptor and enzymatic functions. When a weak electrical or chemical stimulus is sensed, signals are transmitted to the cell's interior along coupling proteins, and this interaction may include non-linear vibrational waves (solitons) in the amide spines of helical proteins."[50]

This is what Prof Adey envisaged when he described cells as "whispering" to one another.[51–53]

## Piezoelectric Qualities

All movements of the body as a whole, or any part, are created by tensions that are carried through connective tissues. Connective tissue is a liquid crystalline material and one of its properties is that it behaves like a semiconductor.

One of the qualities of semiconductors is piezoelectricity—pressure can give rise to electricity and electricity can produce a vibration.[54] So, every movement we make generates a variety of oscillating bioelectric signals or microcurrents.

Piezoelectricity, and the ability of tissue to create electricity when pressure is applied, has been shown in bone,[55–58] the extracellular matrix,[59] teeth,[60] tendons,[61] blood vessel walls,[62] muscles[63] and skin.[64]

These signals spread through the fascia and then pass into cells via integrins that pass through the cell membrane. By passing through the cell wall, integrins anchor the cell wall and the cytoskeleton to the matrix or fascia. These integrins play a key role in communicating information from inside the cell to the matrix outside,[65] thereby establishing a continuum between the cells and the fascia.

Sialic acid–rich extensions of the cytoskeleton from the cell wall are negatively charged and are the sites where cells interact with extracellular proteins. This is so whether they are hormones, cell-to-cell linkers or antigens.[66,67] The sialic acid's negative charge maintains the position of the cell in relation to neighbouring cells by divalent calcium

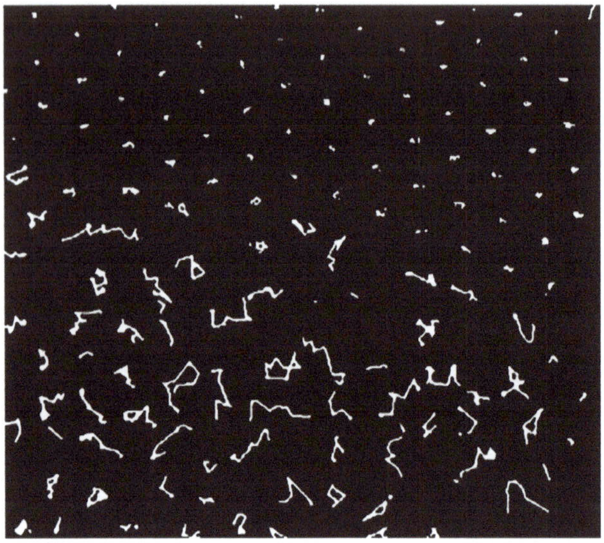

**Figure 5.3 – Ordered and Disordered Regimes of Colloidal Islands.** Trajectories of latex particles in the disordered (bottom) and ordered (top) regimes during 1 second. Reprinted from Hachisu and Yoshimura.[73]

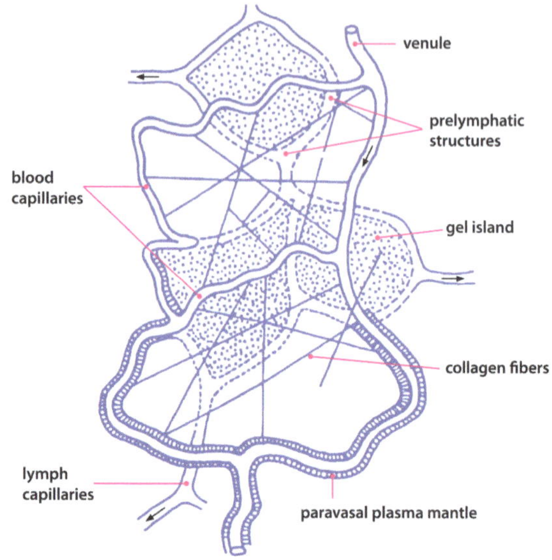


**Figure 5.4 – Outer Peripheral Circulation.** Reprinted from Holdrege.[74] The colloidal medium of the extracellular matrix alternates between a gel-like, island-forming state and a sol-like channel-forming state. Here, the barrier function with regard to the blood is not morphologically determined but is accomplished through flow processes, the so-called paravasal plasma mantle and intervasal edge flow, which interact with the blood clotting system.

bridges. However, these bridges are not stable, allowing them to break and reform as cells change shape and crawl through the matrix or fascia.[68]

Mechanical deformation, acoustical vibrations, electric fields and magnetic fields can act as first messengers by changing the conformational structure of cell membrane receptors, which can lead to modification of ion channels or activation of intracellular enzymes.[69,70]

## Colloidal Properties of the Matrix

Mae-Wan Ho discusses colloids in the context of crystals and self-assembly. Colloids consist of very fine particles suspended in water. Ho points out[71] that colloids can be crystalline and have the ability to form together in an orderly fashion, like a crystal. A variety of colloidal crystalline forms can result, depending on temperature, pH, ionic activity and other additives.

As liquid crystals, with long-range orientational order and electrical dipole interactions, they exist in a state between a liquid and a solid. These liquid crystals can contain within them electrons, protons, phonons and solitons that are free to move within them. They are also responsive to electric and magnetic fields.

In addition, Hachisu and Yoshimura[72] demonstrated that the two ordered (gel) and disordered (sol) regimes of colloidal islands could exist side by side (Figure 5.3). This reminds us of the gel and sol "islands" shown in the illustration of Hauk's paravasal mantle (Figure 5.4).

This is a different perspective and explanation of the same phenomenon proposed by Gabarel and Roques[75] whereby there is a polymerisation and depolymerisation process progressively moving calcium towards its cellular destination. They, along with other authors (Ho, Oschman and Lee), saw calcium moving in waves (of information) through the matrix or fascia.

This movement is the way in which the knowledge that Still suggested was imparted to the blood, moving at the oscillatory rate of the Traube-Hering wave, interfaces with the ionic flux (7 cycles per minute) of the extracellular matrix. This matrix, which is a crystalline colloid, carries this knowledge or information to the cells lying no further than 150 microns from the capillary bed.

As an oscillating dipole, water can orient itself towards an appropriately low intensity electric field. The same can be said for the dipole molecules that are contained in cell membranes. This can be one of the ways in which membrane permeability can be altered as charge can influence channels embedded in the cell membrane.

The fascia or extracellular matrix consists of scaffolds of long linear proteins and polysaccharides, particularly hyaluronic acid, as well as a variety of enzymes. Mixtures of hyaluronic acid with other bipolymers are electronically interactive.

Cell membranes are electrically charged and participate in internal and external cellular communication as well as storage of energy. Normal cells have integrins arranged in symmetrical patterns. The alteration in tensile forces across the cell membrane changes cytoskeletal geometry. Cellular biologist and bioengineer Donald Ingber theorised that "Changing the cytoskeletal geometry and mechanics could affect biochemical reactions and even alter the genes that are activated and thus the proteins that are made."[76]

Neuroscientist and psychopharmacologist Candace Pert's recent research provides support for the hypothesis that pressure waves, frequencies and phonons can drive metabolic processes. Previously, it was believed that molecules—chemical messengers such as peptides—need to attach themselves, or dock, on cell receptors to initiate actions, like activating or deactivating the cell. However, Pert and others reported that sound can activate the receptors on cells: Sound can initiate or deactivate any action needed from the cell, as precisely as a biochemical molecule does...only faster! Pert refers to music in her work, but her point can be applied to any type of coherent sound.[77]

Pert's research highlights just how fast sound is communicated through the body. By the time blood from a systolic event reaches the aortic bifurcation, sound from that same event has already arrived at the feet.

## Applications to Osteopathic Practice

In osteopathic practice, it behooves us to constantly keep in mind Still's emphatic statement regarding the fascia: "By its action we live and by its failure we wither and die."[78]

It is very important for osteopaths to learn to perceive and work with the Traube-Hering wave or oscillation. It has already been pointed out that the research of Surgueef and colleagues has shown that not only is it possible for osteopaths to accurately report the Traube-Hering oscillation, it is also possible to positively influence it through osteopathic treatment.[79]

Nordenström found that, at the capillary bed, groups of ions pass across the capillary and group in the extracellular matrix.[80] These groups of ions pass cyclically across the capillary wall and consistent with this movement, Nordenström measured a cycling alteration of potential between 5 mV and 1 mV in the extracellular matrix that he recorded with microelectrodes. Nordenström found this electrical potential to be both consistent and reliable and thus established a new technology using microelectrodes to record cellular and extracellular matrix activity.

The reliable variation in electrical potential was

at a rate of 7 to 8 cycles per minute, which is very close to the Traube-Hering oscillation and is also consistent with primary respiration. This constant shift in electrical potential within the matrix is what provides the electromotive force for the transfer of electrolytes, oxygen and nutrients from the capillary to the cells. As observed by Hauk, Pischinger and Ho, there are islands of gels that are either more or less viscous and electricity drives the phasic transitions from gel to sol as water shifts from being free or bound. A loss of charge will result in the persistence of gels so the tissues become thickened—what earlier osteopaths have referred to as "drag".

The piezoelectric quality of the extracellular matrix means that squeezing or stretching it gives rise to electricity. Using balanced ligamentous tension or balanced membranous tension, osteopaths can slightly increase the stretch or compression of tissues that have become dysfunctional and thereby supply electricity to areas of the matrix or fascia just as the old doctor envisaged: "As an electrician controls electric currents, so an Osteopath controls life currents and revives suspended forces."[81]

## Chapter 5 Endnotes

1. Irving Dardik, "The Origin of Disease and Health, Heart Waves: The Single Solution to Heart Rate Variability and Ischemic Preconditioning," *Frontier Perspectives* 6, no. 2 (Spring/Summer 1997): 18–32.

2. A.T. Still, *Philosophy and Mechanical Principles of Osteopathy* (Kansas City, MO: Hudson-Kimberly Publishing Co., 1902), 60.

3. Kenneth Saladin. *Human Anatomy*, 6th ed. (New York: McGraw-Hill, 2020).

4. James Oschman, "Fascia as a Body-Wide Communication System," in *Fascia: The Tensional Network of the Human Body*, ed. Robert Schleip et al. (Churchill Livingstone, 2012), https://doi.org/10.1016/B978-0-7020-3425-1.00049-0.

5. Andrew Taylor Still, *Osteopathy: Research and Practice* (Kirksville, MO: A.T. Still, 1910), 318.

6. Paul Pearsall, *The Heart's Code* (New York: Broadway Books, 1998).

7. Avtar S. Ahuja and William R. Hendee, "Effects of Particle Shape and Orientation on Propogation of Sound in Blood," *The Journal of the Acoustical Society of America* 63 (1978): 1074–80.

8. Kenneth E. Nelson et al., "Cranial Rhythmic Impulse Related to the Traube-Hering-Mayer Oscillation: Comparing Laser-Doppler Flowmetry and Palpation," *Journal of the American Osteopathic Association* 101, no. 3 (March 2001): 163–73.

9. James L. Oschman, *Energy Medicine: The Scientific Basis* (Churchill Livingstone, 2000), 223–5.

10. Robert O. Becker and Gary Selden, *The Body Electric: Electromagnetism and the Foundation of Life* (New York: William Morrow, 1998).

11. Traube-Hering wave: In the 1860s Traube and Hering independently measured oscillations of pressure at a rate of about 6-10 times per minute.

12. J.M. Woods and R.H. Woods, "A Physical Finding Relating to Psychiatric Disorders," *Journal of the American Osteopathic Association* 60 (1961): 988–93.

13. Nelson et al., "Cranial rhythmic impulse."

14. Nadia Aalling Jessen et al., "The Glymphatic System: A Beginner's Guide," *Neurochemical Research* 40, no. 12 (December 2015): 2583–99, https://doi.org/10.1007%2Fs11064-015-1581-6.

15. Tsutomu Nakata, "Virchow-Robin Space and Aquaporin-4: New Insights on an Old Friend," *Croatian Medical Journal* 55, no. 4 (August 2014): 328–36, https://doi.org/10.3325/cmj.2014.55.328.

16. Alan W.J. Morris et al., "Vascular Basement Membranes as Pathways for the Passage of Fluid into and out of the Brain," *Acta Neuropathologica* 131 (May 2016): 725–36, https://doi.org/10.1007/s00401-016-1555-z.

17. G. Hauk, "Physiologische Aspekte der Hämorheologie," *Hämostaseologie* 4, no. 1 (1984): 9–12.

18. Still, *Philosophy and Mechanical Principles of Osteopathy,* 55.

19. Still, *Philosophy and Mechanical Principles of Osteopathy,* 55.

20. A.T. Still, *Autobiography of Andrew Taylor Still* (Kirksville, MO: A.T. Still, 1908).

21. A.T. Still, *Osteopathy: Research and Practice* (Kirksville, MO: A.T. Still, 1910).

22. Still, *Osteopathy: Research and Practice,* 318.

23. Björn E.W. Nordenström, *Biologically Closed Electric Circuits: Clinical, Experimental, and Theoretical Evidence for an Additional Circulatory System* (Nordic Medical Publications, 1983).

24. Björn E.W. Nordenström, "Impact of Biologically Closed Electric Circuits (BCEC) on Structure and Function," *Integrative Physiology and Behavioral Science* 27, no. 4 (October 1992): 285–303, https://doi.org/10.1007/BF02691165.

25. Björn E. Nordenström, "The Paradigm of Biologically Closed Electric Circuits (BCEC) and the formation of an International Association (IABC) for BCEC Systems," *European Journal of Surgery Supplement* 574 (1994): 7–23.

26. Nordenström, "Impact of Biologically Closed Electric Circuits."

27. A. Pischinger, *Matrix and Matrix Regulation: Basis for a Holistic Theory in Medicine*, ed. Hartmut Heine (Brussels, Belgium: Haug International, 1991).

28. R. Paul Lee, *Interface: Mechanisms of Spirit in Osteopathy* (Stillness Press, 2005), 214, 212–53.

29. Robert O. Becker, *Cross Currents: The Perils of Electropollution* (Los Angeles: Penguin Publishing Group, 1990), 147.

30. Lee, *Interface,* 214.

31. Gerald H. Pollack, *Cells, Gels and the Engines of Life: A New, Unifying Approach to Cell Function* (Seattle, WA: Ebner & Sons, 2001), 70–101.

32. Nicette Sergueef, Kenneth E. Nelson, and Thomas Glonek, "Changes in the Traube-Hering Wave Following Cranial Manipulation," *The American Academy of Osteopathy Journal* (Spring 2001): 17.

33. Kenneth E. Nelson et al., "Cranial Rhythmic Impulse Related to the Traube-Hering-Mayer Oscillation: Comparing Laser-Doppler Flowmetry and Palpation," *The Journal of the American Osteopathic Association* 101, no. 3 (March 2001): 163–73.

34. Sergueef et al., "Changes in the Traube-Hering Wave."

35. Y. Bouligand, "Liquid Crystals and Their Analogs in Biological Systems," *Solid State Physics*, Supplement 14 (1978): 259–94.

36. A. Szent-Györgyi, "Towards a New Biochemistry," *Science* 93 (June 1941): 609–11, https://doi.org/10.1126/science.93.2426.609.

37. Herbert Fröhlich, ed., *Biological Coherence and Response to External Stimuli* (Berlin: Springer Verlag, 1988).

38. James L. Oschman, *Energy Medicine in Therapeutics and Human Performance* (Butterworth Heinemann, 2003).

39. K.J. Pienta and D.S. Coffey, "Cellular Harmonic Information through a Tissue Tensegrity-Matrix System," *Medical Hypothses* 34, no. 1 (January 1991): 88–95.

40. Herbert Frölich, "Bose Condensation of Strongly Excited Longitudinal Electric Modes," *Physics Letters A* 26, no. 9 (March 1968): 402–3.

41. Pischinger, *Matrix and Matrix Regulation.*

42. Lee, *Interface.*

43. Ana Carolina de Paula, "História Natural de Pacientes com Mucopolissacaridoses" (master's dissertation, University of São Paulo, 2006), https://doi.org/10.11606/D.5.2006.tde-16102014-092555.

44. Oschman, *Energy Medicine in Therapeutics and Human Performance.*

45. Oschman, *Energy Medicine in Therapeutics and Human Performance.*

46. Ove Christiansen, "Mediation of Cell Volume Regulation by Ca2+ Influx Through Stretch-Activated Channels," *Nature* 330, no. 6143 (November 1987): 66–8, https://doi.org/10.1038/330066a0.

47. A. Stutzin and E.K. Hoffman, "Swelling-Activated Ion Channels: Functional Regulation in Cell-Swelling, Proliferation and Apoptosis," *Acta Physiologica* 187, no. 1–2 (May 2006): 27–42, https://doi.org/10.1111/j.1748-1716.2006.01537.x.

48. Laurent Blanchoin et al., "Actin Dynamics, Architecture, and Mechanics in Cell Motility," *Physiological Reviews* 94, no. 1 (January 2014): 235–63, https://doi.org/10.1152/physrev.00018.2013.

49. "Seifritz on Protoplasm," The Lowen Foundation, posted on YouTube, https://www.youtube.com/watch?v=_ihSxAn4WR8.

50. Jerry I. Jacobson, "A Quantum Theory of Disease, Including Cancer and Aging," *Integrative Molecular Medicine* 3, no. 1 (2016): 524–41, https://doi.org/10.15761/IMM.1000200.

51. Bengt Nordén and Claes Ramel, eds., *Interaction Mechanisms of Low-Level Electromagnetic Fields in Living Systems* (Oxford: Oxford University Press, 1992): 44–77.

52. W. Ross Adey, "Whispering Between Cells: Electromagnetic Fields and Regulatory Mechanisms in Tissue," *Frontier Perspectives* 3, no. 2 (1993): 21–5.

53. W. Ross Adey, "Physiologic Signaling Across Cell Membranes and Cooperative Influences of Extremely Low Frequency Electromagnetic Fields," in *Biological Coherence and Response to External Stimuli,* edited by Herbert Frölich, 148–70. (Springer-Verlag, 1988), 148-70.

54. Oschman, *Energy Medicine in Therapeutics and Human Performance.*

55. C. Andrew L. Basset and Robert O. Becker, "Generation of Electric Potentials by Bone in Response to Mechanical Stress," *Science* 137, no. 3535 (September 1962): 1063–4, https://doi.org/10.1126/science.137.3535.1063.

56. Jonathan Black and Edward Korostoff, "Strain-Related Potentials in Living Bone," *Annals of the New York Academy of Science* 238 no. 1 (October 1974), 95–120, https://doi.org/10.1111/j.1749-6632.1974.tb26781.x.

57. Eiichi Fukada and Iwao Yasuda, "On the Piezoelectric Effect of Bone," *Journal of the Physical Society of Japan* 12, no. 10 (October 1957): 149–54.

58. J.H. McIlhaney, "The Charge Distribution on the Human Femur Due to Load," *Journal of Bone and Joint Surgery* 49, no. 8 (December 1967): 1561–71.

59. Pau Urdeitx and Mohamed H. Doweidar, "Enhanced Piezoelectric Extracellular Matrix to Promote Cardiomyocyte Maturation and Tissue Formation: A 3D Computational Model," *Biology (Basel)* 10, no. 2 (February 2021): 135. https://doi.org/10.3390/biology10020135.

60. M. Braden et al., "Electrical and Piezo-electrical Properties of Dental Hard Tissue," *Nature* 212, no. 5070 (December 1966): 1565–6, https://doi.org/10.1038/2121565a0.

61. Eiichi Fukada, "Piezoelectric Properties of Organic Polymers," *Annals of the New York Academy of Sciences* 238, no. 1 (October 1974): 7–25.

62. Eiichi Fukada and Kiyoshi Hara, "Piezoelectric Effect in Blood Vessels," *Journal of the Physical Society of Japan* 26, no. 3 (March 1969): 777–80.

63. Eiichi Fukada and Hiroyoshi Ueda, "Piezoelectric Effect in Muscle," *Japanese Journal of Applied Physics* 9, no. 7 (1970): 844.

64. Leroy S. Levine, Irving Lustrin, Morris H. Shamos, "Experimental Model for Studying the Effect of Electric Current on Bone in Vivo," *Nature* 224 (December 1969): 1112–3.

65. Alan F. Horowitz, "Integrins in Health," *Scientific American* 276 (May 1997): 68–75.

66. J.F. Mannery, "Calcium Ions and Nucleotides at Cell Surfaces," *Experimental Biology & Medicine* 3 (1968): 24–39.

67. James Oschman, *Morphological Correlates of Transport in Membrane Transport in Biology*, Vol 3 (Giebisch G Springer, 1978).

68. A.C. Rapraeger, "An Integral Membrane Proteoglycan Can Bind the ECM Directly to the Cytoskeleton," *Journal of Cell Biology* 96 (1982): 125.

69. J. Bereiter-Hahn, A.G. Matoltsy, and K.S. Richards, *Biology of the Integument* (Berlin: Springer-Verlag,1986).

70. R. Bruce Martin and David B. Burr, *Structure, Function, and Adaptation of Compact Bone* (New York: Raven Press, 1988).

71. Mae-Wan Ho, "Water and Colloid Crystals," *Science in Society* 32 (October 2006): 19–20.

72. Sei Hachisu and Shigekuni Yoshimura, "Optical Demonstration of Crystalline Superstructures in Binary Mixtures of Latex Globules," *Nature* 283 (January 1980): 188–9, https://doi.org/10.1038/283188a0.

73. Hachisu and Yoshimura, "Optical Demonstration."

74. Craig Holdrege, *The Dynamic Heart and Circulation* (Fair Oaks, CA: The Association of Waldorf Schools of North America, 2002).

75. B. Gabarel and M. Roques, *Les Fasciae en Medecine Osteopathique* (Paris: Maloine, 1985).

76. Donald E. Ingber, "The Architecture of Life," *Scientific American* 278, no. 1 (January 1998): 48, https://doi.org/10.1038/scientificamerican0198-48.

77. Candace B. Pert, *Everything You Need to Know to Feel Go(o)d* (Carlsbad, CA: Hay House, 2006), 109.

78. Still, *Philosophy and Mechanical Principles of Osteopathy.*

79. Sergueef et al., *Changes in the Traube-Hering Wave.*

80. Nordenström, *Biologically Closed Electric Circuits.*

81. Still, *Autobiography*, 224.

# Chapter Six

# The Development of the Vasculature

*"A full and complete supply of arterial blood must be generated and delivered to all parts, organs and glands by the channels called the arteries. When it has done its work, then without delay the veins must return all to the heart and lungs for renewal."*[1]

– Andrew Taylor Still, 1899

We turn now to a brief review of the development of the vasculature and the embryology of the venous structure and function.

The cell is a metabolic field. An embryo does not just begin as a fully developed human. Instead, there is a metabolic field occurring at the cellular level within an organ, a limb or the whole body. Each cell has a coherent metabolic field that is expressed as a series of structured metabolic movements that coalesce to form each segment of the embryo developing into a fetus, which develops into an infant and so on.

The liver itself, for example, is a discrete metabolic field of function with structured metabolic movements. These metabolic movements are ordered submicroscopically, but they are also ordered microscopically as well as at a level that can be detected visually.[2]

The circulation starts in the cell as a system of metabolic movements from the membrane towards the nucleus and back to the membrane. There is a constant expression of the primary respiratory mechanism in the cell and then in the whole.

Figure 6.1, from *Biokinetics and Biodynamics of Human Differentiation,* describes the intracellular circulatory pathways in every living cell.

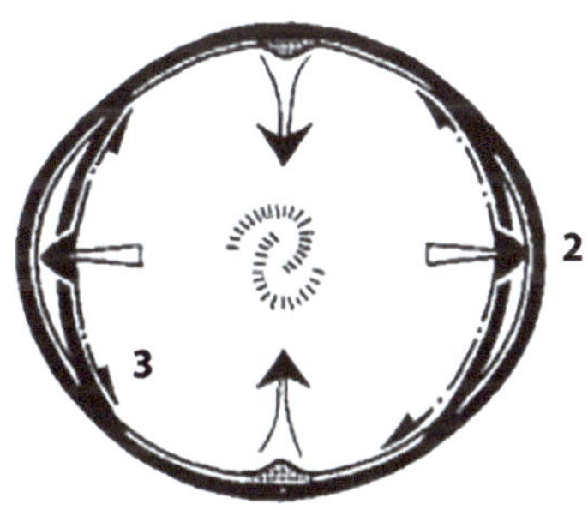


**Figure 6.1 – Intracellular Circulatory Pathways in Cells.** Reprinted from Blechschmidt and Gasser.[3]

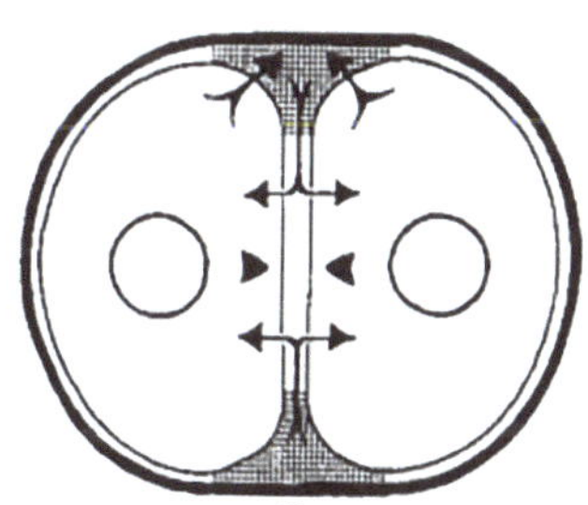


**Figure 6.2 – Reciprocal Biomechanical Cohesion via Metabolism.** Reprinted from Blechschmidt and Gasser.[4]

Reciprocal biomechanical cohesion via metabolism is expressed in subcellular structures in all different forms within the cell and matrix (Figure 6.2). Rippling through the tissues like spectators at a sporting stadium doing a synchronised wave, it allows communication between trillions of cells, throughout metabolic respiration so that, where the primary respiratory mechanism is healthy, all cells are respiring synchronously. It is a biomechanical connection that is made by metabolism, so mechanotransduction (ie, metabolism driven by mechanics) is happening all the time.

## Source and Sink

All circulatory dynamics are based on two simple principles: nourishment and a nutritional source. If you have these two, you have everything. The need for nourishment requires direct connection to a nutritional source. As Prof Blechschmidt put it, "Vascular development is an excellent example of why differentiations of cells do not begin from within."[5]

In Figure 6.3, in the image on the left, the strands in region 1 represent mesoblast cells, which provide pathways for nutrients, lining the chorionic sac and developing into blood islands (the precursors of blood vessels).

The first signs of blood vessel formation occur on days 17 and 18 in the splanchnopleuric mesoderm of the yolk sac, the connecting stalk and the chorion. The right image in Figure 6.3 shows the early stages of the process of blood vessel formation called vasculogenesis.

Blechschmidt promoted the concept of the nutrients flowing parallel to the membrane (**parmeation**) and nutrients flowing perpendicular to the membrane (**permeation**) (Figure 6.4). He emphasised the morphokinetic importance of the fluid-filled chambers formed by these membranes on the development of the embryo.

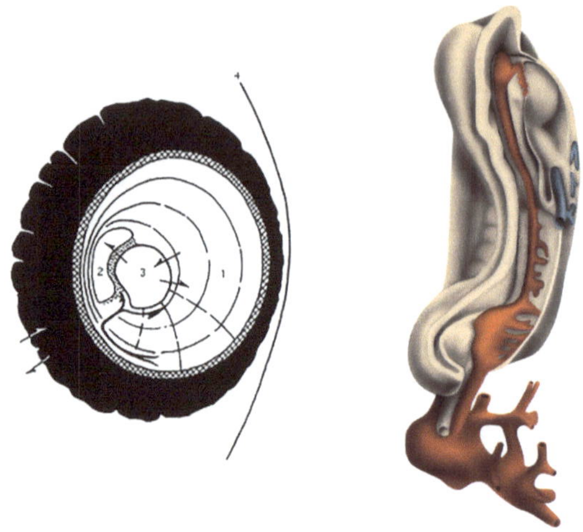

**Figure 6.3 – Early Vascular Formations and Vasculogenesis.** Left image: Human conceptus approximately 0.8 mm in diameter. The stippled region, which is the future embryo is developing between the growing amniotic sac (2) and yolk sac (3). The chorionic sac (1) envelops the whole developing embryo. The tailed arrows represent the flow of nutrients, parallel to the developing membranes. The small, half arrows represent the flow of nutrients perpendicular to the developing membranes. Extra-embryonic mesodermal cells follow the flow of nutrients and coalesce around the embryo to form blood islands that are embryonic vascular structures. Left image reprinted from Blechschmidt.[6] Right image: Early Stage Vasculogenesis: The neural tube is on the left, the amniotic and yolk sac cavities have been cut away, on the right you can see early aortic development in relation to where the heart is starting to bulge (Ht). Illustration by Hugh France.

The side view of the embryo in Figure 6.5 shows how flow that is parallel to the surface it flows past is reduced and is said to **parmeate** that tissue, whereas flow at a right angle to the tissue surface results in increased absorption, described as **permeating** the tissue.

## Canalisation, Blood Islands and Angiogenesis

Figure 6.5 illustrates a side view of the neural tube with the adjacent aorta. The future heart develops

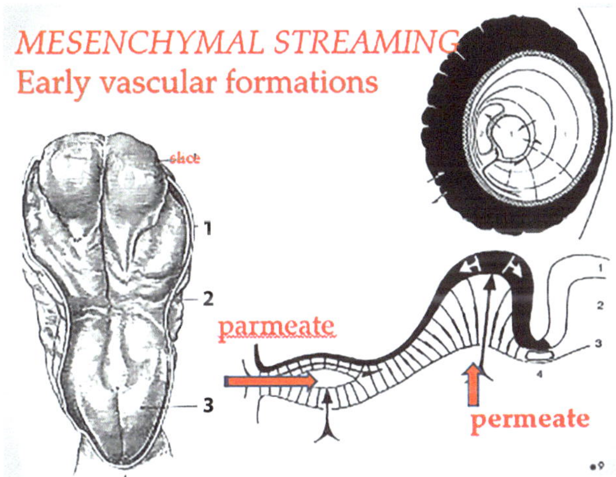


**Figure 6.4 – Mesenchymal Streaming in Early Vascular Formations.** Left Image: Dorsal aspect of the "Ludwig" embryo showing its (1) cranial, (2) cervical and (3) trunk subdivisions, viewed from dorsal side, amnion cut away. Left image reprinted from Blechschmidt and Gasser.[7] Top right image: See Figure 6.3 for legend. Reprinted from Blechschmidt.[8] Bottom right image: Parmeation and permeation. (1) Ectoderm, (2) mesoderm, (3) endoderm, and (4) axial process. Reprinted from Blechschmidt.[9]

here, and as this space expands, function fills the space.

Blechschmidt found in his studies that the vasculature forms in zones that are bound into three-sided configurations by other structures. He called these zones *canalisation zones*. These canalisation zones can be seen before the vessels are visible. In Figure 6.5, the developing head area of a 26-day-old embryo shows only the dorsal aspect. One side has been sectioned off to reveal the endoderm, the adjacent ectoderm and the neural tube. The space enclosed by those three structures is the canalisation zone for the formation of the dorsal aorta, with one forming on each side. As the ectoderm lifts away from the endoderm, some loose space develops within those cells. That loose space is an opportunity for nutrients to flow through the embryo, and where that space opens up is where an artery forms.

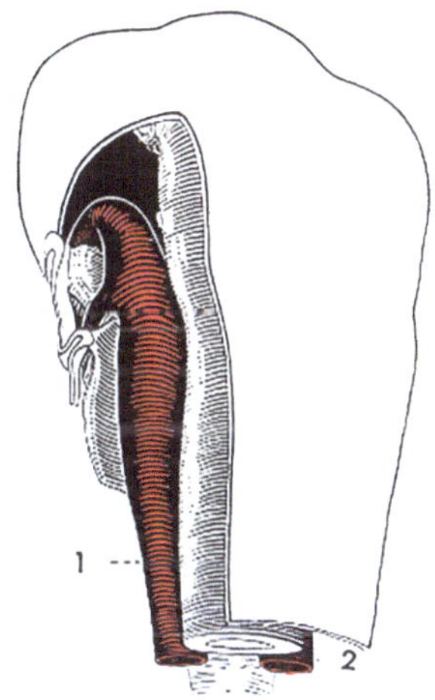


**Figure 6.5 – Neural Tube With Adjacent Aorta.** Part of a serial reconstruction of the head region of a 2.57-mm embryo showing the canalisation zones and left (1) and right (2) dorsal aortae. Reprinted from Blechschmidt and Gasser.[10]

We see the neural tube where the first two pharyngeal arches are, and there, adjacent to the neural tube, spaces open up to allow that trickle of many rivulets that coalesce to form one stream. Because they are heading in that same direction, they form a corrosion field between them, and all these little streams merge to form one big stream, just as they do in nature (Figure 6.6).

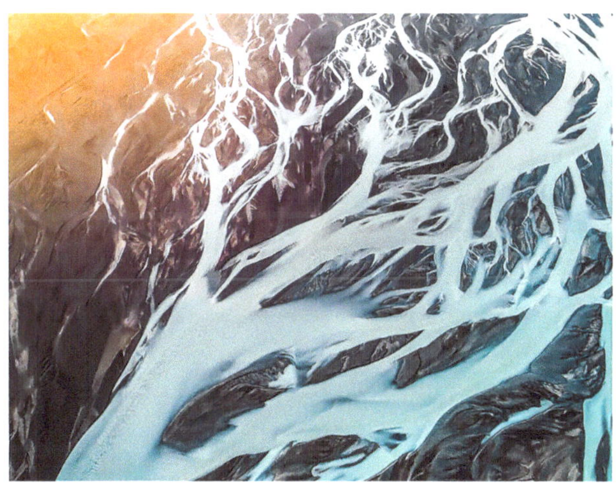

**Figure 6.6 – Rivulets to Streams to Rivers.** Aerial view of a braided river.

The three-sided canalisations coalesce to form fluid vacuoles within interstices between the cells. Mesenchymal streaming represents metabolic flow of nutrients and cells, which lead to the formation of blood islands. From here, early arteries sprout in a process called angiogenesis. A video titled "Angiogenesis" shows this process over an 8-hour time lapse.[11] You can view the video at https://www.youtube.com/watch?v=DlBaNiC2b_w or by scanning the following QR code:

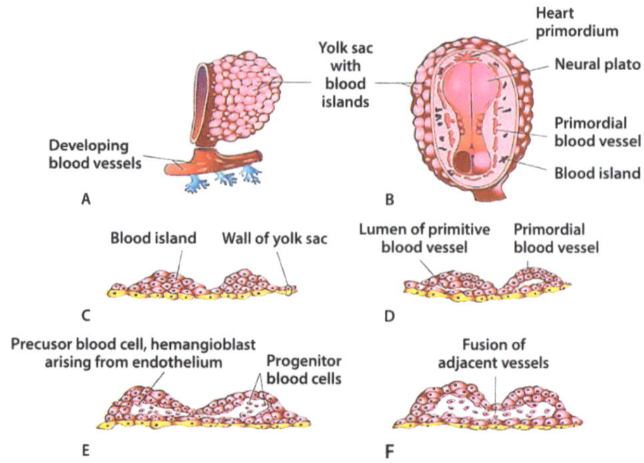


**Figure 6.7 – Mesenchyme Transitions.** Reprinted with permission from Khan.[12]

Whether an artery or a vein develops simply depends on the gradient. Where there is a lot of flow creating a lot of force against the surrounding cell membranes of those lining cells, an expanding space develops and the vessels develop and condense a thicker, more muscular wall, eventually developing into arteries. Where there is less pressure, a less condensed wall develops into veins. So, most small veins do not have a significant muscular component to their media.

This process all happens around the end of the third week of gestation. Some mesenchyme cells are in a position where they get flattened by the flow adjacent to them. Because they have pressure on them from both the outside and inside, they get sculpted into endothelial cells with the fenestrations between them (Figure 6.7).

Basically, fluid starts to trickle through the mesenchyme. Some of the cells get carried with that fluid, and they will become red blood cells and white blood cells. Some of the cells get pressed by the pressure of that flow, and they start to form canals within the mesenchyme, which will develop to become arteries or veins depending on the gradient and the pressure of the flow.

All of this happens with no pump. It is the flow of life, as seen in protoplasm. Dr Viola Frymann, during a 1995 lecture, showed a video on slime mould made by Prof Seifritz. The protoplasm flowed in one direction for some time and then reversed itself and flowed in the opposite direction for several seconds. However, there are **no muscular agencies** in slime mould. Interestingly, injecting anaesthetic into the slime mould caused the protoplasmic streaming to stop. As the anaesthetic dispersed, the streaming resumed. This is another example of fluid flow without a pump.

Slime mould is a plasmodium, an amoeba-like life form that is essentially blobs of protoplasm held together only by a cell membrane, unlike a fungi, which has cell walls.[13] Protoplasm is an example of mesenchyme, which is undifferentiated, responding to flow (Figures 6.8). It is another example of fluid-filled spaces causing early differentiation of cells and of outside fluid compartments causing inside cellular differentiation.

In 2020, *NOVA*, a long-running science series by the United States' Public Broadcasting Service (PBS), produced *The Secret Mind of Slime*[14] examining the research on a creature that has no brain

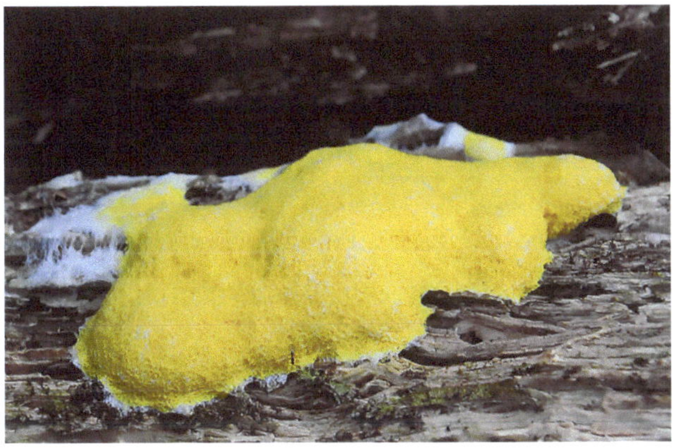

**Figure 6.8 A – Example of Protoplasm.** Fuligo septica, also known as scrambled-egg slime mould. Image courtesy of Henk Monster.

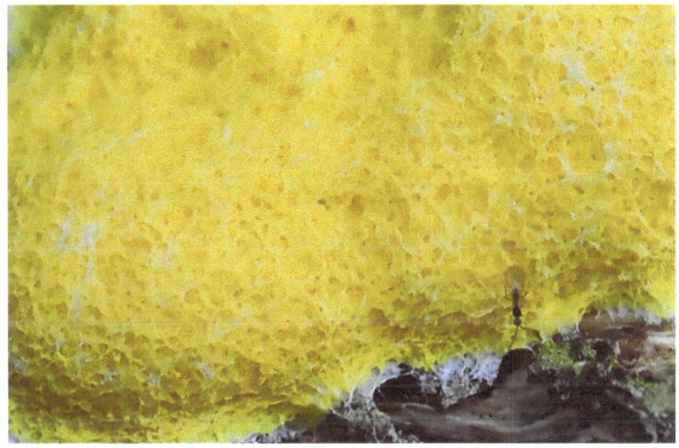

**Figure 6.8 B – Intricate Slime Mould Fabric.** Close-up of Fuligo septica. Image courtesy of Henk Monster.

yet seems to make exceptionally good decisions. In one segment, they showed how slime can traverse mazes. In another segment, they put a slime mould in the middle of an area representing Tokyo and put food in various places to represent surrounding cities. The slime mould mapped the most efficient way to get to that food, which very closely matched the train routes humans devised to enhance travel in and out of the region surrounding Tokyo. Thus, the slime mould exhibits an intelligence that is phenomenal.

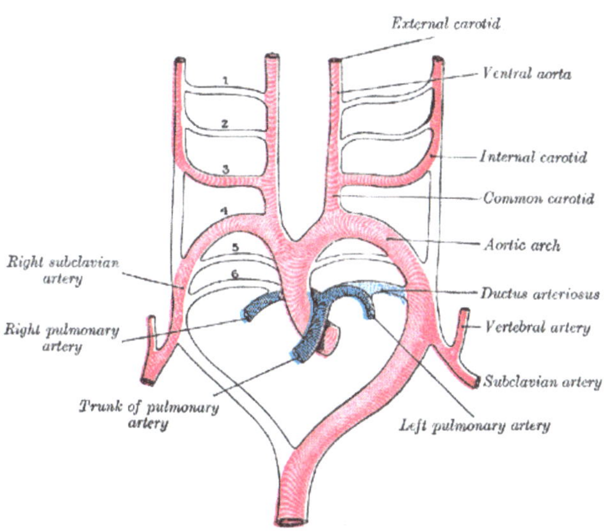


**Figure 6.9 – Embryonic Aorta.**

## Nitric Oxide and Flow

Figure 6.9 is an illustration of the embryonic aorta, demonstrating the dorsal branches of the aorta splitting into left and right dorsal branches and feeding the growth for the somites.[15]

The stimulus for the development of this vasculogenesis is a combination of genetic factors, chemical factors, such as vascular endothelium growth factor (VEGF), and epigenetic factors.

Most importantly, a metabolising cell that isn't getting enough oxygen (hypoxia) generates **nitric oxide**, which leads to the release of the VEGF and results in vascular endothelial growth in the tissues, stimulating changes in the blood vessels that improve delivery of oxygen. Nitric oxide also acts as a neurotransmitter, changing the permeability of the endothelial cell to release its nutrients. This extravasation of nutrients stimulates those growing tissues.

The release of nitric oxide, combined with haemodynamic factors such as increased flow, leads to further development of the vessels.

Most importantly, these haemodynamic factors represent outside to inside differentiation of vascular walls and represent the differentiation of the vascular walls into their adult form. The increasing haemodynamic factors lead to the condensation of vascular smooth muscle cells in the walls of the arteries, and this growth is from proximal to distal.

## Haltefunktion: Permeation, Parmeation and the Restraining Function

A question has frequently arisen when presenting this material in different countries: "What is the difference between laminar and vortical flow?" Laminar flow is what appears in two dimensions while vortical flow is what appears in three dimensions, and they are the same thing. Additionally, laminar flow relates to the friction along the wall that slows down the peripheral flow while down the centre there is faster flow because there is less peripheral resistance. So laminar flow does exist, when viewing it two dimensionally, whereas vortical flow is three dimensional.[16]

Laminar flow can be viewed in Gerald Pollack's video "The Fourth Phase of Water: A Central Role in Health", which you can access by visiting https://www.youtube.com/watch?v=3YyJKqpWKPo (a discussion of the exclusion zone, explored in depth in Chapter 3, begins at 54:50) or by scanning the following QR code:

As previously mentioned, Blechschmidt used two words to describe fluids in relation to the blood vessel wall: **parmeation** and **permeation**. As blood flows into branched capillaries, it flows slowly and the nutritive substances pass via the vessel wall into their target tissues *perpendicularly*, **permeating** them. However, in vessels with a larger lumen, blood flow is faster and runs more *parallel* to the vessel wall and nutrients feed the vessel wall by **parmeation**. As a result, endothelial cell growth is relatively slower in larger vessels and retards the lengthening of the vessel as well. This retarded lengthening has a **restraining effect** on target tissues. The metaphor for this is that the larger vessels are like a cord at the end of which a large sponge is anchored—the cord provides the restraint and the sponge provides the nutrition.

The flow of nutrients is constantly parallel to the cell membrane, and that is one of the forces that maintains quiescence of endothelial cells to stop them from reacting to other factors that we discussed in Chapter 2. Clearly there is a difference in the way nutrients flow along the membrane.

To describe the growth principle developed by Blechschmidt based upon permeation and parmeation, he coined the word *haltefunktion*, emphasising the morphogenetic influence of each on our development. Blechschmidt observed that "after a blood vessel has grown sufficiently in any tissue, it then appears to have a restraining function on the structure it supplies."[17]

To emphasise this very important concept, once blood vessels develop sufficiently, they appear to have a restraining function on the structures they supply. The longitudinal growth of a vessel stem is retarded when compared to the total length of its branches. The reason for this is that as blood passes through the main stem of the vessel, it flows more rapidly than through the capillary networks more distal to it.

The blood and its nutritive substances move faster along the walls of the larger part of the vessel but are less able to permeate through the vessel. As the blood moves distal into the branched capillaries, the flow of the blood apparently slows down and the nutrients are then able to permeate through the capillary walls. As a result, the vessels and capillaries where the blood is moving slower grow faster because they are getting more nutrients, whereas the larger vessel stem gets less nutrition and its growth is relatively retarded. This retardation manifests itself as a restraining function against the tissues/organs that it supplies, which have profuse capillary networks and a greater rate of growth.

Consider Figure 6.10, which shows a longitudinal section of an embryo at day 26. The restraining function of the dorsal aorta against the longitudinal growth of the neural tube is represented by the converging arrows ventral to the neural tube. The lower arrow shows the growth pull of the right aorta. Bending of the neural tube (cephalic flexure) is shown by the curved arrow. Convergent arrows dorsal to the neural tube show the delicate, two-dimensional resistance of the ectoderm (1) on the dorsal surface of the embryo's heart (2).

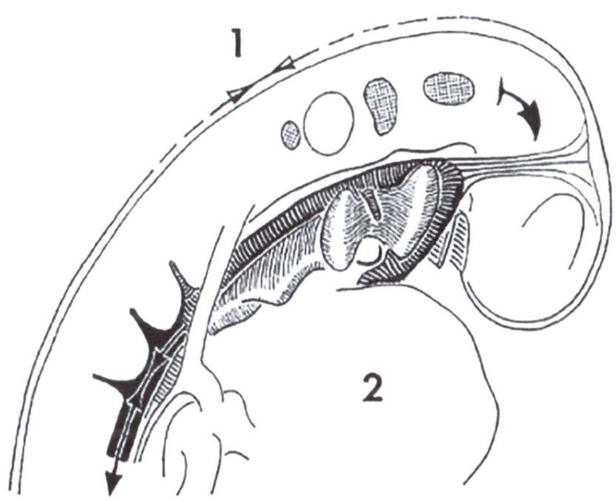


**Figure 6.10 – Longitudinal Section of a 26-Day Embryo.** Reprinted from Blechschmidt and Gasser.[18]

Note the area of the developing head and, below it, the developing heart (numbered 2). We know that the embryonic disc starts to fold during the fourth week, and most embryological texts note that the longitudinal folding occurs due to different growth rates between the anterior structures and that of the neural tube. Figure 6.10 shows us that the vascular and nervous systems are connected by tissue in a mesenchymal continuation and that the retarded growth of the dorsal aortae is restraining the ventral aspect of the expanding brain. This restraint causes the developing brain to bend over the developing heart. You can see that where it bends is exactly where the aorta restrains it.

*Metamerism* is a term used embryologically to describe how geometrically precise the development of the segmental arteries are. Each artery growing from the dorsal aorta, left and right, responds to the growth of the somites, and each artery precisely feeds as many cells as it can. When it can no longer supply a group of cells, another artery starts to sprout. The sprouting of those arteries matches the sprouting and the coalescing of the venous and lymphatic drainage (Figures 6.11 and 6.12).

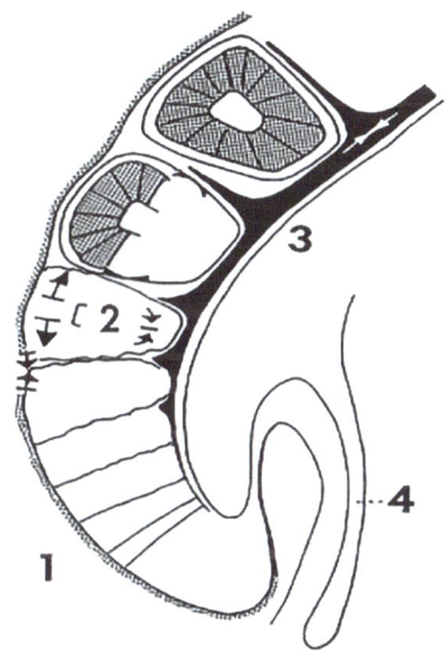


**Figure 6.11 – Diagram of a paramedian section through a reconstruction showing some of the biokinetic features of somite development.** Diagram of the position, shape and structure of the somites as they arise from unsegmented paraxial mesenchyme. Divergent arrows with base lines represent growth near the ectoderm. Convergent simple arrows indicate cells compressed between the metameric aortic branches. Convergent arrows with base lines show retarded growth. Convergent arrows indicate the restraining function of the somite capsule and aorta. 1, Still unsegmented dorsal region deficient in blood vessels; 2, segmentation furrow; 3, gut region with neighbouring aorta (black); 4, allontois. Reprinted from Blechschmidt and Gasser.[19]

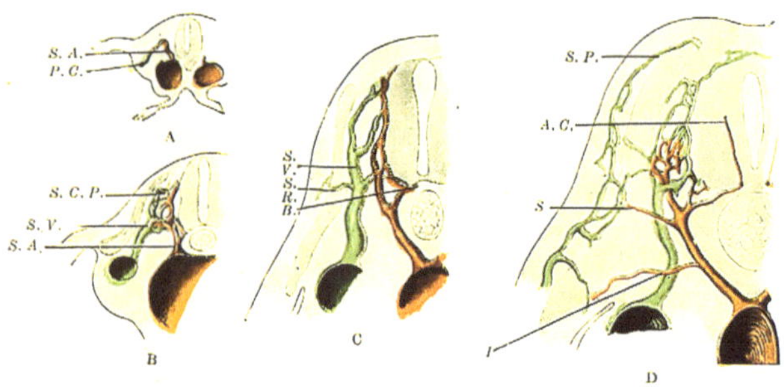


**Figure 6.12 – Segmental Arteries and New Arteries Coalescing With Venous and Lymphatic Drainage.** Reprinted from Gailloud.[20]

The longitudinal growth of a vessel stem is retarded when compared to the total length of its branches. The reason for this is that as blood passes through the main stem of the vessel, it flows more rapidly than through the capillary networks more distal to it.

In Blechschmidt's haltefunktion principle, growth can affect spinal segmental function. The segmental arteries of the aorta may influence the diagnosis and treatment of a segmental dysfunction because each one of those segmental arteries is a branch of the aorta that responds to the growth of the somites. So it functions in relation to the development of the disc, the vertebra and the neural structures.

## Embryological Development of the Vertebral Vascular System

The dorsal branches of the aorta are the main segmental suppliers—except for certain areas. For example, above the clavicle and below L4 there is a different arrangement, which is referred to in the next paragraph. Additionally, the posterior and the lateral branches become part of the intercostal supply in the thorax. There are also anterior branches that supply the viscera.

In the developing embryo, dorsal aortae appear from T4 to L4. Thoracic vertebrae four is often identified as a fulcrum of vascular function. Research by Dr Jane Carreiro focussed on the integration of the respiratory midline and the vascular midline at T4.[21] The bifurcation of the trachea also coincides with the level of T4. These important functions relate to T4, and at L4 the aorta bifurcates into the left and right iliac arteries.

Turning to the development of the venous structures, these relate to a low-pressure mode of function that reflects the relatively lower suction exerted by the lungs compared to the suction of arterial blood by every parenchymal cell of the body. This difference in flow accounts for the fact that arterial blood comprises 20% of blood in circulation while venous blood comprises 80%; this fact is emphasised in Figures 6.13 A-E.

**Figure 6.13 A-E – Circulating Blood, Posterior View of the Cervical Region.** Reprinted from Ento Key.[22]

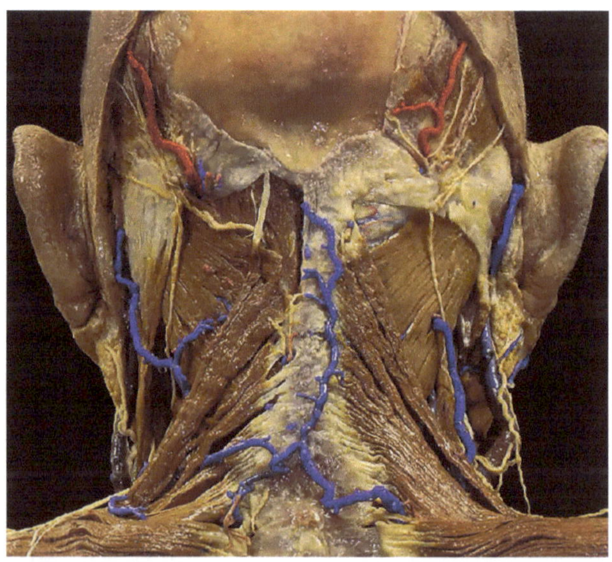

**A.** The skin and subcutaneous tissue have been removed. The sternocleidomastoid muscle has been removed on the right side.

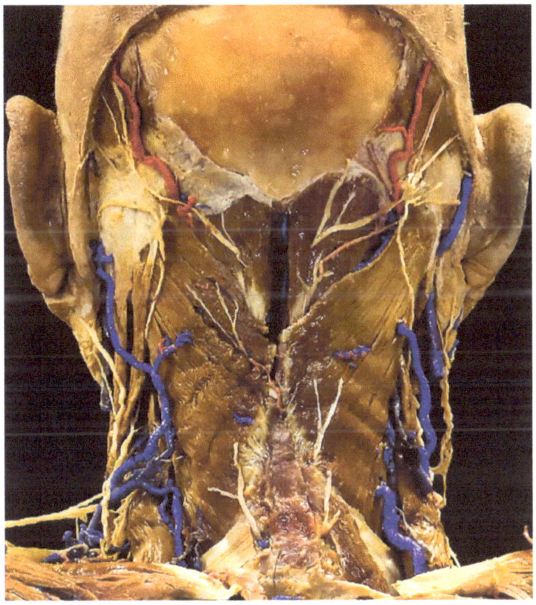

**B**. The trapezius muscles have been removed to expose the splenius capitis muscles.

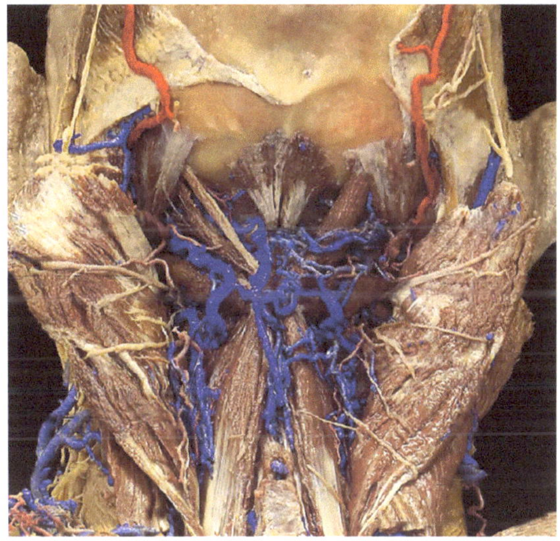

**D.** The deep muscular plane has been exposed bilaterally.

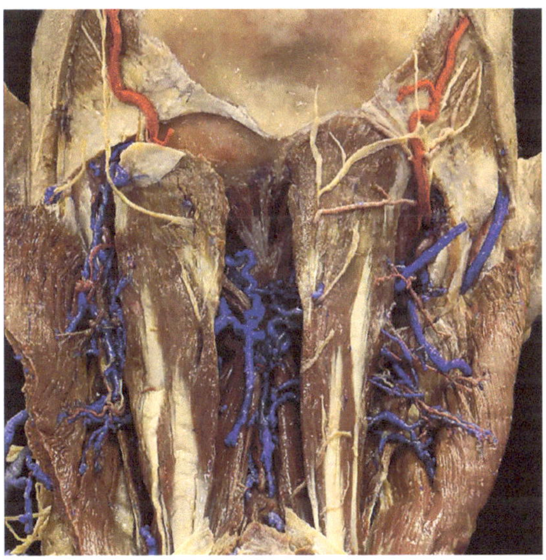

**C.** Both splenius capitis muscles and the left semispinalis capitis have been reflected laterally to partially expose the deep muscular plane.

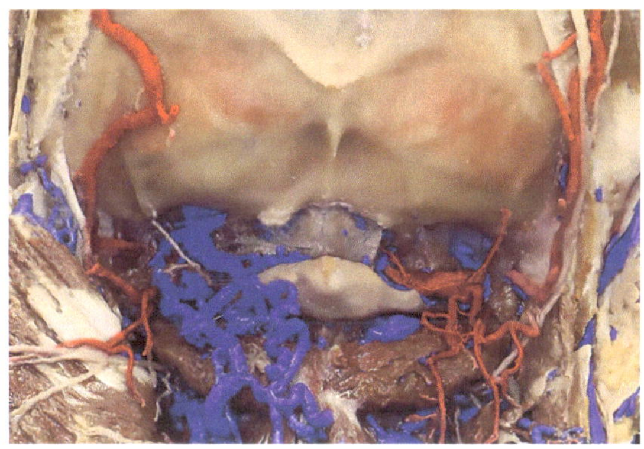

**E.** Subocciput.

In the forearms and in the lower half of the legs, extensive drainage predominantly occurs through the venae comitantes, illustrated in Figure 6.14. These venae comitantes are also present in the vertebral venous plexus surrounding the vertebral artery.

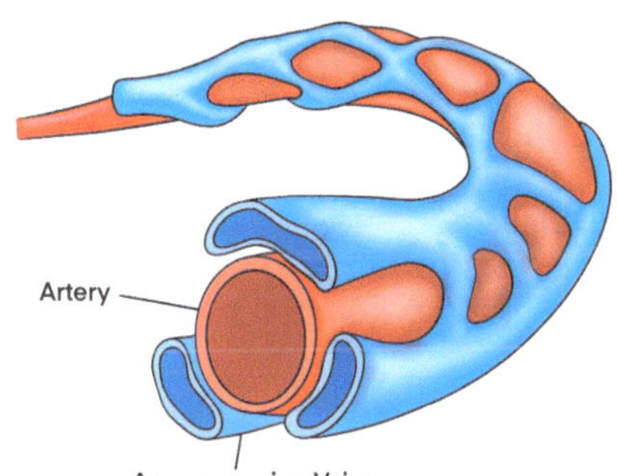


**Figure 6.14 – Venae Comitantes.** Although most veins of the trunk occur as large single vessels, the veins in the limbs occur as two or more smaller vessels that accompany an artery in a common vascular sheath. Illustration by Hugh France.

This low-pressure development of venous function needs to be constantly kept in mind. Note that vortical propulsion and capacitance of the artery will impact venous return: with every arterial pulse, there is an accentuation of the sound of the heart in these venous structures.

The development of the lymphatic system relates directly to the development of the venous functions, which will be discussed in greater depth in Chapter 8.

In the schematic diagram of a developing embryo in Figure 6.15, note that the intersegmental arteries in the thoracic, lumbar and sacral regions give off a dorsal branch, which vascularises the developing neural tube and the epimeres that form the deep muscles of the back. These also give off cutaneous branches that supply the skin. The image to the right in Figure 6.12 illustrates the segmental arteries that are responsible for the supply to the cervical somites, and you can see that they are above the clavicle.

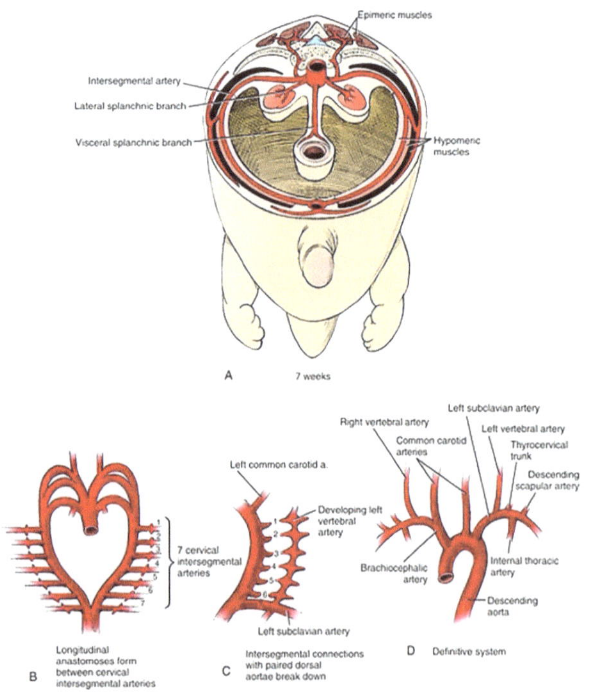


**Figure 6.15 – Development of the Lateral Branches of the Abdominal Aorta.** Reprinted from Schoenwolf et al.[23]

Below the bifurcation of the aorta, similar branching happens. From the subclavian artery, the vertebral artery and the two carotid arteries are derived. Below L4 are the lateral sacral arteries and median sacral artery, which is the termination of the spinal vasculature.

The lateral branch of the aorta nourishes the bone, the vertebral discs, the dorsal root ganglia and the spinal cord itself. It reaches back to the posterior musculature and the posterior elements of the vertebra. They relate very closely to the intervertebral foramen of the vertebra.

The complex of arteries is matched by an equal, if not greater, complex of veins.

The study by Labropoulos et al provides an example of the importance of venous drainage. The study, which investigated the role of venous drainage on the sciatic nerve, showed that venous congestion of that lumbar nerve root is directly related to chronic pain.[24]

Where there is a segmental dysfunction in the blood supply, we emphasise that, as Dr Still said, renovation begins with the veins. The importance of this concept in terms of disc disease requires the drainage and nourishment of the nucleus pulposus and prevents an immune response, including chronic inflammation, which contributes to chronic pain.

The venous system (Figure 6.16) is described as having a valvular system to reduce backflow. However, in Batson's plexus of veins within the spinal canal, only 34% of the number of valves are found generally within the veins systemically. That is one of the reasons why the Batson's plexus is such a good conduit for the transmission of metastatic tissue through the venous system.[25]

Another important point to understand when treating a patient to reduce venous congestion and the related pain is that appropriate and optimal movement of the vertebral column will augment the movement of blood through the veins.[27] Equally important is breathing, because it is the breath

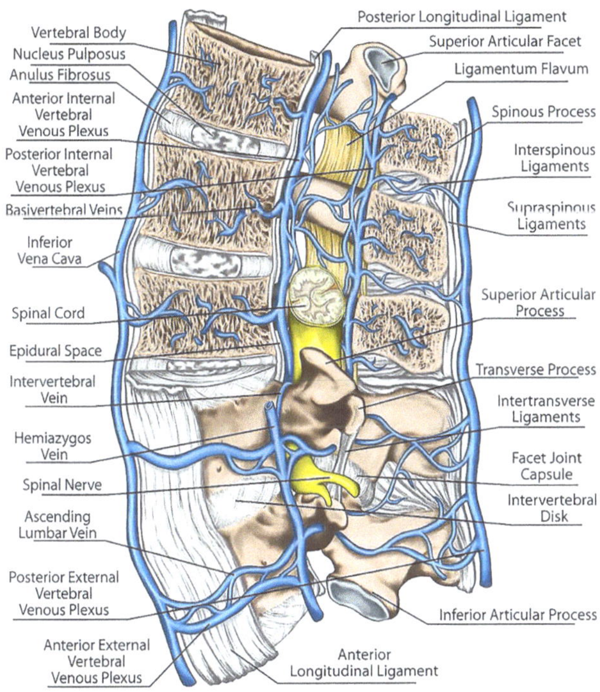


**Figure 6.16 – Vertebral Venous System.** The vertebral venous plexus comprises an interconnected and richly anastomosed system of veins that run along the entire length of the vertebral column. Reprinted from Thibault.[26]

that draws and sucks blood towards the heart.[28]

The denseness of the blood vessels, as seen in Figure 6.17, must be constantly kept in mind.[29] It emphasises the fact that a cell cannot survive if it is positioned farther than 150 μm from its nutritional source.

The median sacral artery is the last dorsal branch of the aorta and is considered the continuation of the aorta. It descends in the midline in front of the fourth and fifth lumbar vertebrae along the anterior aspect of the sacrum to the coccygeal body, which is anterior to the apex of the coccyx. It supplies the ganglion impar where, as Dr Fulford observed, the two sympathetic chains meet.

Dr Richard Koss, long time student of Dr Fulford, confirmed (personal communication) that in many lectures, Dr Fulford emphasised the ganglion impar, a sympathetic bundle of nerves located anterior to the coccygeal junction, particularly in relation to respiratory function.

Fulford stressed the importance of the sacrococcygeal junction and the position of the ganglion impar. He referred to the rectal-respiratory reflex at the ganglion impar. This is a solitary ganglion that connects both halves of the sympathetic chain, so it is called the *imperfect ganglion* or the *ganglion impar*.

When children learn how to walk, sometimes they take a couple of steps and fall backwards, landing on their coccyx. That trauma can be transferred all the way up the sympathetic chain and irritate all the respiratory tissues, creating dysfunction, particularly asthma, otitis media, sinus problems, and so on. In a lecture Fulford gave in the last decade of his life, he said that children with unresolved trauma at the sacrococcygeal junction frequently had

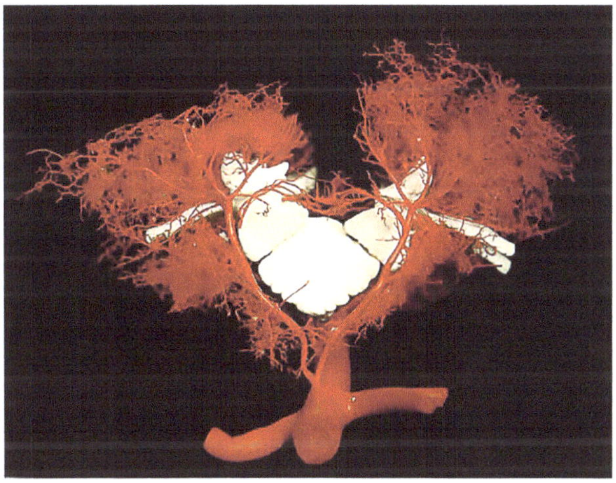

**Figure 6.17 – Density of the spinal blood vessels.** The perfusion of the spinal cord depends upon a vascular network which also provides flow to the paraspinal muscles, whose needs dwarf the flow to the spinal cord. In this view, the aorta is seen giving off paired segmental arteries which course around the vertebral body to supply the paraspinal muscles and, in the midline, the small anterior spinal artery. Reprinted from Griepp et al.[30]

"an energy sink" locked in there. That, in turn, Fulford averred, influences upper respiratory diseases and illnesses (Figure 6.18).

It is possible to see Dr Fulford's emphasis of the ganglion impar in a vascular context.

The dorsal aorta relates to T4 but also to the coccyx as well as the functional midline of the embryonic body, the cartilaginous notochord (discussed in Chapter 4). The coccyx also relates to the longitudinal fluctuation that we feel rising from that area[31] (Figure 6.19 – Carnegie Stage 16).

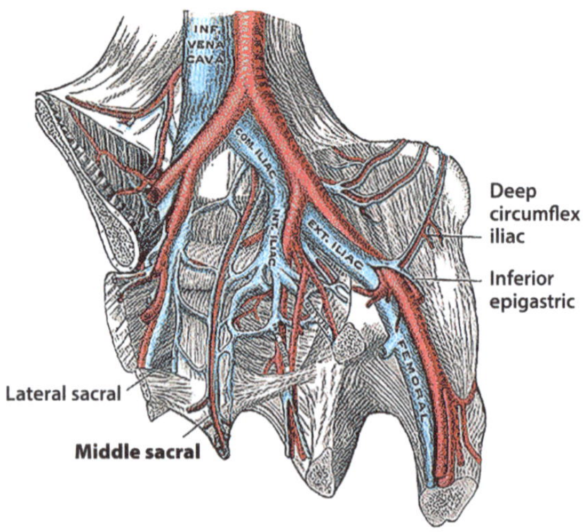


**Figure 6.18 – Middle sacral vein.** Reprinted from Gray. [32]

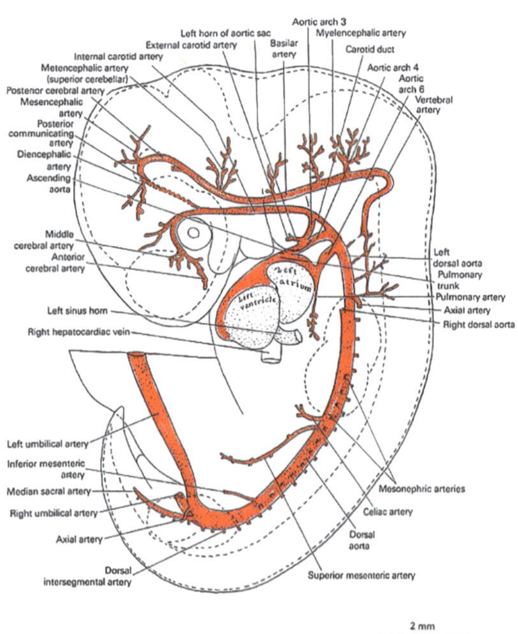


**Figure 6.19 – Carnegie Stage 16.** Reprinted from Gasser.[33]

## Applications to Osteopathic Practice

This chapter supports the osteopathic recognition of the importance of T4 as a reference point for the vasculature. Using T4 as an observation point, the osteopath can assess function occurring above and below that point. For instance T4 can relate below to the vertebral arteries and veins to the function of the aortic bifurcation and to the pelvic arteriovenous plexus. Above T4, it often references the cervical fascia, to the ampulloglomerular organ and the fourth ventricle and structures in its floor.

Blechschmidt's haltefunktion growth principle resulting from his observation that "after a blood vessel has grown sufficiently in any tissue, it then appears to have a restraining/guiding function on the structure it supplies", has practical significance. The osteopath works to eliminate turbulent blood flow and restore normal vortical flow. This results in less shear stress, the reduction in autonomic nervous system activity with de-facilitation and the restoration of normal biomechanics (see Chapter 13, including references). It epitomises the reality of Dr Still's "rule of the artery and vein."

As discussed earlier, the intervertebral disc's nucleus lies at the centre of each somite. In clinical practice, the osteopath strives to restore normal blood flow and drainage of each pair of vertebrae. This ensures nutrients to support repair of the annulus and nucleus of the disc and the removal of waste via the veins. The osteopath needs to assess arterial inflow or venous return, bearing in mind Still's aphorism that **renovation starts with the veins**.

## Chapter 6 Endnotes


1. A.T. Still, *Philosophy of Osteopathy* (Kirksville, MO: Published by the Author, 1899), 28.

2. Erich Blechschmidt and R.F. Gasser, *Biokinetics and Biodynamics of Human Differentiation: Principles and Applications* (Berkeley, CA: North Atlantic Books, 2014), 20.

3. Blechschmidt and Gasser, *Biokinetics and Biodynamics of Human Differentiation*, 6.

4. Blechschmidt and Gasser, *Biokinetics and Biodynamics of Human Differentiation*, 20.

5. Blechschmidt and Gasser, *Biokinetics and Biodynamics of Human Differentiation*, 21.

6. Erich Blechschmidt, *The Ontogenetic Basis of Human Anatomy: A Biodynamic Approach to Development from Conception to Birth* (Berkely, CA: North Atlantic Books, July 2004), 37.

7. Blechschmidt and Gasser, *Biokinetics and Biodynamics of Human Differentiation*, 42, Fig. 5-3.

8. Erich Blechschmidt, *The Ontogenetic Basis of Human Anatomy,* 37, Fig. 2.10.

9. Erich Blechschmidt, *The Ontogenetic Basis of Human Anatomy,* 43, Fig. 2.18.

10. Blechschmidt and Gasser, *Biokinetics and Biodynamics of Human Differentiation*, 83, Fig. 8-2.

11. "Angiogenesis," Derm Pharm, posted July 11, 2014, on YouTube, https://www.youtube.com/watch?v=DlBaNiC2b_w.

12. Mujahid Khan, "Mesodermal Derivatives" (SlideShare), https://slideplayer.com/slide/7500588/.

13. Thomas J. Volk, " IV.B.6.b Myxomycota: True Slime Molds," in *Encyclopedia of Biodiversity,* Ed. Simon Asher Levin (2001), https://www.sciencedirect.com/topics/earth-and-planetary-sciences/slime-mould.

14. Jennifer Robinson, *NOVA: Secret Mind of Slime Mould,* kpbs, September 15, 2020, https://www.kpbs.org/news/arts-culture/2020/09/15/nova-secret-mind-slime.

15. Henry Gray, "Aortic Arches of the Human Embryo," *Anatomy of the Human Body.* (New York City: Bartleby; 1918).

16. Peter A. Stonebridge, "Three Dimensional Blood Flow Dynamics: Spiral-Helical Laminar Flow," *Methodist Debakey Cardiovascular Journal* 7, no. 1 (January–March 2011): 21–6, https://doi.org/10.14797/mdcj-7-1-21.

17. Blechschmidt and Gasser, *Biokinetics and Biodynamics of Human Differentiation*, 20.

18. Blechschmidt and Gasser, *Biokinetics and Biodynamics of Human Differentiation*, 84.

19. Blechschmidt and Gasser, *Biokinetics and Biodynamics of Human Differentiation.*

20. Phillippe Gailloud. "Isolated Aortic Origin of the Intersegmental Spinal Branch," *Journal of NeuroInterventional Surgery* 5, no. 4 (2013): e19, https://doi.org/10.1136/neurintsurg-2012-010306.

21. Jane Elizabeth Carreiro, *An Osteopathic Approach to Children,* 2nd ed. (Churchill Livingstone, 2009).

22. "8 Posterior Aspect of the Neck," *Entokey: Fastest Otolaryngology & Ophthalmology Insight Engine*, https://entokey.com/.

23. Gary C. Schoenwolf et al., *Larsen's Human Embryology*, 6th ed. (Elsevier, Philadelphia, PA: 2022).

24. Nicos Labropoulos, et al. "Veins Along the Course of the Sciatica Nerve," *Journal of Vascular Surgery* 49, no. 3 (2009): 690-6, https://doi.org/10.1016/j.jvs.2008.09.061.

25. R.C. Brook, K. Tung, and R. Oeppen, "Batson's Plexus and Retrograde Venous Spread of Malignancy – A Pictorial Review," *Cancer Imaging* 14, Suppl. 1 (2014), 40, https://doi.org/10.1186/1470-7330-14-S1-P40.

26. Paul K. Thibault, "Cerebrospinal Venous Obstruction: Anatomy, Clinical Presentation, Diagnosis, and Treatment of Chronic Infective Cerebrospinal Venulitis," in *Cerebral Circulation - Updates on Models, Diagnostics and Treatments of Related Diseases,* eds. Alba Scerrati, Luca Ricciardi, and Flavia Dones (IntechOpen, 2022), https://doi.org/10.5772/intechopen.102685.

27. Meridel I. Gatterman, "Functional Anatomy of the Cervical Spine," *Whiplash* (2012): 9–43, https://doi.org/10.1016/B978-0-323-04583-4.00002-3.

28. Oh-Yun Kwon et al., "Effects of Ankle Exercise Combined With Deep Breathing on Blood Flow Velocity in the Femoral Vein," *Australian Journal of Physiotherapy* 49, no. 4 (2003): 253–8.

29. Eva B. Griepp et al., "The Anatomy of the Spinal Cord Collateral Circulation," *Annals of Cardiothoracic Surgery* 1, no. 3 (September 2012): 350–7, https://doi.org/10.3978/j.issn.2225-319X.2012.09.03.

30. Griepp et al., "The Anatomy of the Spinal Cord Collateral Circulation."

31. Raymond F. Gasser, "Carnegie Stage 16-Arteries," *Atlas of Human Embryos* (R.F. Gasser, 1975), Fig. 9, reprinted in *The Endowment for Human Development,* https://www.ehd.org/virtual-human-embryo/figure.php?stage=16&figure=9.

32. Henry Gray, *Anatomy of the Human Body* (Lea & Febiger, 1918), https://commons.wikimedia.org/wiki/File:Iliac_veins.gif.

33. Gasser, "Carnegie Stage 16-Arteries."

# Chapter Seven

# The Heart as a Generator

*"From the heart as the center of force, electricity carries on the process of delivering blood by way of the arteries and other fluids and gases by way of the excretories."*[1]

– Andrew Taylor Still

## The Heart as a Generator of Heat

As we saw in Chapter 3 on water, Viktor Schauberger paid particular attention to water's variations around the temperature of +4°C (39°F). Schauberger saw that water was composed of many strata, or layers, with subtle variations in temperature and electric charge that influence the water's motion, its form of flow and its physical properties, inside a vortex.

Blood circulating within the heart and large arteries maintains a temperature of near 38.0°C, slightly elevated above the average core body temperature near 37.0°C.[2] So, an important role of the heart is to generate and maintain body warmth. At rest, 70% of the heart's oxygen usage is for the creation of heat, and that heat is very carefully controlled within narrow limits.[2] This significant variance of blood temperature from the mean human body temperature induces rhythmic thermal fluctuations in blood cells according to their cyclical transport from the warm heart to the slightly cooler extremities and skin capillaries. This dynamic itself is subject to a diurnal fluctuation and is mediated by the arteriovenous anastomoses opening and closing, thereby controlling the amount of blood getting to the periphery. There exists a drive for blood to be held centrally in the day, which reinforces consciousness, with this dynamic being overridden as activity requires.[3]

It is notable that only warm-blooded animals—mammals and birds—have four-chambered hearts.[4] In the Dynamic Heart and Circulation, Craig Holdrege noted that the internal temperature differentiation between the heart and the rest of the body "corresponds to the organism's ability to maintain a high constant body temperature despite radically fluctuating inner and outer conditions. The heart muscle itself is a source of warmth for the blood, while the peripheral circulation can expand and contract to release or contain warmth."[5]

## The Heart as an Electrical Generator

If the heart were to be considered a pump, the pump, as a machine, would require a motor to provide the energy for the pump to run. A motor takes energy from a fuel source and converts it into mechanical energy using induction. This model of a pumping heart requires it to be both motor and pump.

As stated above, the vast majority of energy consumption in the heart is related to heat production. In health, very little is expended in mechanical work. The metabolic requirements of the peripheral tissues as the real driver for blood movement have been given scant consideration since William Harvey's description of the heart (discussed more fully in Chapter 8), yet it would seem to be the most reasonable description of blood movement through the circulatory system given the amount of work the heart would have to do to propel blood through the system. Recall our discussion of the heart's purpose from Chapter 1, in which we stated that "If the primary or even sole purpose of the heart is a pump, one would expect all of the oxygen to be used to fuel muscular activity. Yet, we find that at rest, of the 250 cc/min (of oxygen) available to it, only 10% of the total consumption is used by the heart. Of that 25 cc/min, 20% is used for basal metabolism, 5% is used in the exertion of the beating heart and 70% (more or less) is used in the creation of heat."

A generator converts mechanical energy into electric energy using electromagnetic induction. The generated electrical energy passing through the coil that is the myocardial band, as first described by Steno, then Pettigrew, and more recently Torrent-Guasp and Buckberg, comes from the coordinated depolarisation of the myocytes along the length of the band. This creates the associated electromagnetic field, which is inducted into the electromagnetically responsive blood being held in the left ventricle. The inducted electric current then flows throughout the body via the blood, which, because of its high salt content and the high electron affinity of the hemoglobin in the red blood cells, makes it an extremely good conductor of electricity.

The question arises as to why the high charge we observe in the left ventricle is not matched in the aorta or in the lungs. The probable answer to this lies in the construction of the heart with its layers of myocardial fibres lying against each other in different orientation, each layer surrounded by a fascial sheath creating a double layer of connective tissue with a potential space between. The fascial double layer acts as an insulator between the layers of myocardial fibres and maintains the contractile impulse within the myocardial band, thus ensuring propagation along the band and limiting any potential for trans-layer charge transfer. This limits any potential to short circuit the contraction propagation along the myocardial band that would distort the shape change of the heart and the associated effective filling/ejecting function.

The three layers of the myocardium and associated fascial double layers, as seen in the interventricular septum, provide a functional electrical shield between the right and left ventricles. The importance of this shield relates to the lower charge maintained in the right ventricle, the low charge arterial return to the lungs, and the high charge information encoding of the blood from the lungs in the left ventricle.

The fascial dynamic, with respect to charge insulation, is further evidenced at the valves of the heart. The valves are formed within and are supported by the fascial endoskeleton of the heart that is particularly condensed at the site of the valves to form the annular rings that hold the valves. The connective tissue condensation limits the wholesale transmission of the charge that is built up in the left ventricle from spreading into the wall of the aorta, which operates at a considerably lower charge level.

The condensation of connective tissue acting as an insulator is seen in dysfunction in the periphery, where the lesion, which was called an "energy sink" by Dr Robert Fulford, distorts the normal charge dynamic of the tissues.

Recall that in Chapter 1 we mentioned that the heart had several ways of using the blood to imprint and transfer information. Adrenalin can increase blood conductance. Electrical currents in the blood stream flow throughout the body. With the advent of SQUID technology, it has been possible to show that the currents generated by the heart create biomagnetic fields detectable in the space around the body.

Nobel laureate Albert Szent-Györgyi recognised that "If a great number of atoms is arranged with regularity in close proximity, as for instance, in a crystal lattice, the terms of the single valency electrons may fuse into common bands"[6] and the structures made of proteins can be electronic semiconductors. This observation meant that the protein frameworks found in cells and tissues around cells may act as electronic "circuits" that can rapidly move energy/information throughout the organism.

Later, Mark Bretscher at Cambridge University in England found that there are proteins extending across cell surfaces, which connect the cell interior with its surroundings. These protein structures came to be called *integrins*. They connect the cytoskeleton of every cell with that of neighbouring cells and with the extracellular matrix.

Pienta and Coffey[7] found evidence for physical connections between the nucleus and cell periphery and their alteration by transformation. This showed that the cytoskeletal matrix communicates with the nuclear matrix and also that there was a continuous flow of information between the extracellular matrix and all parts of the cell.

James Oschman, who worked with Szent-Györgyi, drew the research together and recognised that there is a continuous communication system provided by the matrix that reaches into every part of the body; from the circulation via the matrix to every cell and even, via the cytoskeleton, into the nucleus and the DNA. Additional evidence from the Johns Hopkins laboratory revealed that the components of the living matrix network are capable of vibrating in a dynamic, harmonic and measurable manner. Oschman described this as a systemic language that "is spoken in electrical oscillations and the information is encoded as frequencies."[8] Oschman saw this body-wide continuous system as the substrate for an energetic electronic regulatory system, which he named the "Living Matrix".

In the lesion state, the phasic uptake and release of calcium ions by the connective tissue proteins is disrupted, thereby altering the smooth change of the fluid in the extracellular matrix (ECM) to a higher concentration of electrolytes that causes a phase change to a more fluid state. There is a disassembly of glycosaminoglycans (GAGs) to release bound water to flow.

With the disruption in the ECM of electrical oscillations and the information encoded as frequencies, there is a coincident ability of the ECM to pass the charge and information from the perivascular space to their cellular destination.

From thermodynamics, we understand that there is no loss of energy from the system. That begs the question, what happens to all the energy in the left ventricle that is not imbued into the blood and is shielded from being transferred either to the rest of the heart or to dissipate along the aorta? The answer may be that it is used to produce the heat, which allows the dissipation of electrical energy between each heartbeat and thus allows the formation of a completely fresh energetic information environment in which the heart can process information inputs and can modify the electrical information imparted into the blood on a beat-to-beat basis.

Within the electromagnetic spectrum, the heart must encode information across multiple waves and frequencies with each beat. At the same time, it generates and delivers different pressure waves, sound waves, thermal fluctuations, hormonal cascades, neurotransmitters **and** the blood's helical-vortical charged patterns formed within the trabeculae carneae of the left ventricle.[9,10]

Corollary to this development of charge and spiralling of the blood by the heart is the recognition of the combination of suction towards all cells in the periphery and the magnetic qualities of the blood (discussed more fully in Chapter 8), resulting in self-propulsion.

To gain some understanding of this magnetically-driven self-propulsion, consider the construction and action of the World's Simplest Electric Train,[11] which can be viewed by visiting https://www.youtube.com/watch?v=J9b0J29OzAU or by scanning the following QR code:

In Figures 7.1 to 7.3, the "train" is created by placing a round magnet at the positive and negative ends of an AA battery. Next, copper wire is wound around something that is slightly larger in diameter than the magnets you have attached so that the magnets (but not the battery) are very slightly contacting the wire on either end of the battery, but the battery itself is not touching the wire. This sends electrons through the coil and creates a magnetic field that propels the "train" through its track.

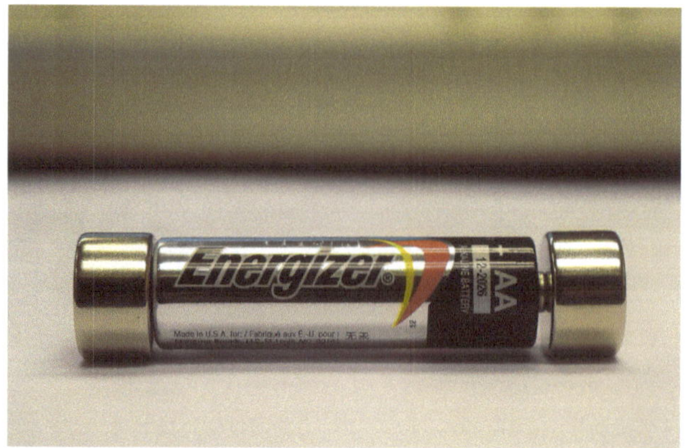


**Figure 7.1 – The Train.** Image courtesy of K&J Magnetics.

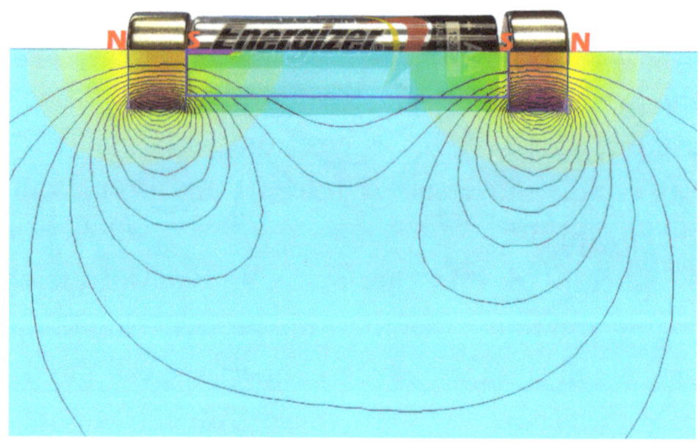


**Figure 7.2 – The Magnetic Field.** Image courtesy of K&J Magnetics.

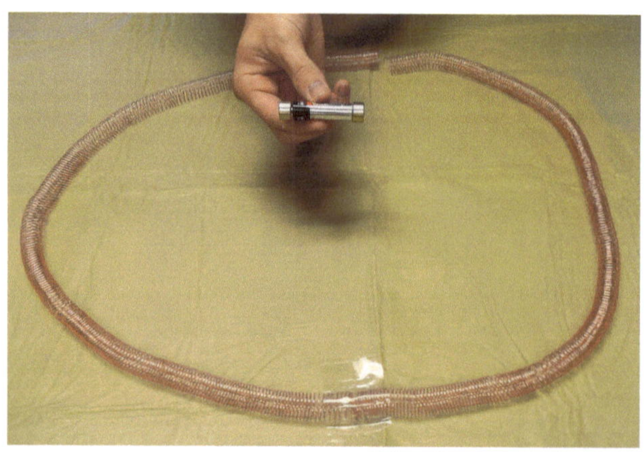

**Figure 7.3 – The Train and Its Track.** Image courtesy of K&J Magnetics.

## Electromagnetism and the Heart

Condensation of electromagnetic function in the midline orientates around and, in the process, creates the heart. The heart is, in fact, a highly complex, self-organised, information-processing centre with its own functional brain (introduced in Chapter 1) that communicates with and influences the cranial brain via the nervous system, hormonal system and other pathways. These influences profoundly affect brain function and most of the body's major organs and ultimately determine one's quality of life.[12]

"In the healthy heart, the varied and complex emotions we experience each day—generated by contact with our internal and external worlds—produces a range of heart rate patterns that are nonlinear and constantly shifting. Communications are embedded within these shifting mixes and patterns, including the communications from and to our bodies, our loved ones, and the world at large. The narrower the range of the electromagnetic spectrum exposure, particularly during major depression and panic disorder, the more regular the beating patterns of the heart become, and the less we are in harmony with ourselves, other people and everything around us. This narrowing and increase in regularity also has direct impacts on our sympathetic and parasympathetic nervous systems.

A constant or increasing state of sympathetic activity increases stress and production of cortisol. While cortisol is an important and helpful part of the body's response to stress, it is important that the body's relaxation response be activated so that the body's functions can return to normal following a stressful event.

Variability in heart rate can be influenced by different states of consciousness and well-being, such as sleeping, resting, working, physical exercise, stress, sickness, etc.

So, it is not surprising that unhealthy emotional states, major anxiety, depression and panic disorders correlate with changes in heart rate variability. As in many pathological heart conditions, the heart's electromagnetic spectrum begins to show a narrower range and beating patterns become very regular."

On the other hand, increasing heart rate variability and heart coherence boosts the body's production of immunoglobulin A, a naturally occurring compound that protects the body's mucous membranes and helps prevent infections.

## The Heart and the Nature of Nature

Heart rate variability was an important clue for Dr Irving Dardik as he strove to understand nature and the way in which it was not linear but a series of waves waving within waves waving. Dardik, a vascular surgeon and educator at the Albert Einstein College of Medicine, concluded that "the way to understand waves waving is to open the mind to the unfamiliar reality that motion has no natural parts."[13] In his conclusion, Dardik sets aside what he calls "the puzzle hypothesis", which assumes that nature is inherently divisible into a series of parts and that breaking it down into smaller and smaller parts will eventually reveal an understanding of the whole of nature. It means seeing motion not as a "thing" that is inherently divisible but as an event in which we see **unity** as a force in nature—a very osteopathic point of view![14]

In his book *The Nature of Nature*, Dardik explains how, in a scientific controlled experiment, attempts are made to ensure that all influences and parts, except for what is being tested, are removed. However, Dardik needed to show that motion across all scales is inherently connected, so nothing could be removed.

Dardik's quest was to discover—knowing that all cellular and molecular motion is cycling—whether those cycles cycle up and down in a continuum. Being a vascular surgeon and an olympic physician with extensive expertise in the functioning of the cardiovascular system, Dardik started his observations with the way in which the heart's function was cycling, beating slower or faster in relation to the movement of the body as a whole. Dardik thought of the whole body as "the body wave" with the "heart's wave" embedded within it. So, the continuum being studied was the heart's and body's exercise-recovery waves.

Dardik strove to retain the recognition that we identify peaks, troughs, and other features as "separate scales" in nested, simultaneously changing waves within waves. He came to see three main facets or principles of waves waving:

1. The continuum of frequencies and amplitudes is nonlinear by nature.
2. The processes of attraction and repulsion come about through the inherent relationship between carrier waves and inner waves, such that the process of attraction is greatest for inner waves as carrier waves come to a peak and repulsion is greatest as carrier waves come to a trough.
3. Scales influence each other simultaneously as waves wave forward, such that there is an inherently continuous relationship between what science has been referring to as separate phenomena of action at a distance and causality.[15]

In relation to the first principle stated above, Dardik affirmed that waves waving demonstrated non-absolute, **relative** frequencies and amplitudes. Waves speed up and slow down. Dardik used the term **frequency** for this quality. Waves also become more or less intense, which Dardik described as **amplitude**. Both frequency and amplitude are always changing.

Dardik pointed out that when waves change substantially in frequency and amplitude, so do the waves with which they nest. For example the more dramatic the sprint, the more dramatic the rise of the heartbeats' frequency and amplitude (Figure 7.4). Additionally, Dardik concluded that "This also means that the sharper the slope of the carrier wave as it rises, the sharper the slope of the rising nested waves within; these become higher frequency–amplitude in their own right."[16]

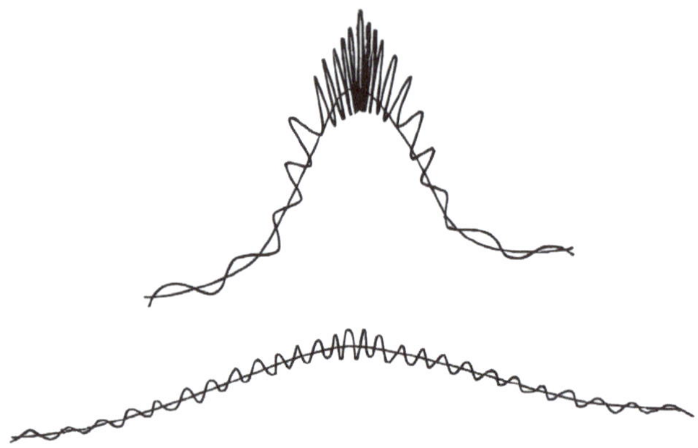

**Figure 7.4 – Frequency-Amplitude Waves.** Above, a sharply sloped wave with more sharply sloped frequency-amplitude waves climbing it and decreasing sharp waves descending it. Below, a less sharply sloped wave with less sharp frequency-amplitude waves climbing and descending it. Both diagrams show that the sharper the slope of the carrier wave, the sharper the slopes of the inner waves (or alternatively, the flatter the slope of the carrier wave, the flatter the slopes of the inner waves). Illustrations reprinted from *The Nature of Nature: The Discovery of Superwaves and How it Changes Everything* by Irv Dardik and Estee Dardik Lichter, copyright © 2017 by Irv Dardik and Estee Dardik Lichter. Used by permission of Rodale Books, an imprint of Random House, a division of Penguin Random House LLC. All rights reserved.

The key idea is that in the complexity of a living human organism, frequencies and amplitudes change together as a continuum across scales. The continuum of frequency and amplitude of a wave is **inherently non-linear**.

The second principle Dardik relates to his observation is that as the heart wave rises to a peak during a burst of exercise, one finds a high-density of fast, forceful heartbeats. He observed that a particular pattern appears such that as the smaller, inner wave climbs the carrier wave, those inner waves speed up and are clustered, swarming, synchronous and dense. With this increase in motion and compression comes an increase in temperature—it's warmer. Then, when the waves come down, they slow down, spread out, and flatten.[17]

Dardik's second principle relates the exercise recovery carrier wave as it crests before the downswing as like a force pulling the inner waves together towards the peak; like a force through which the waves are attracted to one another. By contrast, the heart wave is different when the body is recovering (Figure 7.5).

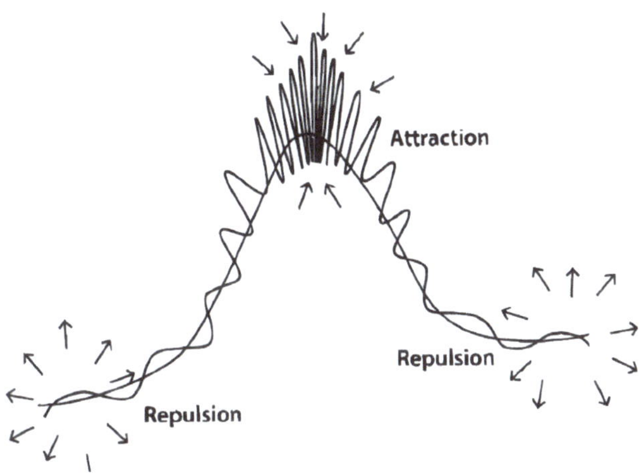


**Figure 7.5 – Attraction, Repulsion and Dispersion.** Attraction naturally happens as carrier waves compress inner waves in a peak. Repulsion, or dispersion, of inner waves naturally happens as carrier waves spread out in a trough. Illustrations reprinted from *The Nature of Nature: The Discovery of Superwaves and How it Changes Everything* by Irv Dardik and Estee Dardik Lichter, copyright © 2017 by Irv Dardik and Estee Dardik Lichter. Used by permission of Rodale Books, an imprint of Random House, a division of Penguin Random House LLC. All rights reserved.

As the heartbeats slow, everything cools down. The waves are not as intense, and their frequency has decelerated.

Dardik's third principle relates to the fact that as individuals, we can directly influence the heart wave with the body wave with a quick sprint followed by sitting down and resting. The heartbeat wave accelerates and decelerates. So, not only can the body wave influence the heart wave as they wave forward together, but within every wave of the heartbeat lie many smaller biochemical waves. These are cycles that are open to influence through this continuum.

Dardik realised that as one layer moves forward, the inherent continuity determines that another layer changes simultaneously with it, regardless of the direction of influence. Thus, the very nature of waves determines that forward moving change occurs on every scale. For Dardik, this means that whereas cause and effect have always been seen as local, linear interactions between parts, change on what we see as one scale inherently "causes" change simultaneously on other scales. Therefore, change is simultaneously causal in both directions, or what Dardik calls *simulcausality*.[18]

However, Dardik regards cause and effect as not the **sole** modus operandi of nature. He points out that the nature of waves waving within waves is both unique and all pervasive as a pattern in nature. Although the pattern is like a fractal in that it is self-similar across scales, it differs from a fractal in that it has nothing to do with points, lines or dimensions. It cannot be broken into parts. So Dardik coined a new phrase for the pattern of the heart wave: an *inherently continuous fractal*. This brings to mind noted science writer Amanda Gefter's observation that "the most profound question in physics today is how to unify the really small with the really big—and when it comes to matters of scale, fractals may turn out to be a key ingredient."[19]

Drawing on both his everyday and Olympic sports medical experiences, Dardik realised that everything in the body is both pulsatile and rhythmic. He points out that the movement of DNA is rhythmic, having been described by researchers as both "breathing" and "dancing".[20]

As Levine and colleagues noted, "Pulsing has been observed in many types of proteins, from alternative bacterial sigma factors to mammalian tumour suppressors such as p53, and has been shown to function in diverse processes from stress response to signalling to differentiation."[21]

Dardik goes on to observe that all hormones are secreted in a pulsatile way. In fact, a recent study found that their cyclic release affects the expression of genes.[22]

Dardik understood that everything is in rhythmic, vibratory motion; rather than being separate layers that are unrelated, they all function through waves that relate as an inherent continuum across scales. He replaces the hierarchical levels going up like a pyramid with dynamically twirling, clustering and disbursing spirals nested inside a fractal-wave continuum as they move forward.

In an earlier article, Dardik described the peaks of waves as areas of intense local activity or densations where mass or particles are generated. (The use of the word *densation* echoes Blechschmidt's description of certain phases of embryology.) With the appearance of particles, **charge** appears concurrently.

These statements relating to rhythm and nested waves strongly resonate with us as we have explored the meaning of Still's insight that the heart imparts knowledge to the blood to enable it to do its work.[23]

## Transmutation

Transmutation involves a change from one form, nature or substance into another and was given a significant role in relation to the cerebrospinal fluid by William Sutherland, DO. He referred to the cerebrospinal fluid as the "juice…that invisible potency"[24] of the body. Thus, transmutation is an adaptive process that occurs in both the cerebrospinal fluid and the blood.

Still stated forcefully: "On whom or what does this engine (man) depend for its motive force?… All must have and cannot act without the highest known order of force (electricity), which submits to the voluntary and involuntary commands of life and mind, by which worlds are driven and beings move."[25]

It appears that the thermal regulation and maintenance of the blood within a narrow range, as mentioned earlier in this chapter, is vital to the transmutational ability of the blood. Recall that Schauberger placed great emphasis on the temperature of water. French scientist C. Louis Kervran proposed that nuclear transmutation, a process whereby one chemical isotope or element converts to another through nuclear reactions,[26] occurs in living organisms; he called this process *biological transmutation*. Kervran reached this conclusion after conducting an experiment with chickens in which there was no calcium in their food or soil yet the chickens were generating calcium in their eggshells. After living for some time with a calcium-deficient diet, the hens began laying eggs with soft shells. When the chickens were later given mica (which contains a significant amount of potassium), they gorged themselves on this and very quickly became able to lay eggs with normal shells.[27]

Extensive interdisciplinary study has revealed that both geological and biological processes induce **low energy atomic nuclear transmutations** at specific resonant temperatures in the presence of specific gases. For instance, Kervran found that during blood circulation, fission of iron atoms releases hydrogen atoms by phonon induction of bound oxygen atoms **only at 37.8°C**. Phonons are responsible for all thermal properties of a solid, such as its heat content and transport.[28]

Kervran defined resonant nuclear reactions as reversible and involving both fusion (joining together) and fission (breaking apart) events between gases, metals, nonmetals and earth metals. His simple in vitro demonstration of the oxygen-dependent low energy atomic conversion of carbon into iron was reported in 1962, wherein ultrapure carbon rods were used as electrodes in an aqueous discharge system. Sediment analysis confirmed the fusion of two carbon atoms with two oxygen atoms to form iron.[29]

Kervran's ground-breaking studies of various other heat-induced atmospheric and lithospheric processes led to his identification of several essential nuclear transmutations, without which such processes cannot be understood. He found that airborne pairs of nitrogen atoms readily combine to form silicon at the edge of the thermosphere (which extends from about 90 km to between 500 and 1,000 km above our planet). A similar fusion event was identified in volcanic reactions where pairs of carbon atoms merged in the formation of magnesium, while pairs of oxygen atoms merged to form sulfur. The natural abundance of elements and the specific isotope ratios produced in thermospheric and volcanic processes provide compelling evidence for low energy nuclear reactions as the unified driving force of nature.[30]

Various researchers have obtained significant evidence for biological transmutation as the origin of calcium from nuclear conversions of sodium, magnesium, potassium and silicon in a wide range of organisms that secrete calcium from one side of a membrane to produce protective shells.[31,32] Experiments showed that avian and reptilian species deprived of dietary calcium were incapable of producing solid eggshells unless provided with a dietary source of silicon, which was then readily converted into the calcium required for normal eggshell development. Similar experiments with crustacean species deprived of environmental calcium sources revealed their ability to supplant calcium with magnesium to facilitate normal shell development.

Kervran also determined that calcium formation during tooth enamel and bone growth processes in all vertebrate species was mitigated by the same substitutive resonant nuclear reactions of magnesium and oxygen fusing to form calcium, as well as another notable reaction: carbon fusing with fluorine to form phosphorus. The reversal of the latter process was identified in the bacterial digestion of bone, with phosphorus undergoing resonant fission into carbon and fluorine daughter isotopes. The constant emission of fluorine gas during bone decomposition is relied upon in the dating of fossil specimens,[33] yet its genesis as a fission product of bacterial digestion remains the only viable explanation.

Kervran further applied his comprehensive findings to resolve many commonly misunderstood biomineral deficiencies in humans involving the biological transmutation of all essential elements as magnesium, calcium, manganese, iron, copper and zinc. In fact, it is known that calcium deficiency and resulting bone depletion cannot be reversed by calcium intake alone. Calcium is now widely supplemented with magnesium, but the underlying mechanism can only be satisfactorily explained by resonant atomic transmutation. Hard evidence for fusion of magnesium and oxygen atoms is found in measurable calcium depletions in all bone. However, calcium requires boron to be metabolised into bones.

Interestingly, a critical part of this conversion process is that healthy blood requires access to light (photons), oxygen, hydrogen, stable blood pH (ie, not too acidic or overly alkaline) and the necessary elements to enable the conversion. The negative charge on the oxygen is a critical factor and therefore must be abundant in the blood to sustain the electrical potential for transmutation.

## The Heart's Field

The electromagnetic field of the embryo condenses in the midline at the heart. The diaphragm then becomes a partition between the two component parts of the field. It separates above from below, a concept that is expressed in the traditional Chinese medicine view of organisation.

As already discussed, the heart is an electromagnetic generator that produces the largest amount of electricity and a greater magnetic field than any other organ in the body. This magnetic field influences embryologic processes and is the reason, for example, that the electrocardiograph preceded the electroencephalogram in development.

In 1887, Augustus Waller recorded the first electrocardiogram with a mercury capillary electrometer at St. Mary's Hospital in London. This was long before there were instruments sufficiently sensitive to measure the electrical activity of the nervous system. As a producer of electricity, it, by definition, must produce a magnetic field. This begs the question: How far out does our field extend and where is the boundary of the individual? Physics tells us that these fields extend indefinitely, but they decrease in strength the further you are from the source. As such, the heart is a significant player in the electromagnetic field relationship with the planet and with each other.

The heart's electromagnetic field—by far the most powerful rhythmic field produced by the human body—not only envelops every cell of the body but also extends out in all directions into the space around us (Figure 7.6 and 7.7). The cardiac field can be measured several feet away from the body by sensitive devices. Furthermore, research conducted at Heartmath Institute suggests that the heart's field is an important carrier of information.

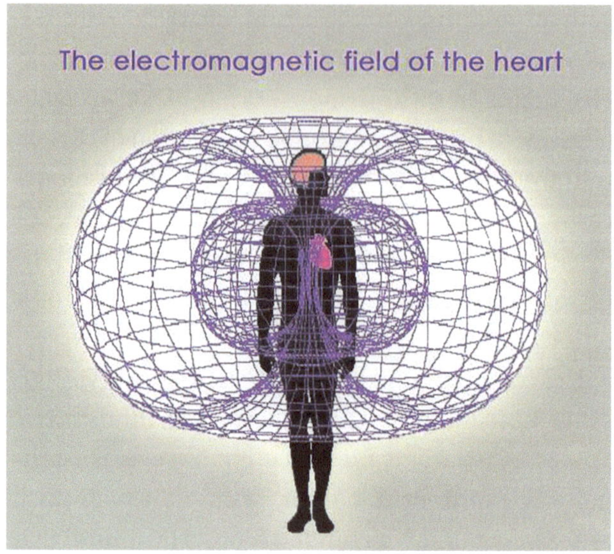


**Figure 7.6 – Electromagnetic Field of the Heart.** Reproduced from https://commons.wikimedia.org/wiki/File:Heart-field.jpg.

The work of Davis and Rawls gives insight into and affirms the positional importance of the diaphragm from an electromagnetic perspective, as illustrated in Figure 7.8.[34]

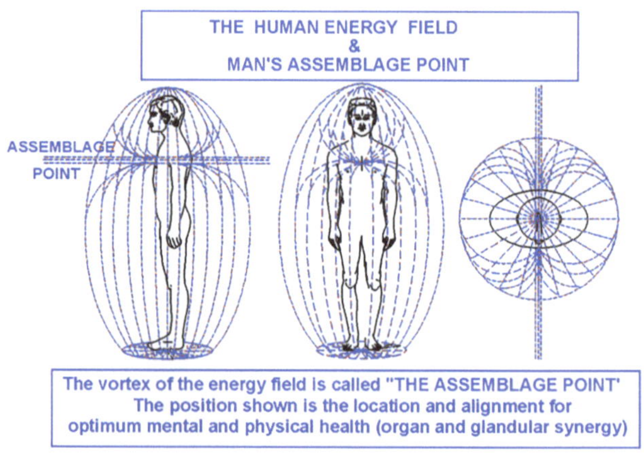


**Figure 7.7 – Assemblage Point**[35]

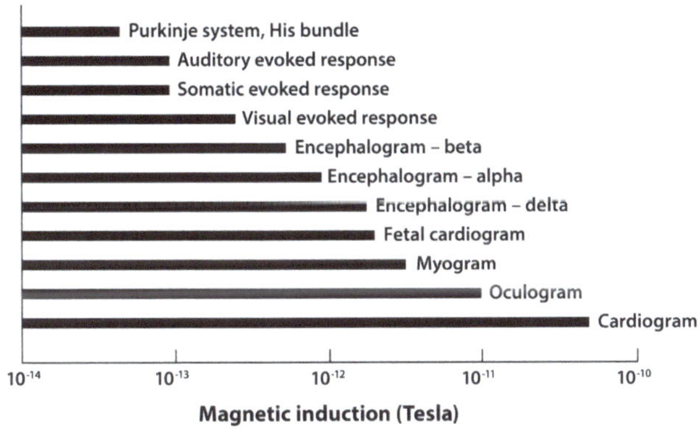


**Figure 7.8 – Magnetic Induction.**[36] The relative strength of the various biomagnetic fields measured in the spaces around the human body.

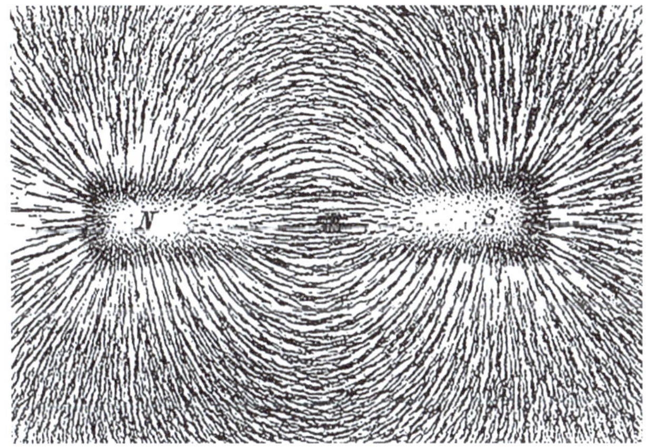


**Figure 7.10 – North-South Magnet With Shavings.** Reprinted from Black and Davis.[37]

Figures 7.9 and 7.10 show the classical views of a magnetic field generated in relation to a north-south magnet.

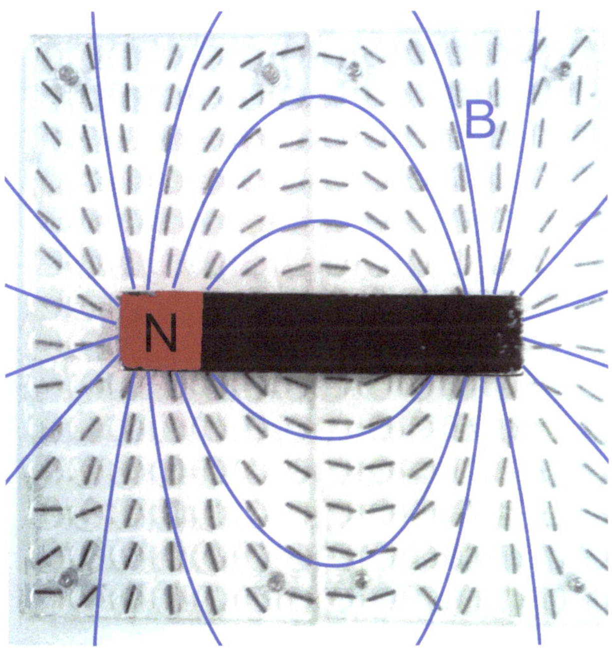


**Figure 7.9 – North-South Magnet With Field Lines.** Reprinted from https://commons.wikimedia.org/wiki/File:Bar_magnet_on_compass_board_with_field_lines.png.

Davis and Rawls showed that the negative energy pull at the north spins to the left and the positive energy poll at the south spins to the right. As a consequence, there is a point of zero magnetism that is known as the Bloch Wall (Figure 7.11) which can be seen in a demonstration using iron filings (Figure 7.12). Using this knowledge, Rob Gourlay was able to create a Magnetized Energized and Activated water device to structure water such that it holds the charge imparted to it on an indefinite basis. He is the first to achieve this accomplishment.

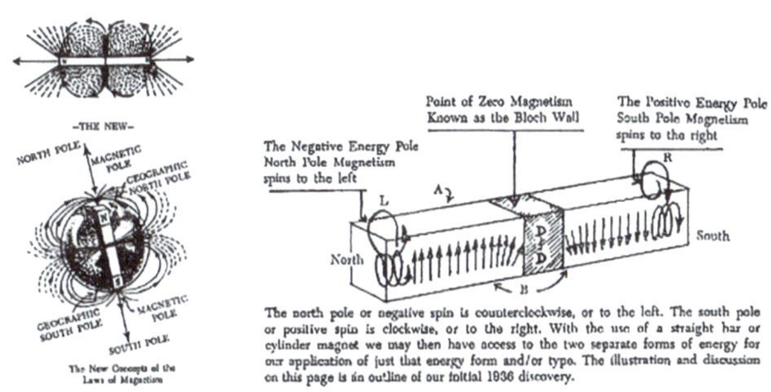


**Figure 7.11 – Magnetism and Its Effect on the Living System.** Images courtesy of Acres USA on behalf of Albert Davis and Walter Rawls' *Magnetism and Its Effect on the Living System.*[38]

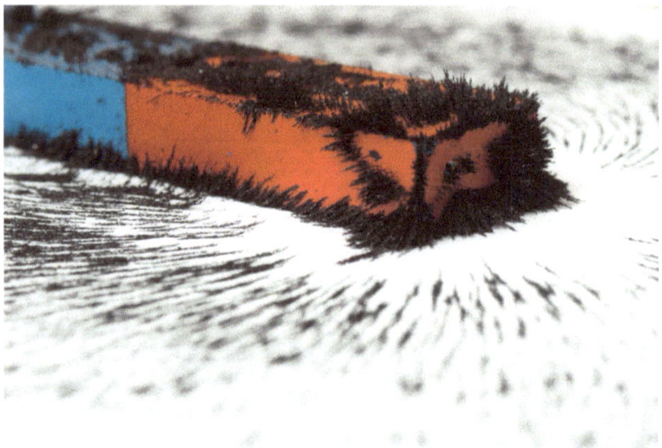

**Figure 7.12 – Electromagnetic Arc Seen in Metal Shavings on Magnet.** Image courtesy of Maciej J. Mrowinski. Reprinted from https://commons.wikimedia.org/wiki/File:Metal_shavings_around_bar_magnet_(close-up).jpg.

## Memory

The attempt to find the particular part of the brain that stores memories has been remarkably unfruitful. Through Pribram's research, it became apparent to him that memory was at least the function of the whole nervous system and that a model of holographic memory storage in the nervous system developed.[39]

Neuropsychologist Paul Pearsall, in his book *The Heart's Code,* provided evidence of an emotional consciousness associated with the heart and that this consciousness was associated with an energy that can be utilised. He named it the L energy. The consciousness component was acknowledged after he interviewed heart transplant recipients who noted, at times, disturbing personality changes and often information about their heart donors that was associated with the traumatic events around their donors' deaths. Some of these stories were amusing, some poignant, and some chilling.

These observations prompted Pearsall to consider that the heart may have a consciousness and a memory.

Obviously, the work of Pearsall has pushed the boundary even further from just the nervous system. The question is whether research in this extension of consciousness has gone far enough. The research relating to this idea proposes that memory is contained in the zero-point field (ZPF) and that each of us accesses the information as required at a personal level and collectively on occasion.[40]

The ZPF has the lowest possible energy that a quantum mechanical system may have. Unlike classical mechanics, quantum systems constantly fluctuate in the lowest energy state as described by Heisenberg's uncertainty principle. Also referred to by physicists as "the vacuum", the ZPF was so-called because fluctuations in the field are still detectable in temperatures of absolute zero. It is the lowest possible energy state, where all matter has been removed and nothing is supposedly left to make any motion. Physicists have understood that, despite the assumption of nothingness, there are fleeting particles known as *virtual particles* generated during a very brief moment in time.[41]

Separately, research of the ZPF/vacuum phenomenon led to some significant alterations on how we perceive consciousness and memory. Through the work of Puthoff[42] and Radin and Nelson,[43] it is now understood that memory is unlikely to be a function of just the central nervous system; neither is it likely to be contained within the cranium.

This concept has been further developed by Pitkanen, who has proposed the idea of a magnetic sensory canvas. His hypothesis is that we are corporal and magnetic selves consisting of magnetic flux tube structures (Figure 7.13).

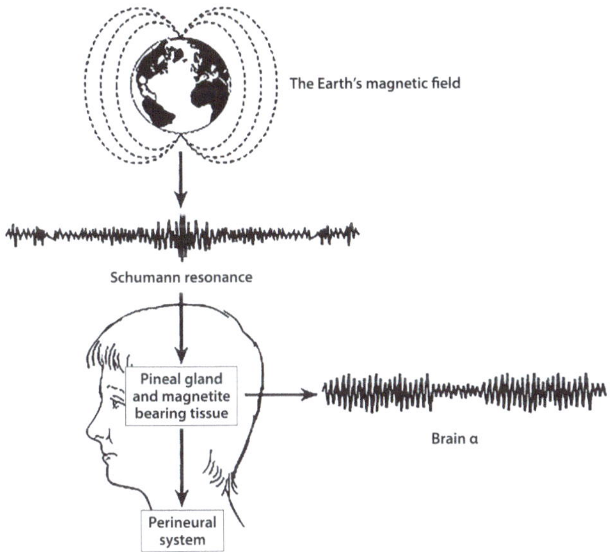


**Figure 7.13 – Magnetic Flux Tubes.** Image courtesy of AcresUSA on behalf of Albert Davis and Walter Rawls' *Magnetism and Its Effects on the Living System.*[44]

These magnetic flux tubes are part of the earth's magnetic field. Sensory representations are realised from oscillations within the flux tubes, resonating harmonically with thalamocortical frequencies that project sensory data into consciousness.

This concept acknowledges that between different electromagnetic fields, interactions take place. If a particular field is greater than another—as is the case with the body's electromagnetic field and Schumann resonances of the earth—the larger does not obliterate the smaller. Rather, there is a mingling of the wave patterns as interference patterns. This model is consistent with the quantum view of electromagnetic field interaction. It is also consistent with the description of Dardik that everything is waves waving within waves.

## Applications to Osteopathic Practice

What all of the researchers of the effects of magnetism are proposing is that there exists another level of interaction amidst the individual, the earth and each other related to the earth's magnetic field. Access to an individual's specific memories is the result of frequency-specific "tuning in" to the field. While the concept sounds like something from the 1990's science fiction television show *The X Files*, the research into this concept of the ZPF holding memory is the basis of the technology of the MRI scanner. Of note, research is coming out of top-tier institutions. Nelson, who has conducted research into the collective memory, is a professor at Princeton University. Pitkanen is in the department of theoretical physics at the University of Helsinki.

In our view, life is there before the moment of conception and continues on after exiting the body at death.

In physics, and in the domain of osteopathy, the electromagnetic field condenses and expresses itself in the midline as the heart, which is the first functional organ in vertebrate embryos. In humans, the heart beats spontaneously at 22 days with blood flow starting by week 3. Condensation of waveforms at conception creates photons and electrons resulting in polarity and an equator. Condensation of waves waving within waves waving results in form, matter, physiology and anatomy.

The condensation of connective tissue acting as an insulator has been observed by many practitioners since the osteopathic profession's attention was drawn to it by Dr Robert Fulford, who called it an *energy sink* that distorts the normal charge dynamic of the tissues. Of interest is the repeated observation that, as a peripheral fascial strain starts to resolve, memories of the event that was the genesis for the strain bubble up and become very vivid in the patient's memory.

As mentioned earlier, the heart is an electromagnetic generator that produces the largest amount of electricity and a greater magnetic field than any other organ in the body.

Assessing the interventricular septum can provide information about the patient's vitality and the response to treatment.

The recognition of the early stage of a change of the septum, which can shift towards the horizontal, can signal an alteration of function.

Dardik describes the peaks of waves as areas of intense local activity or densations where mass/particles are generated. With the appearance of particles, **charge** appears concurrently. In general, we are aiming for an increase in negative charge and a shift towards wellness.

*The Heart's Code* provided evidence of an emotional consciousness that was associated with the heart and with an energy that can be utilised. Restoring charge and an integration of waves within waves can help release memories that otherwise exert a drag on normal patterns of flow.

The author would like to express his sincere gratitude to Natural Resource Scientist and Inventor Robert Gourlay for his invaluable contributions to "The Heart's Field" section of this chapter.

## Chapter 7 Endnotes

1. A.T. Still, *Osteopathy Research and Practice* (Kirksville, MO: The Journal Printing Co, 1910), 328–30.

2. "How Is Body Temperature Regulated and What Is Fever?" InformedHealth.org, Instistute for Quality and Efficiency in Health Care, updated December 6, 2022, https://www.informedhealth.org/how-is-body-temperature-regulated-and-what-is-fever.html.

3. Heinrich Brettschneider, "The Polarity of Center and Periphery in the Circulatory System," in *The Dynamic Heart and Circulation,* ed. Craig Holdrege (Fair Oaks, CA: The Association of Waldorf Schools of North America, 2002), 50.

4. Christiane Liesche, "A Dynamic Morphology of the Cardiovascular System," in *The Dynamic Heart and Circulation*, ed. Craig Holdrege (Fair Oaks, CA: The Association of Waldorf Schools of North America, 2002)

5. Craig Holdredge, "Introduction," *The Dynamic Heart and Circulation*, ed. Craig Holdrege (Fair Oaks, CA: The Association of Waldorf Schools of North America, 2002)

6. A. Szent-Györgyi, "Towards a New Biochemistry," *Science* 93, no. 2426 (June 1941): 609–11, https://doi.org/10.1126/science.93.2426.609

7. Kenneth J. Pienta and Donald S. Coffey, "Nuclear-Cytoskeletal Interactions: Evidence for Physical Connections Between the Nucleus and Cell Periphery and Their Alteration by Transformation," *Journal of Cellular Biochemistry* 49, no. 4 (August 1992), 357-65.

8. James L. Oschman, *Energy Medicine in Therapeutics and Human Performance* (Butterworth-Heinemann, 2003).

9. Aleksandr Goncharenko and Svetlana Goncharenko, "Extrasensory Powers of the Heart," Техника Молодежи *(Technology to the Youth),* no. 5 (2005; translated 2017).

10. Aleksandr I. Goncharenko, "Heartspace as the Basis of Superconsciousness," *Consciousness and Physical Reality* 2, no. 3 (1997; translated 2017): 25–35.

11. "World's Simplest Train," Amazing Science, posted August 26, 2014, on YouTube, https://www.youtube.com/watch?v=J9b0J29OzAU

12. J. Andrew Armour, "The Little Brain on the Heart," *Cleveland Clinic Journal of Medicine* 74, suppl. 1 (February 2007): S48–51. https://doi.org/10.3949/ccjm.74.suppl_1.s48.

13. Irving Dardik and Estee Dardik Lichter, *The Nature of Nature: The Discovery of Superwaves and How it Changes Everything* (Emmaus, PA: Rodale Books, 2017).

14. Dardik and Dardik Lichter, *The Nature of Nature.*

15. Dardik and Dardik Lichter, *The Nature of Nature*, 172–3.

16. Dardik and Dardik Lichter, *The Nature of Nature*, 174.

17. Dardik and Dardik Lichter, *The Nature of Nature*, 177.

18. Dardik and Dardik Lichter, *The Nature of Nature*, 180.

19. Amanda Gefter, "Don't Mention the F Word," *New Scientist* 193, no. 2594 (March 2007): 30–3.

20. "Visualisation of 'Dancing DNA'," University of Leads, published February 16, 2021, accessed March 27, 2023, https://www.leeds.ac.uk/news-science/news/article/4770/visualisation-of-dancing-dna.

21. Joe H. Levine, Yihan Lin, and Michael B. Elowitz. "Functional Roles of Pulsing Genetic Circuits," *Science* 342, no. 6163 (December 6, 2013): 1193–200. https://doi.org/10.1126%2Fscience.1239999.

22. "Hormone Cycling Found to Affect Gene Activity" (news release), National Institutes of Health, August 16, 2009, https://www.nih.gov/news-events/news-releases/hormone-cycling-found-affect-gene-activity.

23. Irving Dardik, "The Great Law of the Universe," *Cycles* (March/April 1994), p275

24. William Garner Sutherland, *Teachings in the Science of Osteopathy* (Sutherland Cranial Teaching Foundation, 2003), 33.

25. A.T. Still, *Autobiography of Andrew Taylor Still* (Kirksville, MO: A.T. Still, 1908), 234.

26. "Nuclear Transmutation," ChemEurope.com, accessed January 25, 2023, https://www.chemeurope.com/en/encyclopedia/Nuclear_transmutation.html.

27. Jean-Paul Biberian, "Biological Transmutations," *Current Science* 108, no. 4 (February 25, 2015): 633–5.

28. Karl W. Böer and Udo W. Pohl, "Phonon-Induced Thermal Properties," in *Semiconductor Physics* (Springer, 2018), 151–79.

29. C. Louis Kervran, *Biological Transmutations*, trans. Michael Abhesera (London: Happiness Press, 1989).

30. C. Louis Kervran, *Biological Transmutation*, trans. Michael Abhsera (Binghamton, NY: Swan House Publishing Co., 1972).

31. M.A. Castañeda Cataña et al., "Knowledge Evolution: Inert Sciences to Living Science," *Global Journal of Ecology* 7, no. 2 (September 2022): 82–9. https://doi.org/10.17352/gje.000066.

32. Jean-Paul Biberian, "Biological Transmutations: Historical Perspective," *Journal of Condensed Matter Nuclear Science* 7, (2012): 11–25.

33. Morgan Isaacs, "Fluorine Dating of Human Bone at the Pre-Columbian Maya Cemetery of Caves Branch Rockshelter, Belize" (master's thesis, The University of Mississippi, 2016), 356, https://egrove.olemiss.edu/etd/356.

34. Albert Roy Davis and Walter C Rawls, *Magnetism and Its Effects on the Living System*, 2nd ed., 12th printing (Fort Collins, CO: Acres USA, 1996).

35. Jon Whale, Human Energy Field and Man's Assemblage Point, Reprinted from https://commons.m.wikimedia.org/wiki/File:AP-Fig1.jpg.

36. S.J. Williamson and L. Kaufman, "Biomagnetism," *Journal of Magnetism and Magnetic Materials* 22, no. 2 (1981): 129-201.

37. Newton Henry Black and Harvey N. Davis, *Practical Physics* (The MacMillan Co, 1913), 242, Figure 200, https://commons.wikimedia.org/wiki/File:Magnet0873.png.

38. Davis and Rawls, *Magnetism and Its Effect on the Living System.*

39. Karl H. Pribram, *The Form Within: My Point of View* (Prospecta Press, 2013).

40. Joachim Keppler, "The Role of the Brain in Conscious Processes," *Frontiers in Psychology* 9 (August 2018), https://doi.org/10.3389/fpsyg.2018.01346.

41. Lynne McTaggart, *The Field: The Quest for the Secret Force of the Universe* (Harper Collins, 2002).

42. "Where does the zero-point energy come from?" *New Scientist*, December 2, 1989, https://www.newscientist.com/article/mg12416932-700-science-where-does-the-zero-point-energy-came-from/.

43. Dean Radin and Roger Nelson, "Meta-Analysis of Mind-Matter Interaction Experiments: 1959–2000," https://www.boundaryinstitute.org.

44. Davis and Rawls, *Magnetism and Its Effect on the Living System.*

# Chapter Eight

# The Venous Return

*"The rule of the artery and vein is universal in all living beings, and the osteopath must know that and abide by its rulings, or he will not succeed as a healer."*[1]

– Andrew Taylor Still

Pulmonary circulation was first described by Ibn Al-Nafis, a physician in the 13th century. He was the first scientist to deduce that all blood that reached the left ventricle flowed through the lungs.[2] Since that time, descriptions of the circulatory system have orientated around the heart and the arteries, while the veins have been considered secondary due in part to their more passive, slower-moving nature.[3,4] However, we have progressively come to understand the significance of what Dr Still knew in 1899 about the massive plexus of veins that accompany the arteries and nerves everywhere in the body:

> "...we see the wisdom just as much in the venous system as in the arterial. The arteries supply all demands, and the veins carry away all waste material. We find building and healthy renovation are united in perpetual effort to construct and sustain purity.... If we go to any other part or organ of the body, we find just the same law of supply, arteries first, then renovation beginning with the veins."[5]

The idea that there must be drainage with renovation, that one cannot be successful without the other, is **very** important. There must be a dynamic equilibrium between the powerful high flow of the arterial blood being drawn towards the tissues, supported by the ability to drain with a substantially slower return flow, so much so that up to 80% of the vasculature carries venous blood. When renovating within an existing house, before you can renovate a room, you first have to empty it and pull out the old or damaged materials, and then you can rebuild. As Still put it, "Arteries first, then renovation, beginning with the veins."[6]

Before the 17th century, there were several theories about what drives circulation, one of which involved suction.[7] However, in 1628 all other theories were silenced when William Harvey, the royal physician to both King James I of England and later King Charles I, published his work *Exercitatio Anatomica de Motu Cordis et Sanguinis in Animalibus*, which proclaimed that the heart was a pump for a system-wide circulatory system. Given Harvey's position, this theory went uncontested formally[8] thus cementing the role of the heart as a pump in Western physiology and anatomy.

However, prior to that point, the historical literature indicates that suction was understood as providing the force necessary to move blood through the system.[9] Interestingly, around the same time Harvey was doing his work, a Danish anatomist named Neils Stensen (also known under his Latin name, Nicolas Steno) was writing about the spiraling myocardial band in his 1666 publication *Elementorum Myologiae*, proclaiming, "The heart is only a muscle."[10] This view contradicted the ethos of the day which viewed the heart as the body's heat generator and/or spirit bringer. His instructor, Professor Thomas Bartholin, an anatomist, a physician and the discoverer of the lymphatic system, enthusiastically supported Stensen's findings, responding by letter:

> "The spirit of Hippocrates will applaud you, because you, through your outstanding observations, revive his view of the heart, which we have moved away from, and provide clear evidence of the fact that the heart really is a muscle. Galenos and his successors will thank you because you have established that the fibers of the heart are of one and the same kind."[11]

So he clarified the understanding of the heart as a muscle, but he also found that the heart's muscle fibres "directed downwards toward the base and from there upwards" and observed that, after death, "the pulsations of the superior vena cava stopped much later than the cardiac beats."[12]

Two centuries later, this information was rediscovered by English anatomist James Bell Pettigrew and published in his widely-acclaimed *Design in Nature* (1908). He was internationally known for his discovery that "throughout the animal and plant kingdoms, at all orders of size, movements were often helical or spiral" (Figure 8.1).[13]

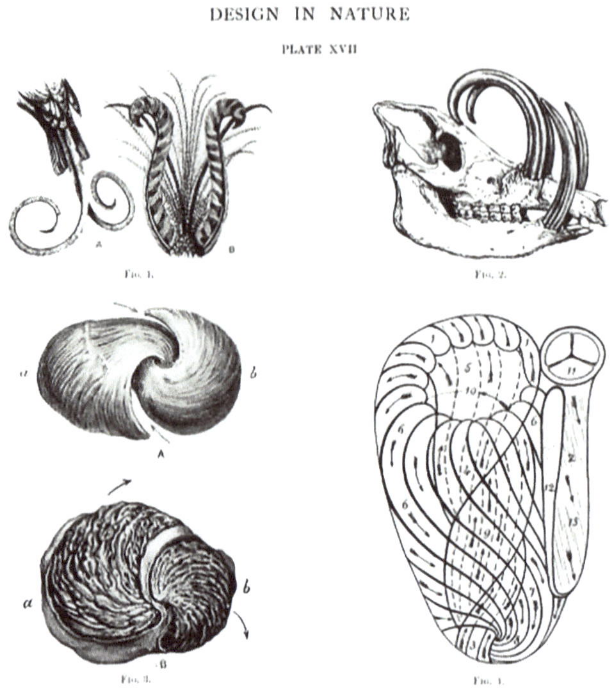


**Figure 8.1 – Spirals in Nature.** Plate XVII from James Bell Pettigrew's 1908 *Design in Nature*, displaying spirals in nature.[14]

This means that the helical ventricular myocardial band that anatomist and cardiologist Francisco Torrent-Guasp proposed and explored over the past few decades was already present in the historical literature, but it kept getting lost or obscured over time.

William Harvey's description of the circulatory system in his 1628 publication *Du Motu Cordis* set the tone for the Western understanding of the heart and laid the platform for the dogma of the pumping function of the heart. Until Harvey's landmark work, physicians of the time believed that the heart was a sucking organ and that it was the lungs that were responsible for the movement of blood through the body.[15] His observation that the heart continued to beat even after excision from animals led him to the conclusion that the heart pumped rather than sucked. This view has been almost universally accepted until the present.

As a consequence of the heart/artery bias in many anatomical illustrations, the venous components frequently suffer a similar fate to that of the connective tissue matrix: relegated to the waste bin of irrelevance. Dr Still, however, understood that the venous system had a significant role in the circulatory dynamic, as evidenced by his quote at the beginning of this chapter from *The Philosophy and Mechanical Principles of Osteopathy*. He acknowledged that the arteries furnish tissues with blood, but he concluded that the homeostatic processes are expressed first in the venous side of circulation.[16] All living organisms undergo continuous renovation. In humans, cells and intracellular components are constantly remodeled and recycled. This occurs, in part, in order to replace old components with fresh, better-quality ones.[17] Dr Still's view implies an integrated role in any consideration of the circulatory system, and any description that fails to develop an understanding of the venous system will be inherently inadequate. This once contentious view is now becoming part of most curriculums as acknowledged succinctly by the National Library of Medicine: "The linkage between total body tissue oxygen demand and resistance to venous return is a fundamental mechanism governing control of cardiac output. This is the basic mechanism by which the cardiovascular system responds to changes in demand for cardiac output as metabolic rate changes."[18]

## Polar Magnetism and Paramagnetism

Some of the properties of the venous blood are commonly understood:

1. It is relatively deoxygenated compared to the oxygenated state of the arterial blood.
2. It doesn't have the same momentum as the arterial blood and so is understood not to be pumped from the centre but rather is **propelled** by pressure from neighbouring structures and adjacent muscular contraction.
3. The absence of a central propulsive mechanism necessitates the presence of valves limiting backflow to aid the return to the heart and lungs.

There are, however, some very important observations and discoveries that are less widely known regarding the vascular system's properties, which we are only beginning to understand.

A discussion of deoxygenated (paramagnetic) blood and oxygenated (diamagnetic) blood follows.

A *paramagnetic* substance is a substance with at least one unpaired electron. The unpaired electron allows it to become magnetised and attracted by the magnet. Paramagnetic fields are oriented parallel to an external magnetic field. A paramagnetic material creates a magnetic field in the same direction as the externally applied magnetic field but does not retain any magnetisation after that field is removed.

Deoxygenated (deoxy-haemoglobin) blood has 4 unpaired electrons and thus is a paramagnetic substance, but it is weakly responsive to external magnetic fields. Venous blood haemoglobin is approximately 70% oxygenated and 30% deoxygenated.

An acute hematoma (12 to 48 hours) contains clotted red blood cells that are predominantly deoxygenated haemoglobin. As a paramagnetic substance, it produces distortions in the local magnetic field that are identified by magnetic resonance imaging (MRI).

Various factors affect the flow of deoxygenated, paramagnetic venous blood, including the following:

1. The paramagnetic quality of deoxygenated blood makes it very weakly attracted by the poles of a magnet but without retaining any permanent magnetism. It is drawn back towards the magnetic field of the heart.
2. The deoxygenated blood is relatively positively charged and thus the blood is drawn back towards the lungs where there is plentiful oxygen and negatively charged blood.[19]

A *diamagnetic* substance (*dia* is Greek for across, as in diameter) is a substance that, like water, has all its electrons paired. Such a substance would not be magnetised and would be repelled by a magnetic field. However, a diamagnetic material produces a magnetic field in opposition to an externally applied magnetic field. This weak opposing field produces a repelling force. Water molecules move away from the stronger magnetic field to a weaker magnetic field. A water surface can be slightly depressed by a nearby magnetic field.

Oxygenated (oxy-haemoglobin) blood has no unpaired electrons and is therefore diamagnetic. Arterial blood haemoglobin is 95% oxygenated and 5% deoxygenated.

Images obtained by functional MRI rely on different contrasts of different materials. One of these contrasts is dependent on the oxygen levels of blood. Metabolic activity of a tissue alters the relative levels of oxygenated and deoxygenated haemoglobin and allows this activity to be visualised. This is known as BOLD (blood oxygenation level dependent) in MRI.[20]

Various factors affect oxygenated blood flow:

1. Diamagnetic oxy-haemoglobin makes an important contribution to flow. The paired electrons in oxygenated haemoglobin are repelled by the electromagnetic activity of the heart, and this electromagnetic repelling force assists in the flow of blood away from the heart. Thus, the haemoglobin molecules are weakly repelled by a magnetic field due to their lack of unpaired electrons. This repulsion reinforces the metabolic suction of the 35 trillion cells at the periphery.[21]

2. Nitric oxide (NO) affects two key aspects of $O_2$ supply and demand by regulating and acting upon smooth muscle and thereby altering blood flow. It also regulates ATP production by acting on the final cytochrome (cytochrome C oxidase).[22]

3. Glycocalyx mediates sensing shear stress, enables balanced signaling, and fulfills a vasculoprotective role.[23]

4. Other humoral and autonomic factors.

This concept of polar and paramagnetic blood has been understood only relatively recently. In the late 1980s, Seiji Ogawa, a researcher at Bell Laboratories in the United States, was looking at how blood responded to MRI. He demonstrated that changes in blood-oxygen levels cause changes in the MRI signal. The technique is called blood-oxygen-level-dependent imaging, or *BOLD-contrast imaging*.[24a]

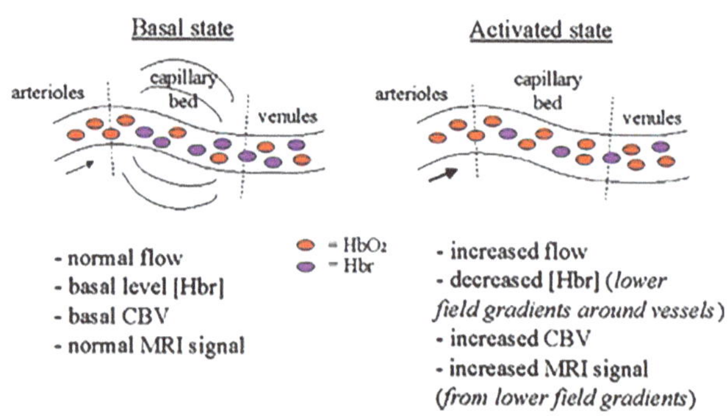


**Figure 8.2 – Physiological Basis of the BOLD Response.** Oxygenated to deoxygenated haemoglobin have different magnetic properties that allow the image to demonstrate function rather than structure.[24b] Abbreviations: CBV = cerebral blood volume; $HbO^2$ = oxygenated haemoglobin; Hbr = deoxygenated haemoglobin; [Hbr] = concentration of Hbr; MRI = magnetic resonance imaging.

Figure 8.2 shows that without a magnetic field, red blood cells arrange themselves rather randomly. In the presence of a magnetic field, red blood cells orientate themselves north to south with respect to each other. When the same thing is done with venous blood, however, no change occurs. In this regard, oxygenated and charged red blood cells function in exactly the same way as any other proteinaceous structure in the body: if a charge is applied to a solution containing tropocollagen molecules, the molecules go from a random mix to an organised state—but venous blood does not behave in the same way.

Oxygenated arterial blood is diamagnetic or polar magnetic.[25] This means if you expose arterial blood to an electromagnetic field, the red blood cells will orientate themselves to that magnetic field. Red blood cells (RBCs) have a functional north pole and south pole that facilitates the aligning of each RBC to the field. Venous blood, however, does not exhibit the same behaviour. It is paramagnetic. It no longer carries the charge required for it to behave the same way in an electromagnetic field, but it retains the **potential** to return to the dipolar state once it returns to the heart and lungs and is reoxygenated. This tells us that blood from the heart, as it gets to the periphery, is not only dropping off oxygen to support the tissues, but it is also delivering charge (Figure 8.3). The nutritive role of blood is as much about its charge as it is about the delivery of oxygen. Given what has been outlined in earlier chapters, this is a very significant point to understand.

The proposed model is based on a movement of blood through the vascular tree that is driven by a hunger in peripheral tissues. This model suggests that metabolic demand throughout the body sucks blood through the vascular tree in a frictionless manner rather than it being pushed by the heart. The video from *Encyclopedia Britannica,* accessible at https://www.britannica.com/video/Red-blood-cells-arteries-capillaries-tissues-oxygen/-18404 or through the following QR code, shows this quite plainly in the first 40 seconds of the video where a single RBC enters a capillary and travels along without being forced from behind.[26]

The venous blood has its own drive for replenishment in the lungs for oxygen and in the heart for charge. While this drive is not as strong as that of the cumulative hunger of all the tissues of the body combined, the interaction between venous blood, the lungs and the heart, in replenishing the depleted venous blood, is another driver for circulatory motion.

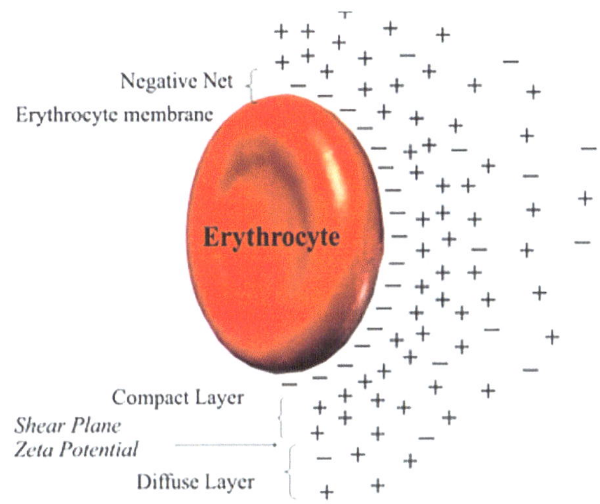


**Figure 8.3 – Charge Dynamic of Red Blood Cell.** Reprinted with permission from *Revista Brasilera de Hemoterapia e Hematolgia.*[27]

The charge dynamic of blood (Figure 8.3) is a modulating dynamic. Research conducted at the HeartMath Institute has shown the difference in electromagnetic signatures of different emotional states as measured by changes in the electromagnetic field generated by the heart.[28,29]

Different emotions have different electromagnetic signatures—they have different frequency signals. The heart is proposed to be involved with the emotional response and, as the primary electrical generator in the body, emits a modulating charge dependent on what we are feeling in any given moment. This modulating charge imprints the haemoglobin molecules in the RBCs, and this message is transferred to the periphery where it alters the functioning of the cells. Consequently, our cellular physiology is different when we are feeling in love versus when we are angry.[30]

The ability of the blood to take on a charge generated by the heart creates the observed phenomenon of the different behaviour of arterial and venous blood in an electromagnetic field that describes venous blood's paramagnetic nature.

Venous blood retains the potential to return to the dipolar state. This occurs once it has taken on the $O_2$/light complex in the lungs and then passes through the electromagnetic field generated by the heart where charge is inducted into and taken up by the electromagnetically responsive $Fe_2$+ ions in the haemoglobin molecules in the RBCs.

The shape change of the haemoglobin molecule (Figure 8.4[31] and the QR code below), when oxygenated/charged versus deoxygenated/uncharged,

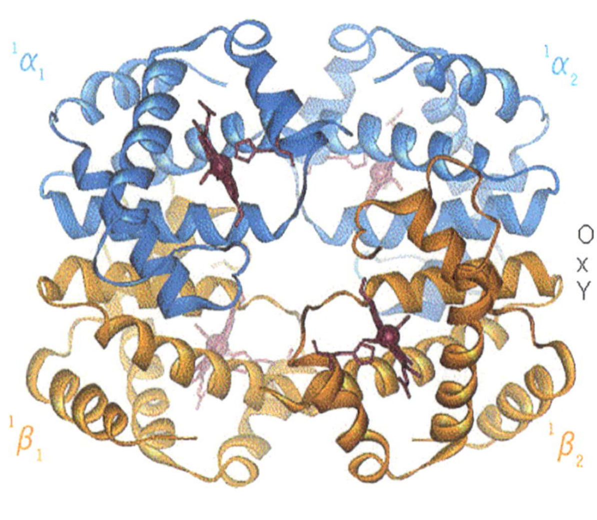


**Figure 8.4 – Haemoglobin t-r State Transformation.**

shows the same flexion/extension pattern of all tissues in response to the primary respiratory mechanism (PRM).

Figure 8.4 represents haemoglobin, which is a more rounded shape when loaded with oxygen and then becomes more like a rugby ball when it has released the oxygen that it carried. You can view a gif[32] of this transformation through the following QR code:

The counter-rotating Dean vortices[33] at each bifurcation of the aorta enhances the flexion phase of the PRM by the arterial system spiraling in counter-rotatory direction in the paired limbs, seemingly to augment the motion of Sutherland's described phenomena regarding the constituent parts of the PRM. The charge dynamic of the arterial blood is part of this augmentation. Conversely, the decreased charge nature of the venous blood is perhaps an explanation for why the external rotation phase of PRM movement in the limbs is easier for many to palpate than the internal rotation phase.

The venous return shows flow organisation at various sites in the body. It is most easily seen in the mixing of the vortical return as seen at the confluence of the superior and inferior caval returns entering the right atrium.

The return from above and below come together not as some random mix; instead, in health, they vortically coil around each other as they merge and flow into the right atrium. The confluence of the superior and inferior vena cavae and the extension into the right atrium assisted by the crista terminalis (shown in Figure 8.12 later in this chapter), is an area of functional anatomy worth much consideration.

## The Venous Reservoir

The first descriptions of veins with their "little doors" came from William Harvey's instructor, Fabricus, in 1603, but it was through Harvey's description of the circulatory system that the role of the valves in the veins was comprehended. In 1819, the continuity of the cerebral and spinal venous systems via anastomoses was described by Gilbert Breschet, but that description was still far from complete.[34]

It was not until the work of Oscar Batson in the early 1940s that there was any differentiation of veins with and without valves. Batson described the continuity of the veins between the cranium and pelvis and the valveless structure of these vessels.[35] This led to the understanding of the channel for the spread of metastases along the cerebrospinal veins. In 1947, William F. Herlihy first proposed that there exist two distinct parts of the venous system. The first part comprises the veins that have valves, and the second comprises the veins *without* valves. The two components are a functionally integrated system with the valveless component acting as a reservoir for venous blood and playing a primary role in the maintenance of intracranial fluid volume.[36] This capacitance nature of the second component part operates differently and outside of Harvey's continuous circular flow model of circulation by permitting venous blood to flow bidirectionally, depending on physiologic need, and to pool until required.

As shown in Figure 8.5, the volume of blood in the venous system far exceeds that within the arterial side of circulation. This allows the interesting physiologic dynamic required for normal, active functioning. If the system was based on an equal distribution of blood on both sides, the speed of blood through the venous system would need to match that of the arterial system during periods of activity and exertion. Because we fluctuate between activity and rest, we require a reservoir of

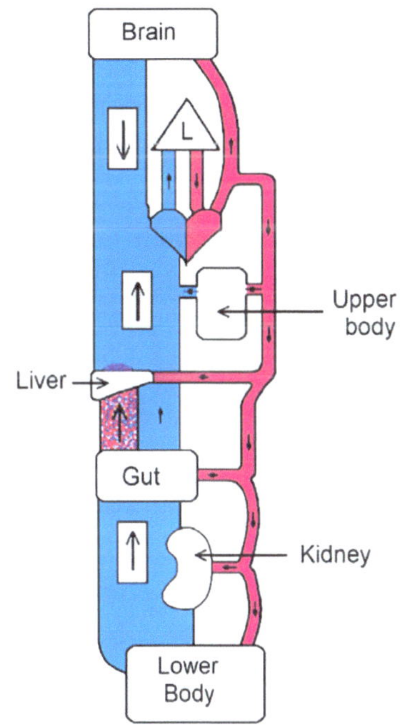


**Figure 8.5 – Blood Volume in Veins and Arteries.** Illustration of the circulation, with the venous system depicted as having a much larger capacity and compliance than arterial system. Arterial blood pressure is intimately related to the arterial blood volume. *Veins blue:* Capacity 5 × that of arteries. *Arteries red:* A small change in venous volume causes a large change in arterial volume—and hence pressure. Arterial volume and hence pressure are sustained by the level of venous tone. Venous tone depends mainly on the intensity of the sympathetic outflow from the brain to venous wall musculature. The portal blood flow is shown stippled red and blue, an intermediate drainage from gut to liver. Apart from the emphasis on the different venous and arterial volumes, the tissues, heart, and lung (L) dimensions are arbitrary.[37]

venous blood to allow for sudden changes in cardiac output required by sudden activity. The whole venous system is a large reservoir, and that includes the veins without valves. The reservoir allows the system to function more like an open system. It also allows the venous system to accommodate variations in lymph volume in response to different states and to return lymph into general circulation.[38] The reservoir model of the low pressure component of the circulatory system allows great flexibility and responsiveness to increased peripheral demand when it is required.

In periods of increased exertion there is an increased peripheral demand for the fuel to drive the increased physiology. With increased peripheral oxygen consumption there is an increase in cardiac output and rate, as would be expected. However, the increase in heart rate alone is not enough to drive the increase in output. Indeed, increasing the heart rate artificially by pacemaker or in tachycardia results in no increase in cardiac output. The only way for cardiac output to increase with heart rate is for the system to be short-circuited by an arteriovenous shunt that eliminates arterial flow to any of the organ systems.[39]

Any increase in cardiac output is achieved by an increase in blood from the venous reserves, which is driven by the need for oxygenated blood from the lungs to fuel the periphery, which literally sucks blood from the venous reservoir to fulfill the demand. This is the view expressed in *The Dynamic Heart* and summarised at the end of the chapter entitled "The Physiology of Circulation: A Review".[40] It should be noted that this view describes normal physiology. However, in response to serious pathology (congestive heart failure or cardiomyopathy), positive inotropes can be given to strengthen the heart's contractions so that it can pump more blood with fewer heartbeats.[41]

The reservoir includes the continuity of the cerebral venous system and its anastomosis with the vertebral venous system (VVS). This system, in turn, comprises the internal vertebral venous plexus (VVP), the external VVP, and the horizontal veins running within the vertebrae. The whole system is known as the cerebrospinal vertebral venous plexus (CSVVP) (Figure 8.6).

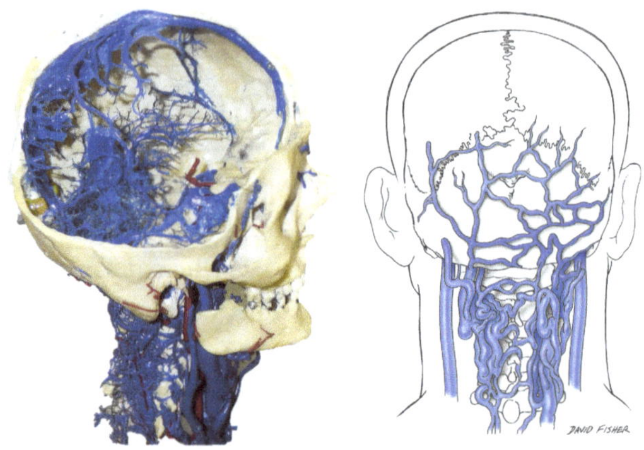


**Figure 8.6a – The Cerebrospinal Vertebral Venous Plexus.** Corrosion cast of the dural venous sinuses and vertebral venous plexus (left) and schematic drawing (right) showing the connections between the emissary veins of the posterior occipital region and vertebral venous plexus.[44]

The internal VVP is made up of an internal component that lies within the spinal column, but it is external to the dura and the external VVP that runs along the vertebral column. A proportion of the external VVPs, which envelope the vertebrae, have valves. The veins with valves are limited to approximately one-third of the total number of veins.

The internal VVPs are valveless and are structured as four main longitudinal channels, anterior and posterior, and have an internal structure like that of the intracranial sinuses with which they are continuous. There are bridging trabeculae containing collagen, smooth muscle fibres and their own arterial and nerve supply.[42] The posterior longitudinal veins are rudimentary in the cervical spine compared to those in the lumbar and thoracic spine. The anterior longitudinal veins lie at the lateral borders of the posterior longitudinal ligament and are connected by transverse veins that lack trabeculae. The transverse veins are connected to the large basivertebral veins that course throughout the vertebral bodies and connect to the external VVP.[43] The absence of valves within the internal VVPs means that movement is dependent on gravity and other physiologic drivers such as respiration and other generators of venous pressure.

The open communication between the internal and external VVPs via the intervertebral veins extends laterally into the following (Figure 8.7):

- radicular veins
- azygous system
- veins of the thoracolumbar wall, including the breast plexus
- parietal pleural veins and posterior bronchial veins to include the lung fields
- ascending lumbar communicating vein
- left renal and suprarenal veins
- sacral plexus
- pelvic and prostatic plexuses

The azygous and hemiazygous veins, the vertebral veins and the upper intercostal veins on the right side of the trunk drain into the brachiocephalic veins (BCVs). In the flow system, the valves first appear in the BCVs. At this point, blood from the VVP flow meets the functional characteristics of venous return from the rest of the body. Additionally, the valves at this point limit the potential for reflux back into the valveless system.

The transverse valveless internal VVP has been

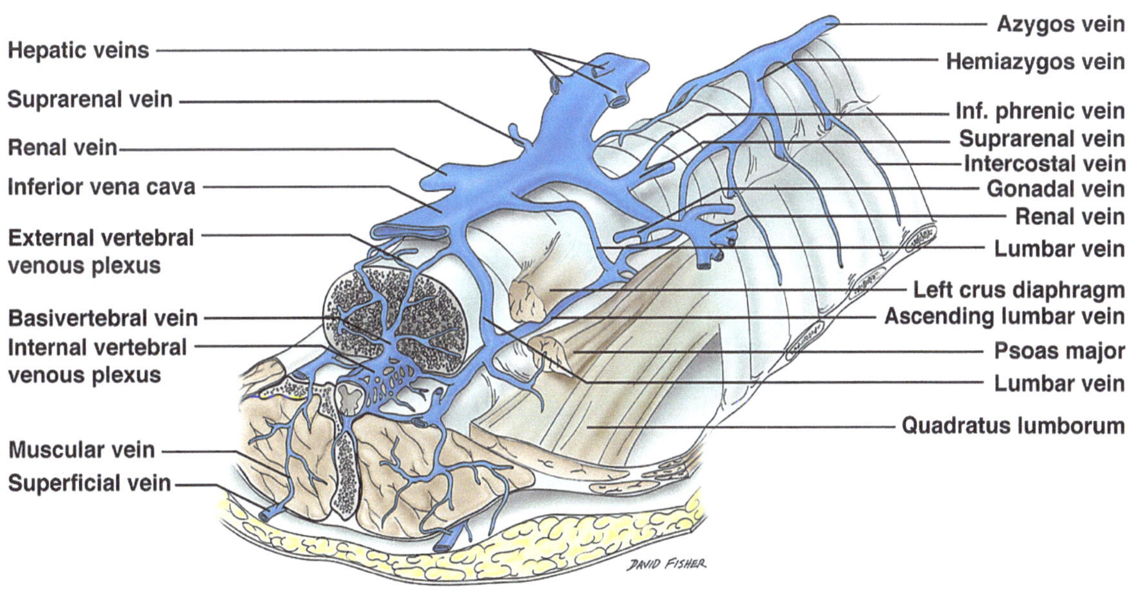


**Figure 8.7 – Schematic drawing of the vertebral venous system.** Note the internal and external vertebral venous plexuses connected via the basivertebral vein.[45]

suggested to be susceptible to distension and varicosity, and there is conjecture that this may be a cause of compression on exiting spinal nerves and a possible cause of radiculopathy other than compression by intervertebral disk protrusion. A procedure known as epidural venography is used to assist in the differential diagnosis of suspected intervertebral disk radiculopathy.[46]

One interesting observation is that when looking at depictions of the superficial veins of the cerebrum, they are generally represented as being inclined anteriorly, sometimes perpendicularly to the sagittal sinus. This makes sense when looking at the growth motion dynamics of the cerebrum embryologically, but it also suggests there are other forces involved in facilitating venous return to the sagittal sinus that overrides any architectural complication. Suction, pulling blood through the system, would prevent any retrograde flow, and this could be achieved by the volume dynamics between the veins and the sinus as well as peripheral demand through the heart-lung complex. The inherent motion of the cerebrum in response to the PRM would also create a more perpendicular orientation of the veins and enhance the drainage potential.

## The Intracranial Venous System

When considering the intracranial venous system, it should be seen, not as a single entity but rather as an integrated part of a functional circulatory unit that is involved in a homeostatic operational complex. The major components of this complex are the four cranial arteries, the choroid plexuses and the cerebrospinal fluid (CSF) that they produce on the arterial side.

The venous side includes the intracranial venous sinuses, the jugular venous complex, the cavernous sinus and the continuation into the ophthalmic veins, the basilar plexus, the foramen magnum cavernous sinus, and the VVP that is continuous with the basilar plexus. As a unit, these form the cerebrospinal vertebral venous plexus (CSVVP). It is important to recognise that venous drainage from the skull can occur through three distinct routes. There is the drainage through the internal jugular system, through the basilar plexus into the CSVVP, and anteriorly through the ophthalmic into the facial and then the jugular veins. The three-route drainage system provides a failsafe mechanism for continual cranial drainage and highlights the importance of the venous system in maintaining the intracranial environment.

Changes in drainage result in pain, but disrupted drainage has also been implicated in the etiology of vascular and Alzheimer's dementia, late-onset depression, benign and secondary intracranial hypertension, communicating and normal pressure hydrocephalus, age-related white matter changes,[47] and multiple sclerosis.[48]

## The Monro-Kellie Doctrine

The Monro-Kellie doctrine, initially described more than 200 years ago by Drs Alexander Monro and George Kellie, indicates the need for input and output to be equal in order to maintain a constant intracranial volume. The extension of this doctrine is the need for a constant intracranial pressure and for input and output to remain, if not at exactly constant levels, at least within certain prescribed parameters. The parameters of the doctrine presume a rigid cranium and that a specified amount of blood entering the cranium forces an instantaneous equal amount of blood out through the jugular bulb.[49] This "adaptive neuronal volume regulation" has been the dominant doctrine since 1783, but recent findings have encouraged researchers to take a second look.[50]

The Monro-Kellie model omits the low pressure, slow transit time of blood through the capillary beds where the blood exhibits relatively long transit times in the vessels.[51] In the capillaries, the flow dynamic is determined by tissue need rather than by upstream pressure in the system. The doctrine also excludes other routes of fluid volume loss from the cranium through CSF movement, including through the cribriform plate and perivascular spaces, then into the cranial lymphatic drainage and general circulation. Additionally, the Monro-Kellie model omits the impact of posture on venous movement from the skull and the impact of organ systems to accommodate venous flow from the VVP.[52]

The doctrine considers the cranium as a stand-alone entity excluded from whole-body physiology. However, the doctrine **does** recognise that a constant intracranial volume and pressure needs to be maintained in order for normal intracranial physiology to be maintained. The ability to maintain this dynamic is the result of complex processes that have yet to be completely explained.

A study by Alperin et al identified a dynamic relationship between the CSF movement from the intracranial space through the foramen magnum in response to a sudden increase in the amount of blood coming into the head.[53] They observed an initial accommodation to the increased intracranial blood that preceded an equal volume of CSF exiting the skull within a time frame of 200-300 ms, by which time the intracranial reserve had resumed its baseline state. Thus, this study identifies how the arterial, venous and CSF systems interact to maintain intracranial pressure during differing physiologic states. It also identifies the speed at which the systems interact to maintain the environment.

There is a volume compliance capability that is achieved by the muscular walls of the arterial system to accommodate both the pressure wave and volume changes associated with cardiac ejection. The pressure wave travels at the speed of sound while the volume change travels considerably slower. The ability to accommodate these volume changes depends on the elasticity of the large arteries entering the cranium. These cardiac pulsations need to be dissipated from the circulatory tree before blood reaches the low-pressure vessels on the venous side. Any volume compliance on the venous side is accommodated by the cerebral and cerebellar veins as the architecture of the venous sinuses—which is limited by the bone of the skull and the tension in the meningeal membranes—and has little ability to assist. This feature of the sinuses is significant in the description of the motion of the cranial bones as described in the PRM model and its relation to circulation as a generator of this motion. This is again discussed in Chapter 14.

## Cranial Pulsations

The observation that all tissues in the cranium pulsate is the result of more than 50 years of study, primarily in relation to neurologic disease. These pulsations are generally accepted as being the result of cardiac activity specifically relating to the arterial pulse wave. However, this view is not universally accepted, and the work of Portnoy and Chopp in the 1980s led them to conclude that the intracranial pulse wave was primarily venous. The implication is that the observed intracranial pressure waves are generated by the brain tissue and are conducted into the compliant venous system. Further studies have shown that there may exist a filter that limits the arterial pulse pressure wave from being transmitted intracranially.[54] These findings challenge the arteriocentric bias when considering cranial dynamics and support the model of the venous system as a significant driver in the development and functional activity of the central nervous system.

With respect to the maintenance of intracranial pressure, both the venous blood and the CSF are conjointly prime agencies of maintaining intracranial volume in response to changing arterial flow in differing physiologic states. There is also the movement of fluid within the glymphatic system, as described in a *Journal of Neuroscience* article by Illif et al,[55] and movement of CSF through the cribriform plate. Both CSF and venous blood have the capability to move across the foramen magnum. The CSF achieves this via the continuity of the subarachnoid space from the intracranial fluid to that contained within the thecal sac. The venous blood capability relies on the continuity of valveless vessels intracranially and into the VVPs.

Real-time MRI studies have shown that there is a flow of CSF into the cranium during forced inspiration with a concomitant caudal flow of venous blood from the cranium.[56] Interestingly, Dreha-Kulaczewski et al identified T4 as an area around which CSF flow is organised. They also postulated that the CSF flow counterbalances the effect of pressure changes in the thoracic and abdominal compartments on the VVP.

## Venous Adaptations

One phenomenon of intracranial drainage is the change in drainage routes in relation to posture. The jugular system has long been taught as the main drainage system for the intracranial space but, since the 1960s, it has been understood that in the upright posture, the jugular vein is not the main route for venous return from the skull. Once the head is raised above 15 degrees, the drainage via the jugular diminishes increasingly until functional collapse of the veins occurs at the vertical position.[57] Multiple studies using various methods of measuring jugular flow have confirmed this phenomenon and have further observed an increase in central venous pressure. For example, with the Valsalva breathing method, the jugular veins start to become effective again. The alternate route for drainage is the CSVVP, and it appears that although posture determines the route, the route is not rigidly fixed. An increase in central venous pressure, and perhaps other physiologic stimuli, allow both systems to act in concert in order to maintain intracranial volume.

While many studies have acknowledged this phenomenon, only one has suggested a mechanism for this switching from the valved jugular system into the non-valved VVP. Parke and Valsamis identified the ampulloglomerular organ (AGO), sitting in the suboccipital cavernous sinus, as having the required neurovascular components to be the switch.[58] Unlike the intracranial sinuses, whose distensibility is limited by boney and meningeal structures that surround them, the thin-walled AGO has the ability to distend easily in response to pressure changes.

This characteristic as well as the abundance of receptor nerve endings and the absence of effector structures (ie., smooth muscle) suggests that the AGO is likely to be a baroreceptor. Its position in the suboccipital cavernous sinus means that it has the ability to respond to intracranial venous pressure changes in preference to the venous sinuses, the veins of the brainstem, the VVP and the thoracic and abdominal walls, by virtue of the valveless connections of the VVP. While there is no published work that further describes this structure, an unpublished research proposal from anatomist Andrew Russell made in 2016 further develops the case that the AGO is indeed the structure involved in the postural modification of drainage pathways.[59] As such, the AGO functions as an integral part of the complex involved in maintaining intracranial volume and pressure.

## Applications to Osteopathic Practice

In clinical practice, it is essential to constantly keep the venous system under review, remembering Still's aphorism "renovation starts with the veins". There are many recurring patterns of pain and dysfunction whose underlying causes are venous. For example, consider the iliac veins (Figure 8.8). A multiparous woman may experience ongoing venous congestion, pain and limitation of movement in the left knee, which is ultimately traced to a common iliac vein compression syndrome, also referred to as May-Thurner syndrome. This syndrome results from a compression of the right common iliac artery compressing the left iliac trunk as it passes from the left side of the vertebral column to descend into the right upper extremity. Osteopathic attention to the left sacroiliac articulation and related myofascial tissues can relieve the pressure on the left common iliac trunk, improve venous drainage of the knee and restore homeostasis to the circulation in that area.

The venous drainage of the pelvis is extensive, as can be seen in Figure 8.9.

Sutherland emphasised the importance of pelvic drainage and taught procedures to lift the pelvic floor. The arcus tendineus fasciae (or fascial white line) is a thickening of the parietal fascia of levator ani muscles along the straight line from the pubic arch to the ischial spine bilaterally. The fascial white lines are the attachment sites for the pubocervical and rectovaginal fasciae. The pelvic fascia provides the point of access and leverage to the treating osteopathic practitioner.

In the abdomen, the portal vein collects blood from the digestive tract via the superior and inferior mesenteric veins. The thermal and acid-base qualities of the descending colon, spleen, stomach and bladder coming into the portal vein allows the two streams (one from the small bowel and one

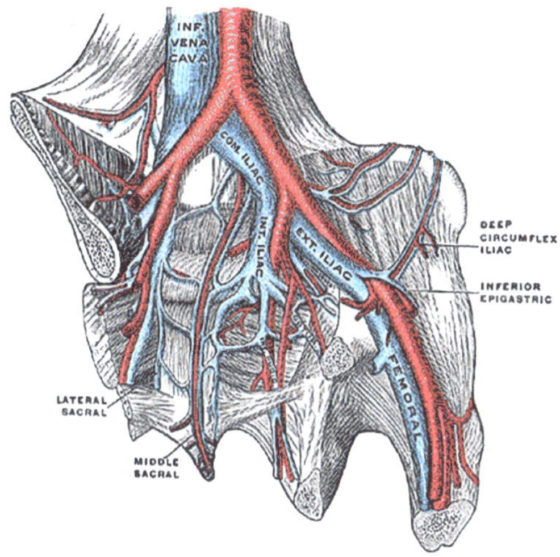


**Figure 8.8 – Iliac Veins.** Reprinted from Gray.[60]

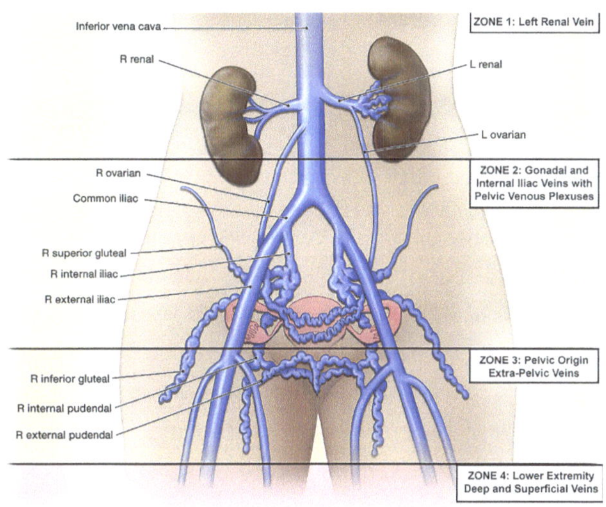


**Figure 8.9 – Pelvic Venous Drainage.** (1) The left renal vein; (2) the gonadal, internal iliac, and pelvic veins; (3) the pelvic origin extrapelvic veins arising in the pelvis and refluxing through the pelvic escape points to the genitalia and lower extremity veins; and (4) the lower extremity veins.[61]

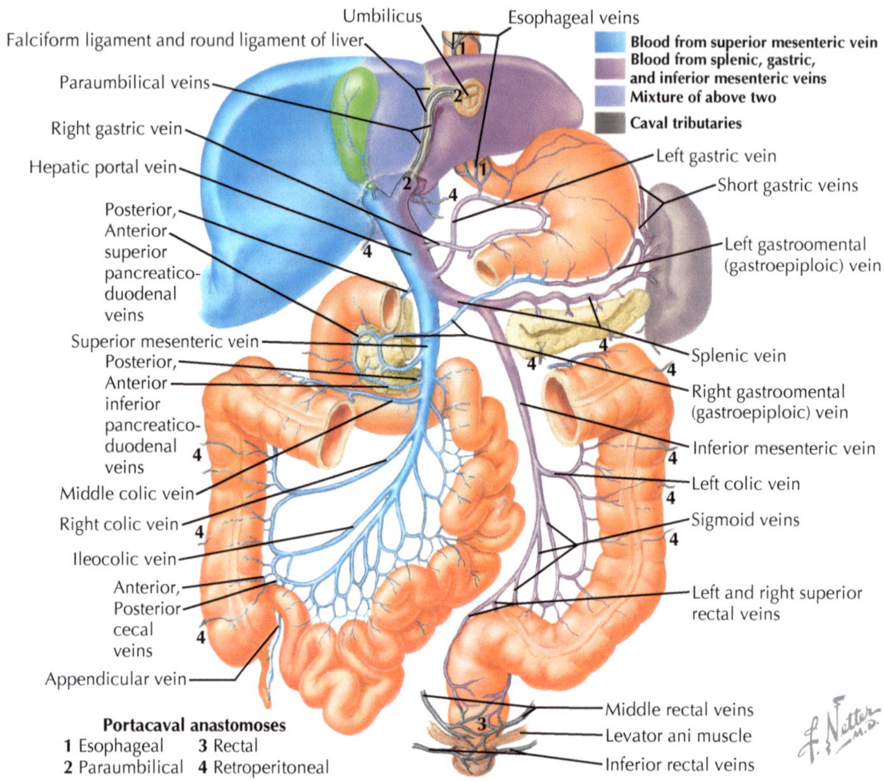


**Figure 8.10 – Abdominal Vascular Supply.** Reprinted with permission from Frank Netter Images.

from the spleen, pancreas, stomach and descending colon) to flow separately such that the blood from the descending colon and spleen go to the left side of the liver for detoxification, whereas the blood coming from the small bowel goes to the right side of the liver for metabolic processing. These two streams can be seen in Figure 8.10. The fulcrum provided by the mesenteric stem allows for an osteopathic approach to support this drainage.

At the confluence of the streams, the separate flows are maintained even though there is no physical barrier. This phenomenon is seen often in the natural world when two bodies of water come together, such as when the Fraser River enters the Strait of Georgia off Vancouver, Canada (Figure 8.11).

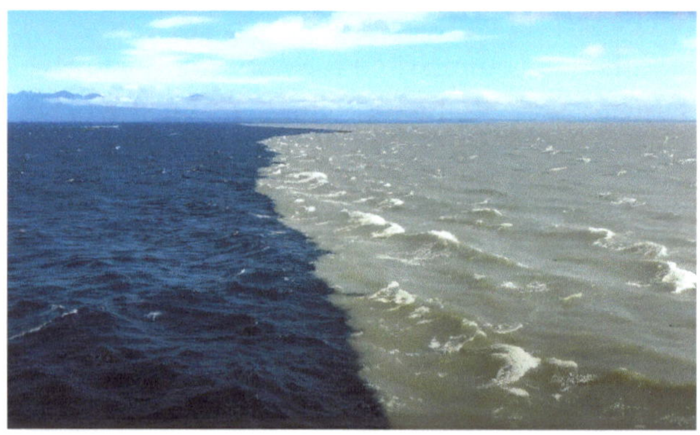

**Figure 8.11 – The Fraser River Entering the Pacific Ocean in the Strait of Georgia.** The silt-laden, tan-coloured Fraser River meets the clear blue waters of the Pacific ocean. For an explanation of this phenomenon see: https://www.youtube.com/watch?v=qRClKxzJX9A

The temperature differences, as well as the differences in dissolved material in the water, establish a clear line of demarcation between the fluid bodies, often for considerable distances, before turbulences create the necessary disruption for mixing to occur. In the example of the Fraser River entering the Pacific ocean, the demarcation extends for many kilometres. Our perception is that the same phenomenon applies to the portal vein.

The venous system, in its structure, is more varied and site specific than is generally perceived. In its function, it is more essential in its role of maintaining the whole body haemodynamics than commonly understood. Its capability as a reservoir supports the fluctuating cardiac output observed between activity and rest. Its relationship with the lungs and the significance of this physiology has not been appreciated in driving circulation since ancient times. Its interface with both CSF circulatory dynamics and the arterial system places it centrally in any whole-body view of fluid circulation. Understanding the role of the venous system as a driver for cranial bone motion as described by Sutherland and explained in Chapter 14 demands that any serious consideration of functional anatomy requires that one must devote much more attention to this system.

The tension of the central tendon of the diaphragm can influence venous flow via the inferior vena cava and often needs to be addressed. A sudden increase in venous return following osteopathic attention may need to be reviewed at the crista terminalis (Figure 8.12), which normalises flow between the superior and inferior vena cava, retaining integrity of vortical flow as blood from above and below enter the right atrium.

Another example of the reward for patients if we pay attention to venous drainage was described in a research report from Poland that highlighted the retrograde flow of dopamine from the cavernous sinus to the internal carotid artery (Figure 8.13).[63] This could potentially increase the availability of dopamine to parts of the brain associated with learning, such as the nucleus accumbens.[64–67]

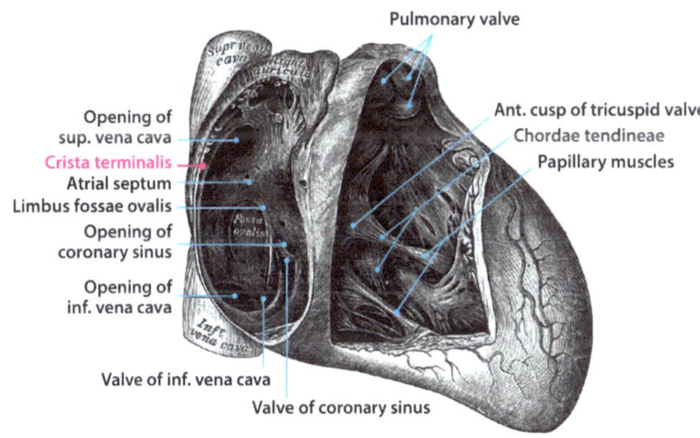


**Figure 8.12 – Crista Terminalis.** Reprinted from Gray.[62]

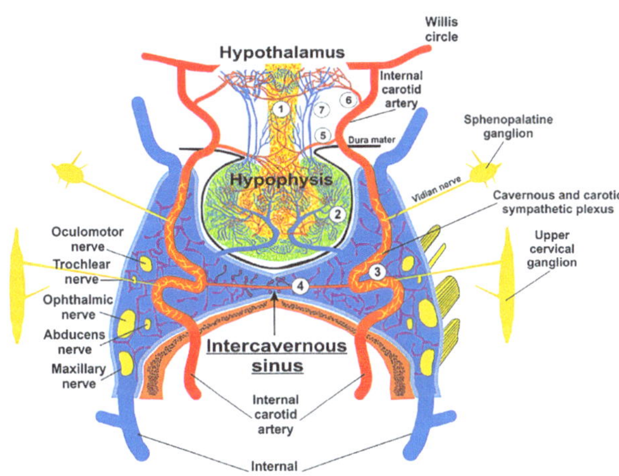


**Figure 8.13 – Cavernous Sinus.** Reprinted from Krzymowski and Stefanczyk-Krzymowska.[68] Scheme of the cavernous sinus occurring in human, rabbit, rat, and many other species without the complex of small arteries and veins lying close to each other in relation to the internal carotid artery in the cavernous sinus: (1) infundibulum-neurohypophysis, (2) adenohypophysis, (3) cavernous segment of internal carotid artery, (4) intercavernous artery; (5) middle hypophyseal artery, (6) superior hypophyseal artery, (7) long portal veins.

The understanding of the CSVVP's role in the processes of disease have been generally limited to descriptions of how metastases can travel in the body, such as from the pelvis to the cranium, with an ease that would not be afforded by a valved structure. However, studies by Zamboni et al developed the hypothesis that chronic venous reflux through the CSVVP preceded pressure changes in the microcirculatory vessel walls leading to a separation of the tight junctions between cells and disruption of the blood-brain barrier. This then precipitated inflammatory processes that were the basis of the pathology involved in multiple sclerosis.[69] The work was controversial for many reasons, including apparent nonreproducibility of the methods and results, but it is interesting in this discussion because it identified potential areas of compromise in the venous drainage sites of the CSVVP. These occurred at the exit of the internal jugular veins from the cranium, either unilaterally or bilaterally, of the azygous system with the superior vena cava, and at the communicating vein between the ascending lumbar vein and the renal artery on the left. The hypothesis proposed flow models for how these blockages modified flow within the system and described the flexibility of the drainage pathways in the system in maintaining intracranial volume.

## The Circulatory Architecture

When considering the CSVVP and circulation as a whole, one striking feature is the asymmetric nature of the circulatory architecture. The comprehension of this architecture is baffling for those trying to understand the mechanics of **how**—when trying to learn the system by rote—in the absence of any clear description of **why**. The answer appears to be that the architectural development of the vasculature is determined by growth and nutrition factors, as explained in Chapter 9.

The presence of a communicating vein between the VVP and the left renal vein would appear to be an anomaly, but consideration of the growth development factors that tie systems together has the potential to provide an answer. The suction forces that stimulate the development and morphology of the lungs are seen in normal physiology as the suction forces that propel blood back to the heart-lung complex. The development of the lungs is asymmetrical as a consequence of the physical constraint of the heart on the left and the mechanical advantage of the liver on the right. The larger space afforded the right lung structurally generates a greater suction field and capability. The drainage pathway of the azygous system is asymmetric and the hemiazygous vein above the diaphragm is relatively deficient compared to its paired structure on the right.

Through palpation, one may observe a contralateral relationship between the lungs and the kidneys. We propose that the increased suction capability of the right lung is likely involved in the asymmetrical architecture of the azygous system.

## Chapter 8 Endnotes


1. A.T. Still, *Philosophy and Mechanical Principles of Osteopathy* (Kansas City, MO: Hudson-Kimberly Publishing Co., 1902), 55.

2. John B. West, "Ibn al-Nafis, the Pulmonary Circulation, and the Islamic Golden Age," *Journal of Applied Physiology* 105, no. 6 (December 2008): 1877–80, https://doi.org/10.1152/japplphysiol.91171.2008.

3. Ajay K. Jain, Elliot J. Smith, and Martin T. Rothman, "The Coronary Venous System: An Alternative Route of Access to the Myocardium," *Journal of Invasive Cardiology* 18, no. 11 (November 2006): 563–8, https://www.hmpgloballearningnetwork.com/site/jic/articles/coronary-venous-system-alternative-route-access-myocardium.

4. K.R. Olson, "Design and Physiology of Arteries and Veins: Physiology of Capacitance Vessels," in *Encyclopedia of Fish Physiology: From Genome to Environment* (Academic Press, 2011), 1111 8, https://doi.org/10.1016/B978-0-12-374553-8.00054-X.

5. Still, *Philosophy and Mechanical Principles of Osteopathy*, 55.

6. Andrew Taylor Still, *The Philosophy and Mechanical Principles of Osteopathy* (Kirksville, MO: published by the author, 1902; Read Books Limited, 2021), https://www.google.com/books/edition/The_Philosophy_and_Mechanical_Principles/338TEAAAQBAJ?hl=en&gbpv=0.

7. Kevin Dann, "The Spiralist," *The Public Domain Review*, August 5, 2021, https://publicdomainreview.org/essay/the-spiralist.

8. Gregory Andrew, "Key Discoveries and Influences of William Harvey," *Brittanica*, May 30, 2022, https://www.britannica.com/biography/William-Harvey/Key-discoveries-and-influences.

9. Dann, "The Spiralist."

10. R. Shane Tubbs, "The Heart Is Simply a Muscle," *Clinical Anatomy* 29, no. 3 (April 2016): 267–8.

11. Tubbs, "The Heart Is Simply a Muscle."

12. Alfredo de Micheli, Raúl Izaguirre Ávila, "A Saint in the History of Cardiology," *Archivos de Cardiología de México* 84, no. 1 (January-March 2014): 47–50, https://doi/10.1016/j.acmx.2013.01.016.

13. *James Bell Pettigrew*, Royal College of Physicians of Edinburgh, https://www.rcpe.ac.uk/heritage/college-history/james-bell-pettigrew.

14. Dann, "The Spiralist."

15. Domenico Ribatti, "William Harvey and the Discovery of the Circulation of the Blood," *Vascular Cell* 1, no. 1 (2009): 3, https://doi.org/10.1186/2040-2384-1-3.

16. Still, *The Philosophy and Mechanical Principles of Osteopathy* (2021).

17. Noboru Mizushima and Masaaki Komatsu, "Autophagy: Renovation of Cells and Tissues," *Cell* 147, no. 4 (November 2011): 728–41, https://doi.org/10.1016/j.cell.2011.10.026.

18. David B. Young, "Venous Return," in *Control of Cardiac Output* (San Rafael, CA: Morgan & Claypool Life Sciences, 2010).

19. Robert M. Davidson and Stephanie Seneff, "The Initial Common Pathway of Inflammation, Disease, and Sudden Death," *Entropy* 14, no. 8 (2012): 1399–442, https://doi.org/10.3390/e14081399.

20. Karla L. Miller et al., "Functional Brain Imaging Using a Blood Oxygenation Sensitive Steady State," *Magnetic Resonance in Medicine* 50, no. 4 (October 2003): 675-83.

21. Matthew Hart, "Magnets Move Blood Like Magneto, But Not in The Way You Think," *Nerdist*, November 10, 2017, https://nerdist.com/article/magnet-blood-magneto-science-experiment-video.

22. Kejing Chen, Roland N. Pittman, and Aleksander S. Popel, "Nitric Oxide in the Vasculature: Where Does It Come From and Where Does It Go? A Quantitative Perspective," *Antioxidants & Redox Signaling* 10, no. 7 (July 2008): 1185–98, https://doi.org/10.1089/ars.2007.1959.

23. Jing Jin et al., "The Structure and Function of the Glycocalyx and Its Connection With Blood-Brain Barrier," *Frontiers in Cellular Neuroscience* 15 (2021): 739699, https://doi.org/10.3389/fncel.2021.739699.

24a. Hideyuki Okano, "Dr. Seiji Ogawa and the Past, Present, and Future of Functional MRI Research," *The Keio Journal of Medicine* 68, no. 4, (2019): 71–2, https://doi.org/10.2302/kjm.68-4_Editorial.

24b. K. Vincent et al., "Blood Oxygenation Level Dependent Functional Magnetic Resonance Imaging: Current and Potential Uses in Obstetrics and Gynaecology," *British Journal of Obstetrics and Gynaecology* 116, no. 2 (2008): 240–6, https://doi.org/10.1111/j.1471-0528.2008.01993.x.

25. Kara L. Bren, Richard Eisenberg, and Harry B. Gray, "Discovery of the Magnetic Behavior of Hemoglobin: A Beginning of Bioinorganic Chemistry," *Proceedings of the National Academy of Sciences of the United States of America* 112, no. 43 (October 2015): 13123–7, https://doi.org/10.1073/pnas.1515704112.

26. "Science: Watch Red Blood Cells Travel Through Arteries and Capillaries to Deliver Oxygen," *Encyclopedia Britannica*, https://www.britannica.com/video/22214/Red-blood-cells-arteries-capillaries-tissues-oxygen

27. Ana Beatriz Barbosa Torino,et al., "Evaluation of Erythrocyte and Reticulocyte Parameters as Indicative of Iron Deficiency in Patients With Anemia of Chronic Disease," *Revista Brasileira de Hematologia e Hemoterapia* 37, no. 2 (March-April 2015): 77-81.

28. R. McCraty and D. Tomasino, "Heart Rhythm Coherence Feedback: A New Tool for Stress Reduction, Rehabilitation, and Performance Enhancement," *Proceedings of the First Baltic Forum on Neuronal Regulation and Biofeedback*, Riga, Latvia, November 2–5, 2004.

29. Glen Rein, Mike Atkinson, and Rollin McCraty, "The Physiological and Psychological Effects of Compassion and Anger," *Journal of Advancement in Medicine* 8, no. 2, (1995): 87–105.

30. Rollin McCraty and Sandy Royall, "Chapter 3: Heart Rate Variability: An Indicator of Self-Regulatory Capacity, Autonomic Function and Health," *Science of the Heart, Volume 2: Exploring the Role of the Heart in Human Performance* (HeartMath Institute, 2015).

31. Animation of hemoglobin t-r state transformation, https://commons.wikimedia.org/wiki/File:Hemoglobin_t-r_state_ani.gif.

32. Animation of hemoglobin t-r state transformation

33. Nivedita Nivedita, Phillip Ligrani, and Ian Papautsky, "Dean Flow Dynamics in Low-Aspect Ratio Spiral Microchannels," *Scientific Reports* 7 (March 2017): 44072.

34. Narenda Nathoo et al., "History of the Vertebral Venous Plexus and the Significant Contributions of Breschet and Batson," *Neurosurgery* 69, no. 5 (November 2011): 1007-14.

35. William F. Herlihy, "Revision of the Venous System: The Role of the Vertebral Veins," *The Medical Journal of Australia* 1, no. 22 (May 1947): 661–72, https://onlinelibrary.wiley.com/doi/abs/10.5694/j.1326-5377.1947.tb94306.x.

36. Herlihy, "Revision of the Venous System."

37. Christopher Bancroft Wolff et al., "New Understanding of Circulatory Blood Flow and Arterial Blood Pressure Mechanisms," *Cardiovascular Research* 118, no. 4 (March 2022): e29-31, https://doi.org/10.1093/cvr/cvab363

38. Heinrich Brettschneider, "The Polarity of the Center and Periphery in the Circulatory System," in *The Dynamic Heart*, ed. Craig Holeridge (Fair Oaks, CA: The Association of the Waldorf Schools of North America, 2002), 38–44.

39. Herman Lauboeck. "The Physiology of Circulation: A Reappraisal," in *The Dynamic Heart and Circulation*, ed. Craig Holdredge (Fair Oaks, CA: The Association of the Waldorf Schools of North America, 2002), 57–8.

40. *The Dynamic Heart*, ed. Craig Holeridge (Fair Oaks, CA: The Association of the Waldorf Schools of North America, 2002), 75–6.

41. Elizabeth S. DeWitt et al., "Effects of Commonly Used Inotropes on Myocardial Function and Oxygen Consumption Under Constant Ventricular Loading Conditions," *Journal of Applied Physiology* (1985) 121, no. 1 (July 2016): 7–14, https://doi.org/10.1152/japplphysiol.00058.2016.

42. Mark D. Stringer et al., "The Vertebral Venous Plexuses: The Internal Veins Are Muscular and External Veins Have Valves," *Clinical Anatomy* 25, no. 5 (July 2012): 609–18, https://doi.org/10.1002/ca.21281.

43. Gregory D. Cramer, "General Characteristics of the Spine," in *Clinical Anatomy of the Spine, Spinal Cord and ANS*, 3rd ed. (St. Louis, MO: Mosby Publishing, 2014).

44. Kennedy Carpenter et al., "Revisiting the Vertebral Venous Plexus--A Comprehensive Review of the Literature," *World Neurosurgery* 145 (January 2021): 381-95, https://doi.org/10.1016/j.wneu.2020.10.004.

45. Joe Iwanaga et al., "Venous Drainage of Lumbar Vertebral Bodies: Anatomic Study with Application to Kyphoplasty, Vertebroplasty, and Pedicle Screw Complications," *World Neurosurgery* 137 (May 2020): e286-90, https://doi.org/10.1016/j.wneu.2020.01.174.

46 Cramer, "General Characteristics of the Spine."

47. Stavros Michael Stivaros and Alan Jackson, "Changing Concepts of Cerebrospinal Fluid Hydrodynamics: Role of Phase-Contrast Magnetic Resonance Imaging and Implications for Cerebral Microvascular Disease," *Neurotherapeutics* 4, no. 3 (July 2007): 511–22.

48. P. Zamboni et al., "Chronic Cerebrospinal Venous Insufficiency in Patients With Multiple Sclerosis," *Journal of Neurology, Neurosurgery & Psychiatry* 80, no. 4 (April 2009): 392–9.

49. William D. Lakin et al., "A Whole-Body Mathematical Model for Intracranial Pressure Dynamics," *Journal of Mathematical Biology* 46, no. 4 (April 2003): 347–83.

50. Anna C.J. Kalisvaart et al., "An Update to the Monro–Kellie Doctrine to Reflect Tissue Compliance After Severe Ischemic and Hemorrhagic Stroke," *Scientific Reports* 10, no. 1 (December 2020): 22013, https://doi.org/10.1038/s41598-020-78880-4.

51. Heinrich Brettschneider, "The Polarity of the Center and Periphery in the Circulatory System," in *The Dynamic Heart*, ed. Craig Holeridge (Fair Oaks, CA: The Association of the Waldorf Schools of North America, 2002), 38–44.

52. Stephen B. Hladky and Margery A. Barrand, "Mechanisms of Fluid Movement Into, Through and Out of the Brain: Evaluation of the Evidence," *Fluids and Barriers of the CNS* 11 (December 2014): 26, https://doi.org/10.1186/2045-8118-11-26.

53. Noam Alperin et al., "Hemodynamically Independent Analysis of Cerebrospinal Fluid and Brain Motion Observed with Dynamic Phase Contrast MRI," *Magnetic Resonance in Medicine* 35(5) (May 1996): 741–54.

54. Mark E. Wagshul, Per K. Eide, and Joseph R. Madsen, "The Pulsating Brain: A Review of Experimental and Clinical Studies of Intracranial Pulsatility," *Fluids and Barriers of the CNS* 8, no. 1 (January 2011): 5, https://doi.org/10.1186/2045-8118-8-5.

55. Jeffrey J. Iliff et al., "Impairment of Glymphatic Pathway Function Promotes Tau Pathology After Traumatic Brain Injury," *The Journal of Neuroscience* 34, no. 49 (December 2014): 16180–93, https://doi.org/10.1523/JNEUROSCI.3020-14.2014.

56. Steffi Dreha-Kulaczewski et al., "Respiration and the Watershed of Spinal CSF Flow in Humans," *Nature: Scientific Reports* 8 (April 2018): 5594, https://doi.org/10.1038/s41598-018-23908-z.

57. Edward Tobinick and Charles P. Vega, "The Cerebrospinal Venous System: Anatomy, Physiology and Clinical Implications," *Medscape General Medicine* 8, no. 1 (February 2006): 53.

58. Wesley W. Parke and Marius P. Valsamis, "The Ampulloglomerular Organ: An Unusual Neurovascular Complex in the Suboccipital Region," *The Anatomical Record* 159, no. 2 (October 1967): 193–8, https://doi.org/10.1002/ar.1091590208.

59. Andrew Russell, "The Ampulloglomerula Organ, Suboccipital Cavernous Sinus and the Vertebral Venous System," unpublished.

60. Henry Gray, *Anatomy of the Human Body* (Lea & Febiger, 1918), https://commons.wikimedia.org/wiki/File:Iliac_veins.gif

61. Mark H. Meissner et al., "The Symptoms-Varices-Pathophysiology classification of pelvic venous disorders: A report of the American Vein & Lymphatic Society International Working Group on Pelvic Venous Disorders," *Journal of Vascular Surgery: Venous and Lymphatic Disorders,* https://doi.org/10.1016/j.jvsv.2020.12.084.

62. Henry Gray, *Anatomy of the Human Body (Lea & Febiger, 1918)*, plate 493, https://commons.wikimedia.org/wiki/File:Gray493.png.

63. T. Krzymowski and S. Stefanczyk-Krzymowska, "New Facts and the Concept of Physiological Regulation of the Dopaminergic System Function and Its Disorders," *Journal of Physiology and Pharmacology* 66, no.3 (2015): 331–41.

64. Ann E. Kelley, "Neural Integrative Activities of Nucleus Accumbens Subregions in Relation to Learning and Motivation," *Psychobiology* 27 (1999): 198–213.

65. Rudolf N. Cardinal and Timothy H.C. Cheung, "Nucleus Accumbens Core Lesions Retard Instrumental Learning and Performance With Delayed Reinforcement in the Rat," *BMC Neuroscience* 6, (February 2005): 9.

66. John T. Gale et al., "Reward and Reinforcement Activity in the Nucleus Accumbens During Learning," *Frontiers in Behavioral Neuroscience* 8 (April 2014): 114.

67. Benjamin P. Gold et al. "Musical Reward Prediction Errors Engage the Nucleus Accumbens and Motivate Learning," *Proceedings of the National Academy of Sciences of the United States of America* 116, no. 8 (February 2019): 3310–5, https://doi.org/10.1073/pnas.1809855116.

68. T. Krzymowski and S. Stefanczyk-Krzymowska, " New Facts and the Concepts of Physiological Regulation of the Dopaminergic System Function and Its Disorders," *Journal of Physiology and Pharmacology* 66, no. 3 (2015): 331-41.

69. P. Zamboni et al., "Chronic Cerebrospinal Venous Insufficiency in Patients With Multiple Sclerosis," *Journal of Neurology, Neurosurgery and Psychiatry* 80, no. 4 (April 2009): 392–9.

# Chapter Nine

# The Heart-Lung Connection

*"Every atom of arterial blood is sent forth as a ripe seed, grown in the garden of life, the lungs."*[1]

– Andrew Taylor Still

From the time of conception, the primary physiologic driver is hunger. It is the need for nutrition that demands the zygote's implantation into the uterine wall, and it is our hunger, whether physiologic, intellectual, emotional or spiritual, that must be satisfied in order for the tissues of our bodies to receive enough food to support all of our endeavors. Our hunger drives us. Our tissues' hunger drives us. While medical science has long held that our heart pushes nutrition through the system, the view that hunger pulls blood though our arteries—that blood is pulled or sucked towards every cell in our body by the unrelenting hunger that began when ovum and sperm first met—has not been seen as the motive driver of fluid motion.

Medical science has been orientated to the significant role of blood as the transporter of oxygen through the body, with the release of metabolic by-products occurring in the lungs before the blood is replenished by the uptake of oxygen in the alveoli.

## Light as "Ripe Seed"

Dr Still considered the lung the "fountain of life". He wrote that "every atom of arterial blood is sent forth as a ripe seed, grown in the garden of life, the lungs."[2] The challenge is to understand what he meant by his assertion that when blood leaves the lungs, it lives and acts as atoms or seeds of life. Was he referring to the oxygen-carrying capacity alone, or were there other **seeds** that he was referring to, only one of which is understood in physiology? If we step outside the limit of what is currently understood in medical literature, we will see that there are hints at other possibilities for consideration.

This chapter explores the dynamic that exists between the heart and the lungs and provides an expanded view of haemoglobin's role based on its ability to carry more than just oxygen. Our proposal is that haemoglobin (Hgb) also has the ability to take on photons and electromagnetic (EM) messages from the heart.

Because we cannot ask, we will never know precisely what Still was referring to in all of his writings, but they contain more than what was able to be understood at the time.

In considering what Still may have meant, a reasonable beginning would be to consider what is currently understood about haemoglobin, beyond that it is a red substance in the blood, it carries oxygen throughout the body, it carries carbon dioxide out of the body, and it contains iron.[3]

It is understood that light drives the functioning of plant life through the activity of the chlorophyll molecule. Chlorophyll belongs to a class of molecules known as porphyrins and is characterised by a magnesium ion in its centre. One quality of porphyrins is their ability to absorb and hold light for physiologic processes. Haemoglobin, or Hgb, also belongs to the porphyrin class of molecules and differs from chlorophyll by the replacement of the magnesium in the centre of the ring with an iron ion as well as differences in the makeup of the ring itself. As a member of the porphyrin group, Hgb shares the ability to absorb and carry photons—light! This process is illustrated in Figure 9.1.

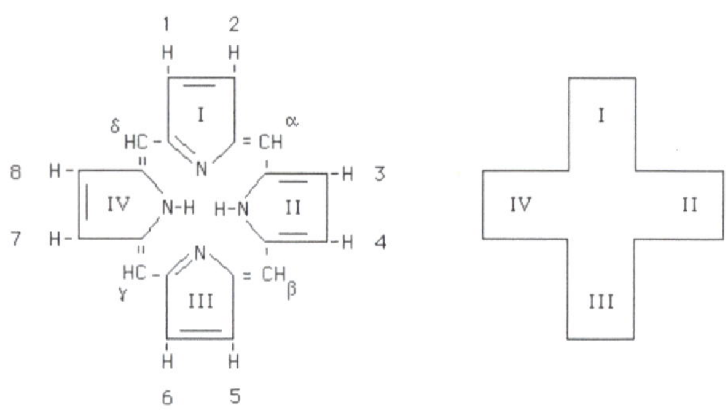


Porphin, showing the four pyrrole rings and the Roman numerals which designate them. Arabic numbers indicate positions at which substituents may be attached. Greek letters denote the methene bridges.

Schematic representation of porphin.

**Figure 9.1 – Haemoglobin Process to Absorb and Carry Light.** Reprinted from Baggott.[4]

The porphyrin ring contains many conjugated bonds (a series of double bonds separated by single bonds), allowing the molecule to absorb light in the visible part of the spectrum. Hgb's colour results from the iron atom and the attached protein chain modifying the wavelength of the absorption (Figure 9.2).[6] There is a differential absorption of

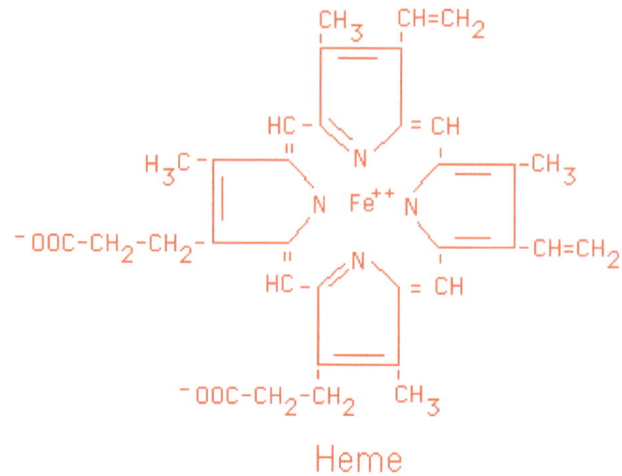


**Figure 9.2 – Porphyrin With Iron Added=Heme.** Reprinted from Baggott.[5]

infrared (800 to 1000 nm) and red light (600 to 700 nm) by blood, depending upon whether it is oxygen rich or poor. Oxygenated blood absorbs more infrared light whereas deoxygenated light absorbs more red light.

This capacity of porphyrin is starting to be used therapeutically, particularly in cancer treatment, because of porphyrins' photodynamic and photothermal properties.[7] Porphyrins are organic compounds that act as "activators" or photosensitisers in photodynamic therapy. When exposed to particular wavelengths of light, porphyrins produce reactive oxygen species as singlet oxygen which can kill the cancer cells that have absorbed the porphyrins.

Different therapies employ the saturation of tissues with porphyrins that are then stimulated with light. It is being used, for example, to treat superficial tumours in the body. The tumour cells scavenge the porphyrins, and, when stimulated by light, the complex produces reactive oxygen, species and increases the local temperature to essentially cook the tumour from the inside.[8] This example demonstrates the prodigious light-absorbing ability of porphyrins, something we argue is important in human physiology.

While the ability of porphyrins to utilise light is recognised, this understanding has not been considered in relation to lung physiology. Our view is that there is an interchange between the porphyrin ring of Hgb in the lungs and sunlight from the external environment embedded in atmospheric water. The potential exists for the lungs to absorb light from the environment and bring it into the system and for it to be involved in our physiology. The lungs then become not only a chemical bridge between the external world and the internal world, but also a conduit, through water, for photons from the external environment. In our view, this may be what Still saw as "arterial blood (that) is sent forth as a ripe seed."[9]

Prior to the digital age, audio recordings were done on tape—a thin film of Mylar that was coated with an electromagnetically responsive material (commonly ferric oxide or $Fe_2O3$). The metal oxide, when exposed to an electromagnetic field, would remember the magnetic message, which allowed it to be read over and over again. Used primarily in audio cassette or reel-to-reel recordings, the message could be erased and rewritten with another.

The electromagnetically responsive Hgb molecule allows blood to function somewhat like the cassette or old reel-to-reel tape, where signals are retained by taking a magnetic imprint that is stored on the magnetically responsive medium. We've concluded that blood, with its haemoglobin-oxygen-light complex, passes through to the heart and is exposed to the electromagnetic field emanating from the coil of the heart muscle. It is here that oxygen and other exogenous information is conjoined with the endogenous feeling state: these states themselves are a response to the external world as perceived by the sense organs.

The Hgb complex is modified by taking on an electromagnetic imprint from the heart that corresponds to whatever we are feeling at that time. This is stored by the electromagnetic responsive Hgb molecule. The recorded feeling, with oxygen and photons picked up by the blood in the lungs, is taken out and transferred into the periphery and then transferred to each cell in the body. However, the audio or videotape analogy breaks down at this point because the same message from the heart is not replayed perpetually. The transference of charge with oxygen and light in the periphery renders the Hgb clean and able to take on a new imprint when it returns to the lungs for replenishment. In health, blood then moves to the heart for a new emotion imprint.

In this way the heart modulates physiology in the cell on a beat-to-beat basis. It should be noted that strong environmental electromagnetic sources have the potential to similarly imprint the Hgb and imprint their own message on the venous blood, and this has the potential to be a cause of dysfunction, if not pathology.[10] Here it takes on yet another message about how we are feeling at that moment.

The significance of light as a physiologic entity was initially developed by Fritz-Albert Popp. Popp identified the light-producing property of DNA. In his extensive work he noticed that the more a DNA molecule is unwound, the more light it emits.[11] He documented how light is associated with different fluctuations of physiology, in particular the menstrual cycle in female humans, how photons catalyse physiologic processes, and how the movement of frequency through fluids can generate light through sonoluminescence, a process in which ultrasound waves are projected upon bubbles suspended in liquid, causing the bubbles to implode and resulting in a flash of light, also known as emission of photons.[12–14] Popp's work and its implications in physiology are discussed more fully in Chapter 1.

Given these discoveries, photons must be considered as physiologically significant. The passageways of photon entry into the body require consideration.

The eyes serve as one such passageway, but does this mean that individuals with impaired or non-functioning visual systems are excluded from this important resource? Research has shown that light-sensitive production of melatonin remains in some blind people, but, it is absent in most.

According to a 2018 article in *Ophthalmology*, it is believed that those who retain the ability to produce melatonin can do so due to the survival of "photosensitive retinal ganglion cells, which project primarily to the circadian pacemaker and are functionally distinct from the rod and cone photoreceptors that mediate vision".[15] Perhaps a similar characteristic ensures continuous photon absorption?

What of all the other physiology that Popp identified as being catalysed by light? Another possible route is acupuncture points and their connections to the meridian system. The use and efficacy of laser acupuncture has been recorded, with many symptomatic and physiologic changes identified as a response to laser acupuncture.

In "Biophysical Bases of Acupuncture", Ding et al acknowledge there is no mechanical stimulation of collagen fibres with laser acupuncture, as with the use of needles, to produce signaling in the matrix, but they suggest that "cross talk between transduction pathways could allow for photon-mediated effects".[16] Others reference the presence of light-responsive chromophores in mitochondria.[17,18] These studies reflect the thinking presented in Chapter 5 on the communication role of the connective tissue matrix, including the role of calcium in signal transduction pathways in the matrix.

The observation of the phenomenon of transdermal light being able to stimulate activity in the connective tissue matrix **and** exert an effect down to the level of cellular mitochondria begs the question, what was the purpose of acupuncture points before needles were invented?

Weber describes how low level laser light causes an enhancement of the proton gradient via the mitochondrial membrane with increased production of adenosine triphosphate (ATP)—an increase of 150%.[19] Tiina Karu showed in several of her publications that red and **infrared laser** light stimulates mitochondrial respiration via cytochrome c oxidase.[20] Yellow light stimulates the mitochondrial respiratory chain at complex III (cytochromes) by stimulating complex III of oxidative phosphorylation. Furthermore, the spectroscopy of copper ions in cytochrome c oxidase enables low-level infrared light to activate the terminal enzyme complex of the inner mitochondrial membrane. As a result, the low level light therapy results in increased mitochondrial ATP production. Due to increased energy metabolism and a reduced rate of apoptosis, neuro-reparative processes are achieved.[21,22]

Given that light stimulation on the acupuncture points produces a response, it is reasonable to assume that the physiological entities known as acupuncture points are portals for light to enter the system.

Oschman[23] pointed out that in 2006, Langevin published a study that suggested the possibility that the connective tissue could provide a ubiquitous information distribution network. She also pointed out that the liquid crystals of connective tissue are known and referred to in acupuncture as a meridian system that functionally interconnects all parts of the body.[24]

She also documented the interaction and integration that exists between acupuncture points and connective tissue planes. In the 1950s, Dr Voll showed that electrical skin resistance was lower at acupuncture points, making it easier for the conduction of electricity.[25] Langevin showed that stimulating a point on one meridian may affect the electrical properties both on the same and on other meridians; she also showed that disease can adversely affect electromagnetic function of acupuncture points and hence disrupt meridian function.[26]

Another passageway for protons revolves around

the proposal that we absorb light into our bodies via water vapor through the lungs and that the light is transported through the body via Hgb as a product of its light-carrying capability.

Popp's observation—that the more the DNA molecules are manipulated the more light they produce—is the reference in this discussion when considering the red blood cells (RBCs).[27] While these cells develop with a nucleus and organelles, these are expelled once the RBCs enter the bloodstream in order for the RBCs to carry more Hgb molecules. It is also the reason for the cell's unique biconcave shape that facilitates movement through capillaries that have a smaller diameter than RBCs.

Because the RBC lacks a nucleus, our hypothesis is that it is therefore the only tissue in the body that does not emit biophotons. Popp showed that the nuclei of cells emit coherent light.[28] However, as mentioned above, once in the bloodstream RBCs do not have a nucleus. Given that nothing in the body happens by chance, consider the likelihood that the absence of an intrinsic light-emitting capability in RBCs empowers them to be completely neutral, passive carriers of light throughout the body. In considering the notion of light entering the body via the lungs, there needs to be a medium that could facilitate the transfer.

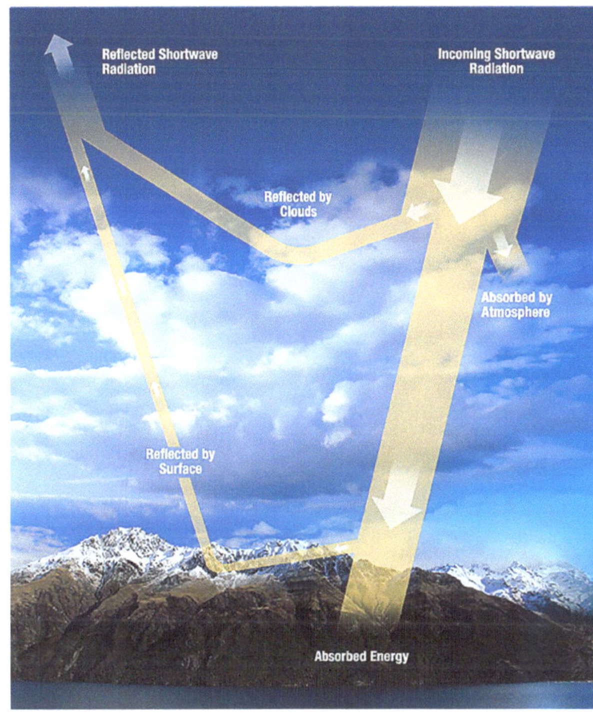


**Figure 9.3 – Incoming Solar Radiation.**[29]

Figure 9.3 is an image created by NASA illustrating earth's incoming radiation. According to their research:

> "Of the 340 watts per square meter of solar energy that falls on the Earth, 29% is reflected back into space, primarily by clouds, but also by other bright surfaces and the atmosphere itself. About 23% of incoming energy is absorbed in the atmosphere by atmospheric gases, dust, and other particles. The remaining 48% is absorbed at the surface."[30]

This creates the possibility that the air we breathe, including the water that generates humidity, brings light and information from the environment into our body system.

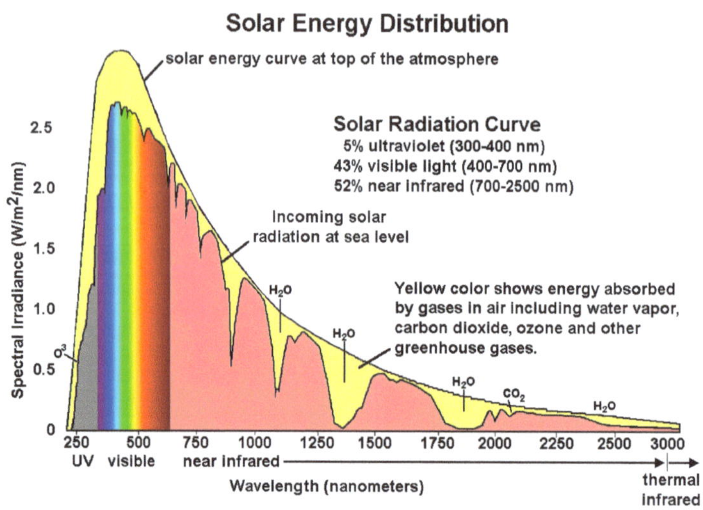


**Figure 9.4 – Solar Energy Distribution.**[31]

Figure 9.4 depicts the absorbency of the atmosphere with reference to different types of incoming solar radiation. The even curve represents the incoming solar radiation at different frequencies without any absorption by the atmosphere. The curve beneath describes the levels of solar radiation measured at sea level. The area between identifies the radiation that is absorbed by the different components of the atmosphere.

Many cultures around the world, particularly ancient civilisations, believed there was something in the air we breathe that was more than the air itself. In ancient Chinese, Hindu, Hebrew, and Greek cultures, air was thought to carry a consciousness, a spirituality that was important for sustaining us. It is not our intention here to explore the principles of Prana, Ruah, Pneuma, Chi and other belief systems that foster similar ideologies, but solely to point out that this measurement of solar radiation absorbed by the atmosphere is akin to a phenomenon recognised in many cultures for centuries: Light carries information,[32] and it is unreasonable to believe that the light coming into the atmosphere does not bring with it information that connects us with the sun and universal electromagnetic frequencies.

## The Importance of Epitaxy

Some of this light/information is absorbed by atmospheric water. The ability of the atmosphere to absorb light is acknowledged as the ability of atmospheric water and other gases to absorb solar radiation.[33] With this absorption there are established pathways for light to enter human physiology: through breathing, through the rods of the retina of our eyes and through the acupuncture meridians mentioned previously. The extension of this concept is to ponder the quality of the absorbed light/atmosphere/water complex and water's ability to be imprinted by the light with information that then potentially impacts physiology. This leads to the vexing question: Does water have the capability to retain information, to have a memory?

The ability of water to retain memory for long periods of time has yet to be explained adequately and is a subject that is "capable of turning a peaceful and intelligent person into a violently irrational one," as observed by Michel Schiff, author of the book *The Memory of Water*.[34] The notion of water having memory has been even more fiercely contentious since Davenas et al started exploring the idea in 1988 following their observation that a solution of antibodies, diluted so much that none of the original antibodies remained, was still able to produce an immune response.[35]

Davenas et al's research was extended by Kröplin, who was looking to develop bio-energetic medicines for astronauts to use. By accident, he discovered that even the weakest magnetic field alterations changed the way water molecules structured themselves and that these changes could be seen under a microscope, specifically using dark field microscopy. His research on water and its memory demonstrated that not only does water contain a memory of a substance or field that it was exposed to, but that the imaging of that memory is further influenced by whomever is capturing the images. The same sample of water, imaged by different people, will alter with each person following the same protocols.[36] Additionally, Nobel laureate Luc Montagnier later reported that radio waves were produced and emitted from bacteria and viruses even when the solutions containing the microbes had been massively diluted.[37]

In the article "Water: The Quantum Elixir", published in the April 2006 issue of *New Scientist*, Robert Matthews stated, "Water functions in a crystalline manner, able to alter its molecular relationships according to the material and energetic environment."[38] This occurs consequent to the ability of the zero point field's weak hydrogen bonds between molecules to break and reform easily. This process is known as *epitaxy*. The zero point field (domain of lowest kinetic energy) refers to the hydrogen bonds or energy between the hydrogen atom of one water molecule and the oxygen atom of a neighbouring molecule. They are relatively weak bonds.

Interestingly, another atom that is also vital to life that has the capacity to change according to its environment (epitaxy) is carbon. With carbon, the same atom can exist as graphite or diamond, depending on pressure and temperature.

Science hasn't fully explained these phenomena, nor their implications, but other researchers have joined Davenas et al, Kröplin and Montagnier in exploring water memory behaviour.

As Prof Szent-Györgyi observed, "There are four dimensions with which the biologist must be concerned: macroscopic (anatomy), microscopic (cells), molecular (proteins) and sub-molecular or electronic. Biology readily followed physics into the first three but took practically no cognisance of the fourth; it stopped at the molecular level."[39]

For electrons to be mobile, a conducting material is necessary, and Szent-Györgyi concluded that proteins were electronic conductors.[40] Mae Wan Ho pointed out that virtually all of the body structure, in the form of the connective tissues or extracellular matrix, is composed of liquid crystals capable of sustaining content coherence.[41]

In the quantum world, the quantum field is not mediated by forces but by the exchange of energy in a dynamic open field. The zero point field (ZPF) is an important part of the subatomic functioning of information transfer. Hal Puthoff showed through his calculations that the virtual particle flux provided the energy input to sustain the motion of subatomic particles and that the motion of all the particles in the universe produces the ZPF.

In effect, this is a self-sustaining feedback loop that occurs in the universe as a whole.[42] As he wrote in one article, "the ZPF interaction constitutes an underlying, stable 'bottom rung' vacuum state that decays no further but reproduces itself on a dynamic-regeneration basis."[43]

## Messages and Images Imprinted in Water

Dr Masaru Emoto was one of the better-known investigators of this property. His research resulted in *The New York Times* best seller *The Hidden Messages in Water.*[44] His work became very popular but was largely discredited by the academic world because of researchers' inability to replicate his findings. Nonetheless, the images he produced are striking and create a visually compelling case for water to take on information from sound, thought, prayer and even electromagnetic sources such as cell phones. His work relies on microscopic crystalline images taken from water that has been frozen after exposure to a signal.

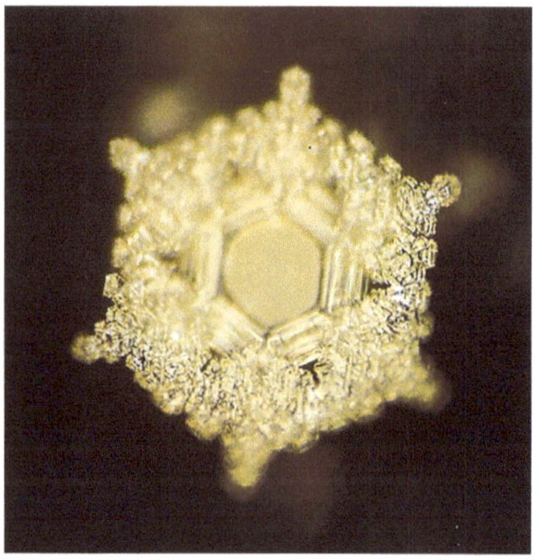

**Figure 9.5 – Frozen Water Crystals: "Gratitude and Beauty"**

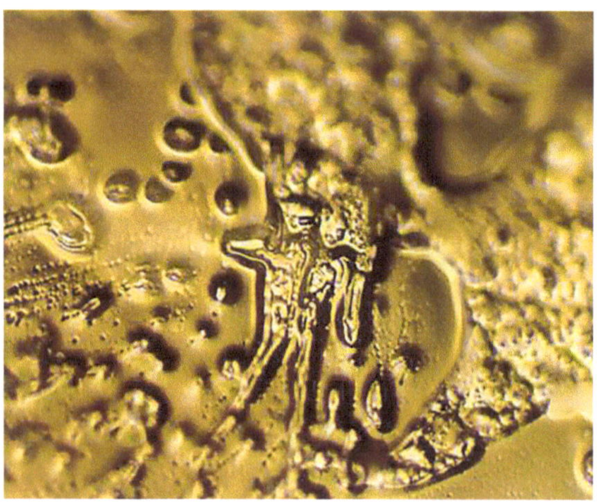

**Figure 9.6 – Frozen Water Crystals: "You Make Me Sick and I Will Kill You"**

Figures 9.5 and 9.6, show water samples placed in bottles where the signals were labels carrying emotional messages taped on the outside of the bottle. In these experiments there were many different messages used but for the images below one bottle carried the message "Love and Gratitude" and the other bottle carried the message "You Make Me Sick and I will Kill You". You can probably deduce which is which even without the captions.

United States photographer Rose-Lynn Fisher has also explored the way water—specifically in the form of tears—alters with differing emotional states. Fisher, who works at the interface between art and science, spent 8 years photographing tears from a wide source of triggers through the lens of a microscope camera. Triggers ranged from biological, such as those induced by chopping onions; emotional tears, such as those from laughter, joy, fury or sorrow; physical tears, triggered by pain; and even tears from unknown sources, perhaps caused by unconscious reasons. Fisher won an international photography award for her collection, *The Topography of Tears.* Figures 9.7 and 9.8 are two photographs from her collection: Redemption (left) and Compassion (right).[45]

There have been many other examples of how water, imaged after being dried post-exposure to other phenomena, changes. Another example of this are images of water containing a homeopathic remedy at different potencies. These are all examples of electromagnetic events that have imprinted information into water with the water conforming to and recording the information.

What is so special about water? The most obvious attribute is that water is critical for life. However, there is much more to what makes it special.

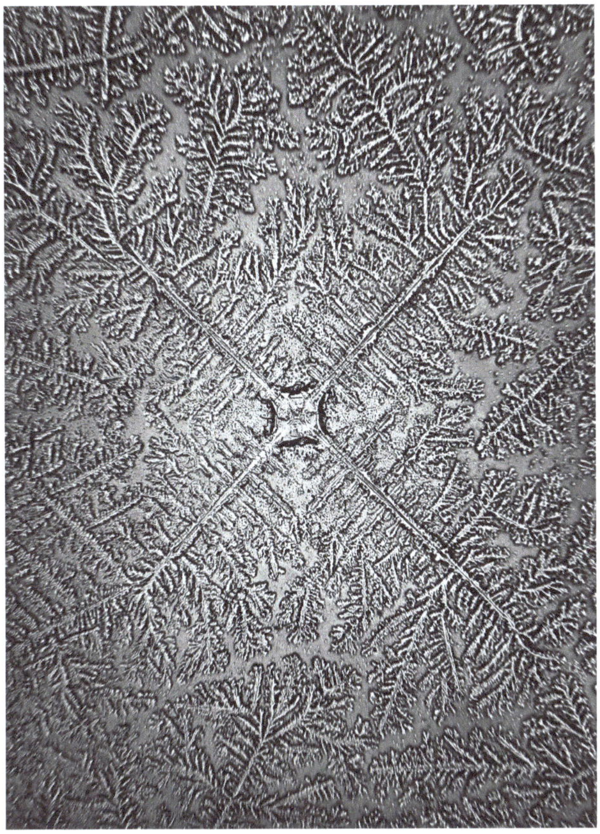

**Figure 9.7 – Photograph of a Tear: Redemption.**
*Redemption* from *The Topography of Tears* © Rose-Lynn Fisher, published by Bellevue Literary Press 2017.

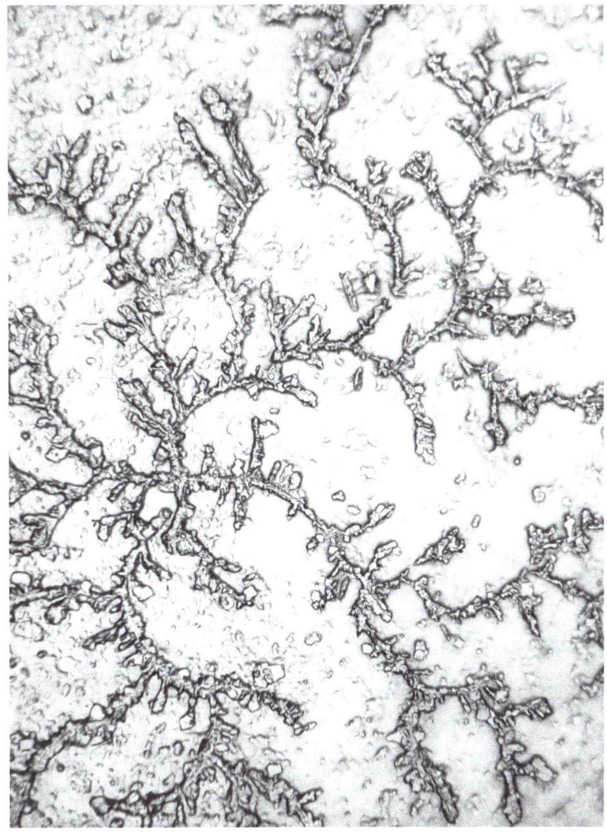

**Figure 9.8 – Photograph of a Tear: Compassion.**
*Compassion* from *The Topography of Tears* © Rose-Lynn Fisher, published by Bellevue Literary Press 2017.

Felix Franks, the physical chemist who changed the way many scientists thought about water, said, "Water is the magic ingredient that transforms lifeless powders on laboratory shelves into living things. Without water, it is all just chemistry, but add water and it becomes biology."[46]

This is, in part, due to it being a dipole molecule and the functional capabilities that are inherent in this structure. The primary capability is the ability to respond to charge. Because of the doubly electronegative and electropositive poles, water molecules organise themselves in relation to charge and electromagnetic fields. In the organisation of exposure of bulk water to any particular field, hydrogen bonds form between adjacent molecules and result in large, complicated, lattice-like structures that could also be suited for information storage,[47] but, because of the instability of water, these lattices fall apart rapidly upon removal of the organising field when water is in its liquid state. This is seen when a drop of water "dances" in response to exposure to a sonic field in the same way that fine particles organise in response to vibrations on a cymascope (discussed with Hans Jenny's pioneering work in Chapter 1).[48]

The idea that water functions in a crystalline manner and is able to respond to the environment is understood. It is also known that water possesses the ability to store information that has been impressed upon it for long periods.[49] This can be measured by specific electromagnetic wavelengths found in the water. As a consequence, water that has been in the proximity of harmful substances will pick up their electromagnetic signature and contain it. Water has the ability to transfer that signature into other environments—including the living system.

This means that even if we filter out the atoms of substances from our water, we are not filtering out the electromagnetic signatures of anything detrimental that the water encountered or contained. In the same way that a homeopathic remedy has an impact on the body, those electromagnetic signatures will have an impact on our physiology. This same capability of water to hold information can also be used for therapeutic purposes, which is the realm of homeopathy and other bio-energetic medicines. The process can go both ways, but for some reason many scientists and others find it much easier to recognise the negative impacts of exposure of water to substances than to recognise that this same dynamic could be used to have potentially beneficial outcomes for the body.

## Temperature Is Critical to Information Transfer

Based on research performed in Germany, the ideal temperature that gives water the maximum structural potential to take on information is 37.5°C, which happens to be the normal human body temperature.[50] This finding suggests that water at this temperature is at its maximal structural point of effectiveness to acquire a large amount of information.[51] The hydrogen bond between water molecules bends and changes shape in response to temperature, and when it is at human body temperature, it has a maximised ability to acquire information coming into its proximity. The human body, therefore, may be uniquely susceptible to the memory and informational capacity of water in view of this temperature factor. Water energised at this temperature with positive emotions would have the best potential to spread its good news throughout the body. Conversely, water energised with negative emotions would be able to spread its bad news with unfortunate efficiency.

The structure of water gives it a great capacity to store information within its matrix. Its ability to do so underpins its potential to mediate between the energetic and material worlds. In other words, water has the capacity to transfer energetic patterns of information to the material plane and physical body. Still talked about the relationship between the celestial and the terrestrial. For example, he wrote, "The mind is asked to find the connection between the physical and the spiritual."[52] The transfer of energetic patterns of information to the material plane from the celestial exactly mirrors that thought.

Researchers at the Aerospace Institute in Stuttgart have done some intriguing studies of the ability of water to hold information. In one experiment, scientists plunged the head of a flower into water, then withdrew the flower after only a few moments and examined droplets from the water sample, recording the images as seen through a powerful microscope. Next they placed the water in an agitator for long enough to obliterate any of the original molecules. However, when examining the water again, the droplets continued to display the same unique constructions.[53]

Thus, water has the capacity to organise around frequency and everything has a frequency because everything is formed from atoms, which are formed by electromagnetic waves. Electromagnetic energy in all of its different forms has the potential to organise water in harmful or beneficial ways. This means that all electromagnetic events such as sound, light, x-rays, MRIs, the protein charge in the extracellular matrix, emotions, thoughts and words have the ability to influence water. Bodies of water, such as lakes, rivers, oceans, and even water in a bowl or beaker, can be affected.

Let us now return to the water contained in our atmosphere, and the primary energetic force that it is exposed to: Light.

One primary and recurring thesis in this book is that the heart does not pump blood through the circulatory tree. The anomalous observations associated with the pumping model are many:

- The work equivalence equations that have been developed throughout previous decades, discussed in Chapter 1
- The observation that cardiac muscle hypertrophies with work in pathology but not in health, addressed in Chapter 7
- The reduction of the radius of the aorta with ejection from the heart vs the expected straightening if under pressure, discussed in Chapter 1
- The observation of blood circulating before the heart develops, addressed in Chapter 6
- The observed negative peripheral arterial pressure observed in health, discussed in Chapter 1 and Chapter 11
- The observation of RBCs moving individually through capillaries rather than being pushed from behind, discussed in this chapter

The alternate view proposed is that blood is sucked through the system and that the process is driven by tissue demand for nutrition. In this model, hunger is the primary driver, the lungs are the pantry, and the heart supplies the flavor and seasoning as it integrates inputs from the environment, via the senses, and modifies the meal accordingly. The blood leaves the heart flush with oxygen and light, as well as psycho-emotionally modulated. The blood is charged electromagnetically and behaves as such in an electromagnetic field. It transfers oxygen, light and emotional information and electromagnetic charges across the capillary walls, at which point it becomes diminished in carried oxygen, depleted of light, the emotional information and electromagnetic charge. It exhibits no organisation when observed in an electromagnetic field but retains the ability to return to its arterial conformation time and time again. When that will occur is dependent on what is happening in the physiology. In sleep it will take some time. When physical demands are higher, such as during work, stress or exercise, the time in the venous reservoir return will be much reduced.

The venous blood has its own drive toward the lungs—the need to eliminate $CO_2$ before resorption of $O_2$ can occur. The waste and gaseous exchange influences the blood to such a degree that it is what drives the return flow of blood in the system—not the heart. It is a fundamental drive in the circulatory dynamic and is paired with the peripheral nutritional need. The pairing of these physiologies drives all of circulation. We breathe not because our heart beats, but rather our heart beats because we *breathe*. Input creates output. Hunger creates input.

Prior to William Harvey's publication of *Exercitatio Anatomica de Motu Cordis et Sanguinis in Animalibus* in 1628, it was believed that blood was sucked through the system. Since that time, medicine has adopted the pump model unquestioningly. It is interesting to note that the challenge to the orthodox view of the model has not come from within medicine but from outside of it. Viktor Schauberger, whose work was an early and ongoing reference to the development of this model, and Rudolf Steiner, a philosopher and the founder of Anthroposophy, both considered the heart not

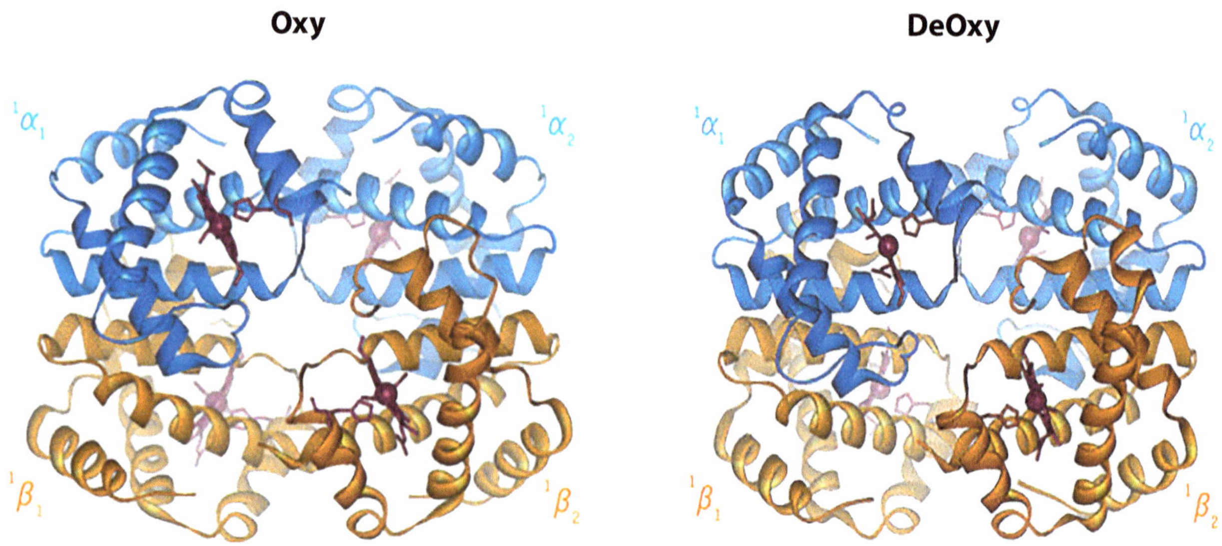


**Figure 9.9 – Haemoglobin in Oxygenated and Deoxygenated State.**[55]

to be a pump. They understood that the pulsatile nature of circulatory flow was the product of the movement of the blood itself. The functioning of the lungs in this dynamic was seen as pivotal, as was the charge differential between arterial and venous blood (discussed in Chapter 8).

Perhaps this provides a better understanding of what Dr Still meant when he wrote "the heart, the fountain of life, is the organ in the human body which imparts the attributes of life and *knowledge* to the blood so that it can proceed correctly with all its work".[54]

The images in Figure 9.9 are of a haemoglobin molecule in its oxygenated and deoxygenated state. In the image on the left, marked "OXY," the overall shape is swelled and round, whereas the one marked "DeOxy" is flatter and thinner in the central area.

This shape change resembles the flexion and extension of primary respiration, suggesting again that patterns are replicated at every level of function.

Returning also to Dr Still's comment that "… when the blood leaves the lungs, it lives and acts as atoms or seeds of life", we can now see the possibility that this is not just about the oxygen in blood,[56] but it is also about the uptake of environmental light that is being brought in to augment the biophotonic dynamic within the body. Popp said that every biochemical process in the body is catalysed by a photon.[57] All of the chemistry of the body requires photonic input to drive it. We have proposed that this whole dynamic is driven by hunger. It is not just hunger for oxygen, or hunger for instruction on how to function in response to our feelings; it is also the hunger to be connected through photons to the external world. We need light. When we eat food, we are absorbing electrons and photons, and when we sunbathe, we are dining on photons.

In teaching the Rule of the Artery, we discuss the functional dynamic within the extracellular matrix where water will bind to protein. This is the fluctuant dynamic that water helps express in response to the primary respiratory mechanism, as well as in response to the energy of life that is in the tide.

## Applications in Osteopathic Practice

In the years following Dr Still, osteopaths taught that T4 is important as a fulcrum for the cardiovascular system and is related to the cardiac neural plexus, the aortic arch and the pulmonary trunk.

We pay attention to the suction of blood into the pulmonary system and out; there is a lower pressure in the lungs compared to the aorta to allow maximum imprinting from the air.

We have perceived the pressure and charge differential between the left and right side of the heart and its importance in health.

The importance of the carena at the pulmonary trunk as a way of maintaining vortical flow has been recognised. We also explore the flow from the right ventricle into the lungs and observe the quality of vortical and helical flow.

Altered or chaotic flow in the lungs is significant and may "mark the beginning to an hour and a minute when disease began to sow its seeds of destruction in the human body."[58]

## Chapter 9 Endnotes

1. A.T. Still, *Osteopathy Research and Practice* (Kirksville, MO: A.T. Still, 1910), 30.

2. A.T. Still, *Osteopathy Research & Practice*, 30.

3. "Hemoglobin," Britannica, updated March 12, 2024, accessed January 13, 2023, https://www.britannica.com/science/hemoglobin.

4. James Baggott, "Structure of Porphyrins," NetBiochem, accessed August 24, 2023, https://library.med.utah.edu/NetBiochem/images/porphin.gif.

5. James Baggott, "Porphyrins," NetBiochem, accessed August 24, 2023, https://library.med.utah.edu/NetBiochem/NetWelco.htm.

6. Paul May, "Hemoglobin," The Molecule of the Month, https://www.chm.bris.ac.uk/motm/hemoglobin/hemoglobv.htm.

7. Xiangdong Xue, Aaron Lindstrom, and Yuanpei Li, "Porphyrin-Based Nanomedicines for Cancer Treatment," *Bioconjugate Chemistry* 30, no. 6 (April 2019), 1585-1603, https://doi.org/10.1021/acs.bioconjchem.9b00231.

8. Jia Tian et al., "Recent Advances of Multi-dimensional Porphyrin-Based Functional Materials in Photodynamic Therapy," *Coordination Chemistry Reviews* 420 (October 2020): 213410.

9. A.T. Still, *Osteopathy Research & Practice*, 30.

10. Grzegorz Redlarski et al., "The Influence of Electromagnetic Pollution on Living Organisms: Historical Trends and Forecasting Changes," *BioMed Research International* 2015 (2015): 234098, https://doi.org/10.1155/2015/234098

11. M. Rattemeyer, F.A. Popp, and W. Nagl, "Evidence of Photon Emission From DNA in Living Systems," *Naturwissenschaften* 68, no. 11 (November 1981): 572–3.

12. A.J. Coleman et al., "Acoustic Emission and Sonoluminescence Due to Cavitation at the Beam Focus of an Electrohydraulic Shock Wave Lithotripter," *Ultrasound in Medicine and Biology* 18, no. 3 (1995): 267–81.

13. Shin-ichi Hatanaka et al., "Influence of Bubble Clustering on Multibubble Sonoluminescence," *Ultrasonics* 40, no. 1-8 (May 2002): 655–60.

14. T.G. Leighton et al., "A Search for Sonoluminescence In Vivo in the Human Cheek," *Ultrasonics* 28, no. 3 (May 1990): 181–4.

15. Joseph T. Hull, Charles A. Czeisler, and Steven W. Lockley, "Suppression of Melatonin Secretion in Totally Visually Blind People by Ocular Exposure to White Light: Clinical Characteristics," *Ophthalmology* 125, no. 8 (August 2018): 1160–71, https://doi.org/10.1016/j.ophtha.2018.01.036.

16. G. Ding et al., "10.15 - Biophysical Bases of Acupuncture," in *Comprehensive Biomedical Physics*, Vol. 10, ed. Anders Bahme (Elsevier, 2014): 299–316.

17. Neville N. Osborne et al. "Visual Light Effects on Mitochondria: The Potential Implications in Relation to Glaucoma," *Mitochondrion* 36 (September 2017): 29–35.

18. Mei-Jie Jou et al., "Mitochondrial Reactive Oxygen Species Generation and Calcium Increase Induced by Visible Light in Astrocytes," *Annals of the New York Academy of Sciences* 1011 (April 2004): 45–56. https://doi.org/10.1007/978-3-662-41088-2_5.

19. Michael Weber, Robert Weber, and Martin Junggebauer, *Medical Low Level Laser therapy – Foundations & Clinical Application* (ISLA Research Group, 2015), 50.

20. Tiina Karu, *The Science of Low-Power Laser Therapy* (Amsterdam: Gordon and Breach Science Publishers, 1998).

21. Tiina Karu, "Primary and Secondary Mechanisms of Action of Visible to Near-IR Radiation on Cells," *Journal of Photochemistry and Photobiology B: Biology* 49, no. 1 (March 1999): 1–17.

22. Hoon Chung et al., "The Nuts and Bolts of Low Level Laser Therapy," *Annals of Biomedical Engineering* 40, no. 2, (February 2012): 516–33.

23. James L. Oschman, "Charge Transfer in the Living Matrix," *Journal of Bodywork and Movement Therapies* 13, no. 3 (July 2009): 215–228.

24. Helene M. Langevin and Jason A. Yandow, "Relationship of Acupuncture Points and Meridians to Connective Tissue Planes," *The Anatomical Record* 269 (2002): 257–265.

25. S. Rosenblatt, "The Electrodermal Characteristics of Acupuncture Points," *American Journal of Acupuncture* 10 (1982): 131-7.

26. David F. Mayor, ed., *Electroacupuncture: A Practical Manual and Resource* (Edinburgh: Churchill Livingstone/Elsevier, 2006).

27. Fritz-Albert Popp, *Biologie des Lichtes* (Hamburg: Verlag Paul Parey, 1984).

28. Fritz-Albert Popp et al., "Biophoton Emission. New Evidence for Coherence and DNA as Source," *Cell Biophysics* 6, no. 1 (March 1984): 33–52, https://doi.org/10.1007/BF02788579.

29. Science Mission Directorate, "The Earth's Radiation Budget," National Aeronautics and Space Administration, accessed June 7, 2024, http://science.nasa.gov/ems/13_radiationbudget.

30. "Earth's Energy Budget," *The Earth Observatory.* Robert Levy NASA Goddard Space Flight Center, published June 14, 2009, https://earthobservatory.nasa.gov/features/EnergyBalance/page4.php.

31. "Atmospheric Processes and Climate," *Introduction to Earth Science*, section 5.3, accessed January 20, 2023, https://gotbooks.miracosta.edu/earth_science/chapter5.html.

32. "Bio photons and the regulation of the body with Prof. Fritz-Albert Popp from the International Institute of Biophysics e. V. in Neuss, Germany," Meth Medura Foundation, https://www.pansori-network.org/testen/test3_en_Popp_biofysics.pdf.

33. "Absorption/Reflection of Sunlight," Understanding Global Change, https://ugc.berkeley.edu/background-content/reflection-absorption-sunlight/.

34. Michel Schiff, *The Memory of Water*, as quoted in Yolène Thomas, "The History of the Memory of Water," *Homeopathy* 96, no. 3 (July 2007): 151–7.

35. E. Davenas et al., "Human basophil degranulation triggered by very dilute antiserum against IgE," *Nature* 333, no. 6176 (June 1988): 816–8.

36. Bernd Kröplin, *The World in a Drop*, 2nd ed. (International Center of Numerical Methods in Engineering, 2016).

37. Luc Montagnier et al., "Electromagnetic Signals Are Produced by Aqueous Nanostructures Derived From Bacterial DNA Sequences," *Interdisciplinary Sciences: Computational Life Sciences* 1 (March 2009): 81–90, https://doi.org/10.1007/s12539-009-0036-7.

38. Robert Matthews, "Water: The Quantum Elixir," *New Scientist*, April 5, 2006, https://www.newscientist.com/article/mg19025461-200-water-the-quantum-elixir.

39. Albert Szent-Györgyi, "Submolecular Biology," *Radiation Research* 2, suppl. 2 (1960): 4–18, https://www.jstor.org/stable/i284210.

40. Albert Szent-Györgyi, "The Study of Energy-Levels in Biochemistry," *Nature,* 148 (August 1941): 157–159.

41. Mae-Wan Ho, *The Rainbow and the Worm: The Physics of Organisms* (Singapore: World Scientific Publishing Company, 2008).

42. H.E. Puthoff, "Source of Vacuum Electromagnetic Energy Zero-Point Energy," *Physical Review A* 40 (November 1989): 4857–62.

43. H.E. Puthoff, "The Energetic Vacuum: Implications for Energy Research," *Speculations in Science & Technology* 13, no. 4 (1990): 247–57.

44. Masaru Emoto, *The Hidden Messages In Water* (The Netherlands: Hado Publishing, 2001).

45. Rose-Lynn Fisher, *The Topography of Tears* (New York, NY: Bellevue Literary Press, 2017).

46. Robert Matthews, "Water: The Quantum Elixir," *New Scientist*, April 5, 2006, https://www.newscientist.com/article/mg19025461-200-water-the-quantum-elixir.

47. Bernd Kröplin, *The World in a Drop*. https://www.worldinadrop-shop.com/en/c/books.

48. Hans Jenny, *Cymatics: A Study of Wave Phenomena and Vibration*, rev. ed. (MACROmedia Publishing, July 2001).

49. Masaru Emoto, *The Secret Life of Water* (Atria Books, Simon & Schuster: 2011).

50. Vandana Gupta, "Water," *NAMAH: Journal of New Approaches to Medicine and Health* 21, no. 3 (October 2013), http://www.namahjournal.com/doc/Actual/Water.html.

51. Emiliano Brini et al., "How Water's Properties Are Encoded in Its Molecular Structure and Energies," *Chemical Reviews* 117, no. 19 (September 2017): 12385–414 (see p. 12392).

52. A.T. Still, *Philosophy and Mechanical Principles of Osteopathy* (Kansas City, MO: Hudson-Kimberly Publishing Co., 1902), 249.

53. "Water Has Memory," Oasis HD, posted April 19, 2011, on YouTube, https://www.youtube.com/watch?v=MZmYcJ0DNBc.

54. A.T. Still, *Osteopathy: Research and Practice* (Kirksville, MO: The Journal Printing Company, 1910), 318.

55. Animation of hemoglobin t-r state transformation. https://commons.wikimedia.org/wiki/File:Hemoglobin_t-r_state_ani.gif.

56. A.T. Still. *Osteopathy: Research and Practice.*

57. F.A. Popp et al., "Physical Aspects of Biophotons," *Experientia* 44 (July 1988): 576–85.

58. A.T. Still, *Autobiography of Andrew Taylor Still* (Kirksville, MO: A.T. Still, 1908), 18.

## Chapter Ten

# The Aorta as a Fulcrum

*"The wisdom of Nature's architect is found in every drop of your blood."**

– Andrew Taylor Still, 1908

This chapter explores the way in which the vasculature, particularly the aorta, acts as a fulcrum in relation to growth and subsequent function. Underlying all is the need for nourishment of all the cells, both in the embryological stage and after birth.

From his research, Erich Blechschmidt concluded that the aorta, with its tributaries, acts and functions as a growth fulcrum.[1] Notice how all of the flexion surfaces in the body are on the side with the majority of the vasculature. We flex to the side of the vasculature. We adduct and protract to the side of the vasculature, and the embryological growth movements reflect an attraction towards the nutrient source.

Consider the forearm (Figure 10.1) as an example. The elbow bends into flexion. Our wrists bend into flexion. Flexion is driven by where the majority of the vasculature resides, towards where the majority of the nutrition flows. Growth movements are structured by the vasculature.

Embryological growth movements reflect the nutrient waves arriving at the cells of the embryo. The arrival of each wave encourages flexion and the growth, in response to that wave, promotes extension. This is how Blechschmidt described the successive bending of the head towards the tail with a

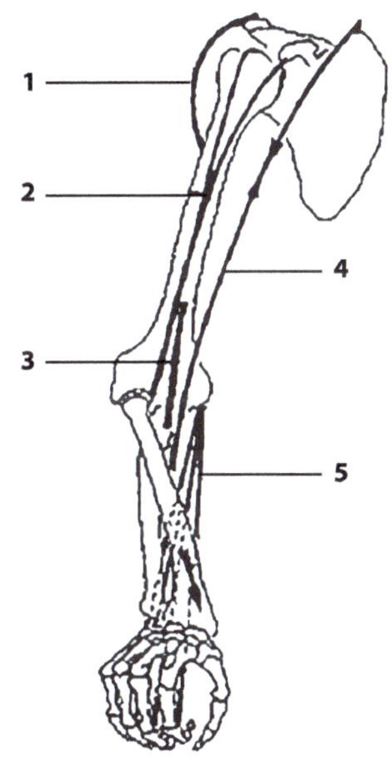


**Figure 10.1 – Dilation Fields.** Directions of important dilation fields of adult right upper limb. Arrow designates preceding growth elongation of radius. Converging double arrow: restraining function of brachial artery (4). (1) Lateral shoulder (deltoid) muscle formed by growth of adduction of arm. Various flexor muscles arise during growth elongation of the skeleton: (2) biceps brachii muscle, (3) brachialis muscle, and (5) flexor digitorum superficialis. Reprinted from Blechschmidt.

*A.T. Still, *Autobiography*, 1908, p. 330.

coincident rotation of the upper part of the body to one side and the lower part to the other side.

So the vasculature acts as a growth fulcrum, and expanding on that, we will also observe how the vasculature amplifies the function of the heart. Next we will look more specifically at the aorta and its ventral and lateral branches, applying that observation to the somatic dysfunction of the viscera.

The circulatory dynamics are seen through the lens of the need for nourishment being met by a nutritional source and the application of that wonderful rule in nature: you either use it or you lose it. Certain areas of the embryo grow asymmetrically, and in those areas the vasculature becomes unnecessary, in which case that particular area atrophies and coalesces with other functions.

During fetal development, Blechschmidt and Gasser[2] give examples of "biokinetic" schemes of human embryos. One such scheme is to take a developing finger where there are some areas being stretched and some that resist stretch, with consequent asymmetry.

Blechschmidt described the conceptus as asymmetric. He suggested that there is a clear difference in surface growth between the conceptus' superficial areas and its more central portions. He called the outer, more rapidly growing tissue of the conceptus the ectoblast and the inner, more slowly growing portion the endoblast. The main source of mesoblast in the conceptus is its most rapidly growing component, which is the ectoblast. Blechschmidt envisaged cells and fluids being squeezed by lateral growth pressure in the ectoblast and being left behind as the more rapidly growing tissue grows away. Asymmetry is innate as a consequence. Blechschmidt called the recapitulation process that repeatedly occurs as **encapsis** in human ontogeny (Blechschmidt, 1960) and also related it to tripartite divisions found in adult anatomy.[3]

During the development of the heart, it changes from a horseshoe shape to a tubular shape, which

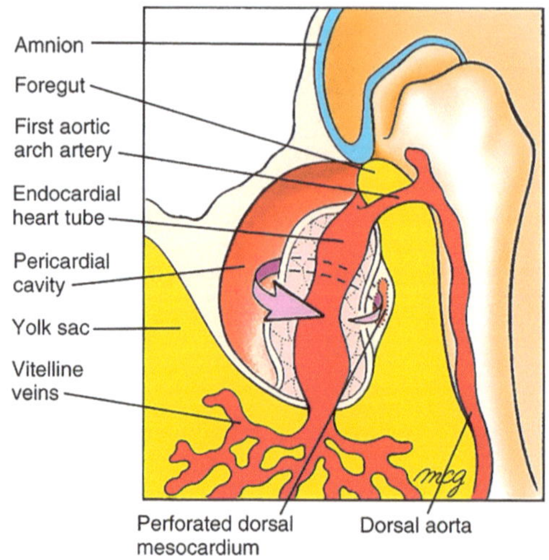


**Figure 10.2 – Dilation of the Chambers Forming Left and Right Ventricles.** Formation of the transverse pericardial sinus of the definitive pericardial cavity by rupture of the dorsal mesocardium early in the fourth week. Arrow passes through the transverse pericardial sinus. Reprinted from Schoenwolf.[4]

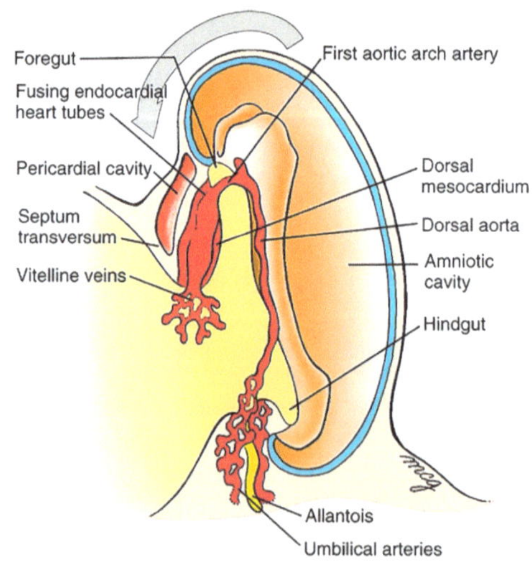


**Figure 10.3 – Formation of the First Aortic Arch Artery and Dorsal Aorta.**

then folds in on itself in relation to the folding of the whole embryo. In Figure 10.2, we see dilation of the chambers forming the left and right ventricles. Development proceeds from a single tube to a chambered heart.

The first aortic arch artery and dorsal aorta form during the third week. The paired dorsal aortae de-

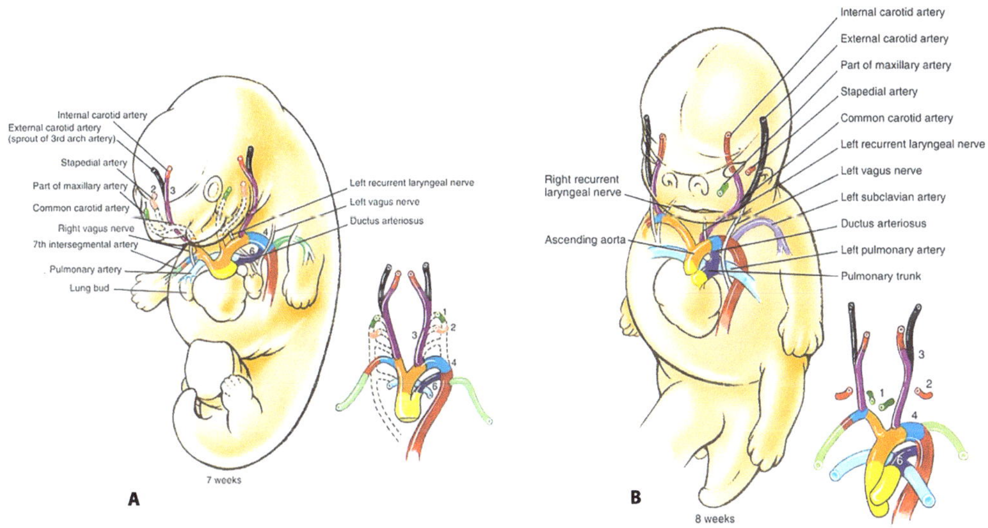


**Figure 10.4 – Arteries of the Pharyngeal Arches.** Development of the aortic system. A, Formation of the first arch is complete by day 24 but regresses as the second arch forms on day 26. The third and fourth arches form on day 28; the second arch degenerates as the sixth aortic arch artery forms on day 29. A, Development of the arches in the second month. Note that the arteries arising from the first three pairs of aortic arch arteries are bilateral, whereas vessels derived from arches four and six develop asymmetrically. B, At 8 weeks. Note the asymmetrical development of the recurrent laryngeal branches of the vagus nerve, which innervate the laryngeal muscles. As the larynx is displaced cranially relative to the arch system, the recurrent laryngeal nerves are caught under the most caudal remaining arch on each side. The right recurrent laryngeal nerve therefore loops under the right subclavian artery, whereas the left recurrent laryngeal nerve loops under the ductus arteriosus. Reprinted from Schoenwolf et al.[6]

velop in the dorsal mesoderm on either side of the notochord and connect to the fusing endocardial heart tubes while body folding ensues. As flexion and growth of the head fold (large curved arrow) and carry the forming primary heart tube into the cervical and then into the thoracic region, the cranial ends of the dorsal aortae are pulled ventrally until they form a dorsoventral loop—the first aortic arch artery. A series of four more aortic arch arteries will develop during the fourth and fifth weeks. Reprinted from Schoenwolf et al.[5]

The arrow in Figure 10.3 highlights how the dorsal aspect of the brain flexes downward and carries the amniotic cavity with it. The dorsal aorta comes off the developing endocardial tube. There is another dorsal aorta on the opposite side of the foregut.

The arteries of the pharyngeal arches and the aorta develop in a cranial-caudal sequence (Figure 10.4). There are six pairs in total, of which the fifth is usually rudimentary. Everywhere an artery folds or twists near another artery, a corrosion field combines the two flows into one. The complex regression and corrosion of the vessels can be seen in the animation at https://www.youtube.com/watch?v=9dBg2yrwv0Y. For your convenience, you may also scan this QR code:

During early development, there is a flow of intercellular fluid towards the developing brain that comes back down towards the connecting stalk, which forms the future umbilicus.

We recommend viewing the video, referred to

above, several times because the process is complicated. What it emphasises is the multidimensional growth of the embryo, which is important because everything that you see with this modelling of the vasculature relates to those embryological flexion, extension and rotational movements. The result is that the heart folds to the left and the liver folds to the right. The development of the vasculature reflects those growth movements. The venous functions tend to coalesce on the right side so we have the predominance of the inferior and superior vena cava on the right, but the arterial functions coalesce mostly on the left.

The embryo bends as a result of the tension and resistance from the dorsal aortae as it forms the pharyngeal arches (Figure 10.5). The aortic arches form in response to the metabolic fluid gradients that develop from the heart. The aortic arches remodel to form the blood vessels that supply the head, neck and upper extremity.

Blechschmidt emphasised that the bending and twisting of the embryo is strictly related to the restraining function of the dorsal aortae. A significant morphogenetic function of the developing embryo is the fulcrum of the vasculature.

In Figure 10.6, we can see that the dorsal aorta has fused between T4 and L4 and is separated above and below.

Also in Figure 10.6, a mass of arteries can be seen sprouting from the ventral aspect of the dorsal aorta, and those arteries go on to form the vitelline arterial plexus to supply the yolk sac. This occurs at about week 4. The arterial plexus forms from a flow of intercellular fluid going up towards the developing brain area, which develop into veins, and a return flow of intercellular fluid back down towards the connecting stalk.

Before the dorsal aortae fuse, there is a plexus on each side. As the dorsal aortae fuse, so do the vitelline arterial plexuses. Then, as the embryo folds laterally, the yolk sac becomes smaller and the vitelline arterial plexuses coalesce and many of the channels regress to form single unpaired arteries that supply the gut tube.

The fusion of the dorsal aortae between T4 and L4 resolves the midline between the respiratory

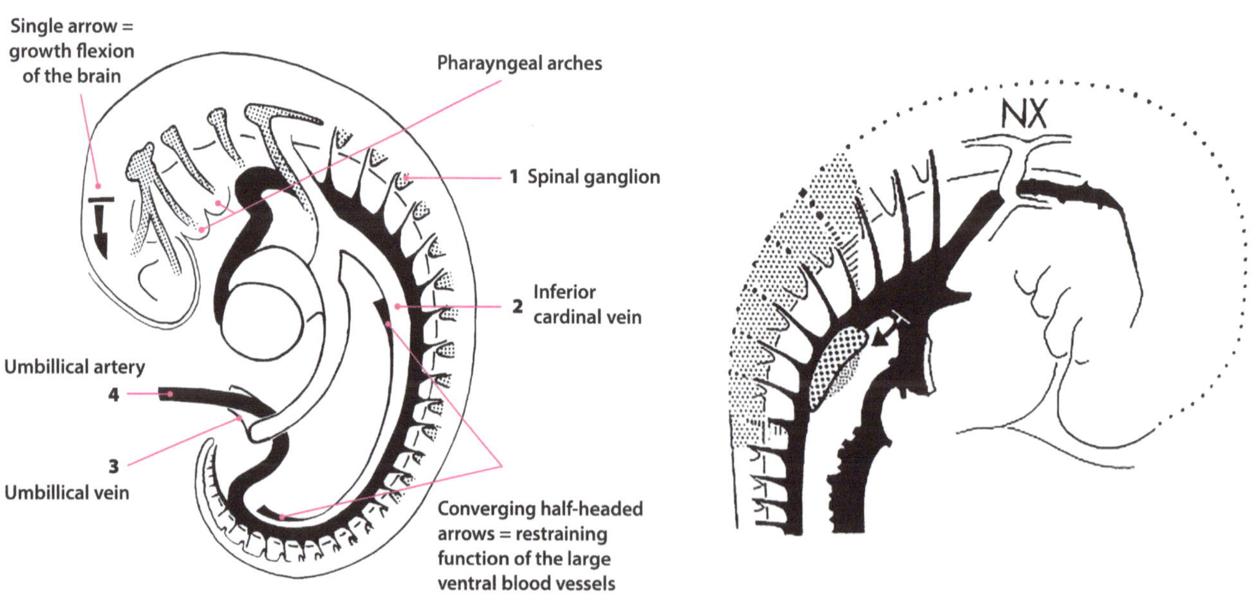


**Figure 10.5 – Embryo Bends Forming Pharyngeal Arches.** 1: Spinal ganglion. 2: Inferior cardinal vein. 3: Umbilical vein; 4: Umbilical artery. NX = Cranial nerve ten. Reprinted from Blechschmidt.[7]

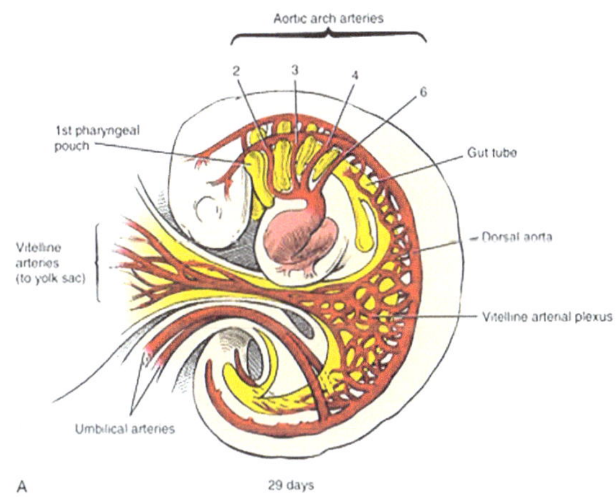


**Figure 10.6 – Fusion of the Dorsal Aorta at 29 Days.** Reprinted from Schoenwolf et al.[8]

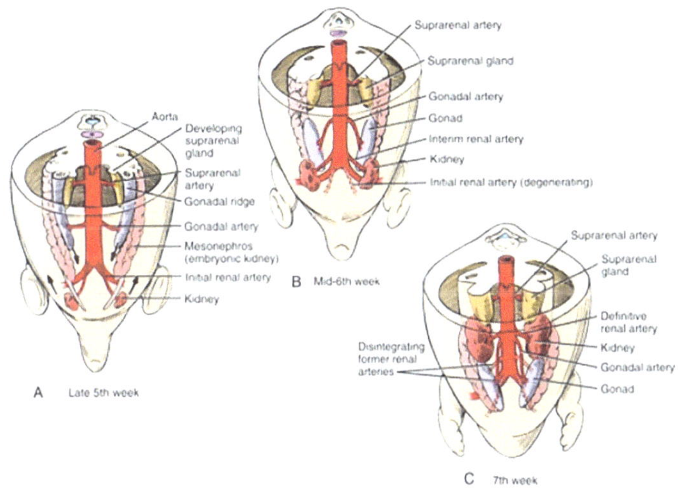


**Figures 10.7 – Development of the Lateral Branches of the Aorta.** A, Lateral sprouts of the dorsal aorta vascularise the suprarenal glands, gonads and kidneys. During the sixth week, the gonads begin to descend while the kidneys ascend (arrows). B and C, The gonadal artery lengthens during the migration of the gonad, but the ascending kidney is vascularised by a succession of new, more cranial aortic sprouts. The suprarenal arteries remain in place. Reprinted from Schoenwolf et al.[9]

functions and the circulatory functions. The fusion also coincides with the function of the ductus arteriosum, which detours the circulation of blood away from the lungs until birth at which time it closes, becoming the ligamentum arteriosum.

In Figure 10.7, the lateral arteries of the aorta are the suprarenal, renal and gonadal arteries, which are paired.

The metabolic flow of fluids, or the fluid fields, were already present before the arteries developed. The source of nutrients is the dorsal aorta and the sink absorbing it all are somatic and visceral tissue development.

In Figure 10.7, you can see the discontinuous lines. This is meant to represent a succession of renal arteries developing as the kidney apparently migrates from a sacral position upwards to about the second lumbar position. From Blechschmidt's studies it appears that this migrating model is inaccurate. The kidney does not ascend, nor does the aorta sprout different arteries as it goes. The branches are tough and restraining like the dorsal aorta and **do not** migrate.

The kidney does start in a very low position. The renal artery is short and has a degree of tension, and the kidney remains in close relation to it during its development. Remember that arteries become retarded in their growth due to all their nutrition being absorbed by the end organ. The artery itself and its walls have less nutrition to grow on. However, the rest of the embryo is growing both in width and in length, so it is not that the kidney ascends upwards but that everything else is growing longitudinally down, therefore giving the perception that the kidney ascends. As for the gonad, it has a restraining band of tissue—the gubernaculum—that remains close to its original length throughout the growth process. It restrains the organ as the embryo grows; its influence is stronger than that of the artery so it remains relatively stationary and the rest grows away from it, thus giving the illusion of descent.

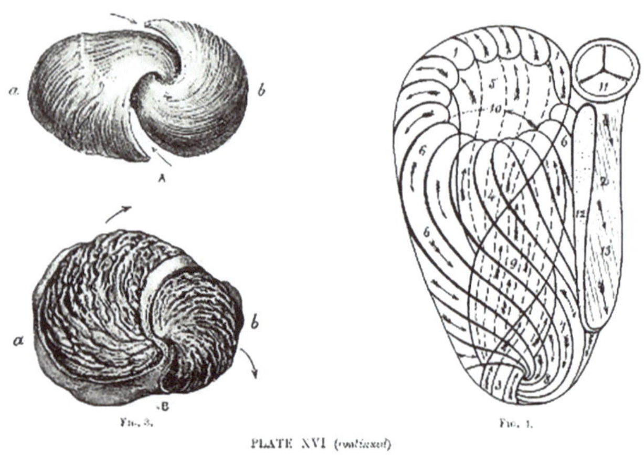

**Figure 10.8 – Pettigrew's Design in Nature (1908).** Left, Interior plaster cast of heart ventricles and spiral whirls. Right, Left ventricle diagram of Muscle Fibres' left-handed ("involute" into apex) and right-handed ("evolute" at the base) spirals with enumerated sequence. Reprinted from Pettigrew.[10]

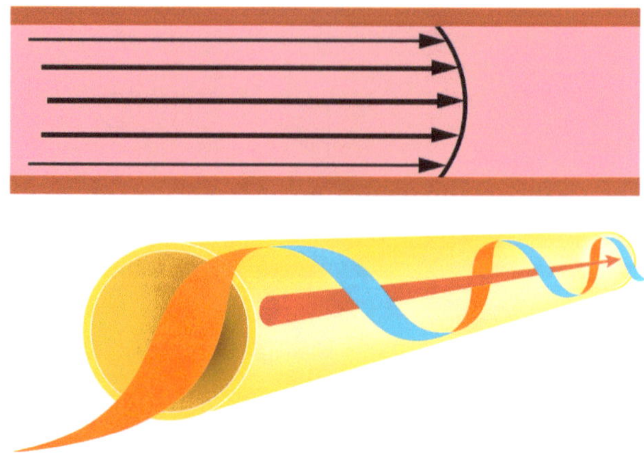

**Figure 10.9 – Spiral Laminar Flow.** Two-dimensional versus three-dimensional representation of laminar flow in a tube. Image courtesy of Peter Stonebridge and *Methodist DeBakey Cardiovascular Journal.*[13]

Relative to vortical flow, a vortex is a spiral with vectoral quality; it contains fractal characteristics with purpose, direction and power. The images in Figure 10.8 are drawings from Anatomist James Bell Pettigrew's 1908 work *Design in Nature*, a three-volume compilation of more than 2,000 figures and illustrations. The images illustrate the innate spiral form of the heart in multiple layers.

Vortical flow is a spiral with purpose. It carries information in fractal form.

Recent work in cardiac and peripheral vascular blood flow[11] has shown evidence, in elegant complexity, of how blood flows within the heart and large to medium arteries. Using the technology that was available at the time, blood flow was described as laminar, meaning that blood was observed to travel smoothly with some apparent layering for ease of flow. At each point the blood was viewed, where factors like temperature, pH, speed of flow and related pressure all remain constant, an apparent layering is seen. With the more recent availability of magnetic resonance imaging and colour Doppler flow imaging it has been possible to move from a two- to a three-dimensional representation of flow within the blood vessels. The more recent imaging has suggested a more spiral and rotational property to blood flow rather than the more linear, laminar description.

Peter Stonebridge, professor of vascular surgery at the University of Dundee, termed this blood flow *spiral laminar flow*, an equally valid term (Figure 10.9).[12]

Figure 10.9 depicts both a two-dimensional and a three-dimensional representation of what you have learned. It is a three-dimensional phenomenon, and it has a spiral quality to it. In the image from Viktor Schauberger's *Hidden Nature* in Figure 10.10, it is a vortex coming towards you.[14]

Often we relate to earth in terms of how we have perceived it in the past. When we traditionally think about laminar flow, it is regarding water passing through a pipe; because of the friction that exists between the water and the pipe, the outer rings of water flow much slower than the internal rings. However, that is what happens in standard fluid dynamics.

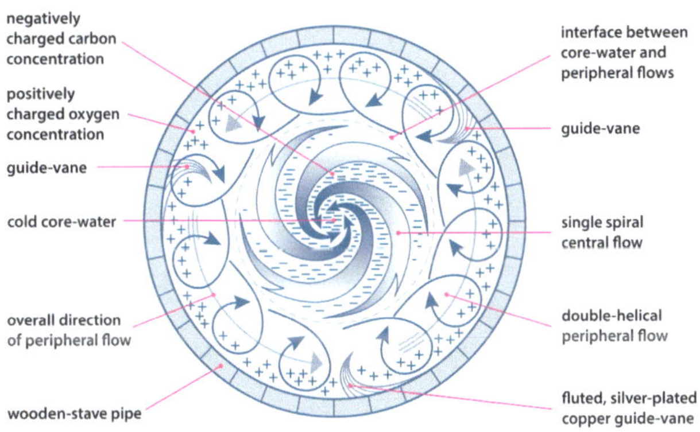


**Figure 10.10 – Flow Dynamics of the Double-Spiral Pipe.**

The vortical flow of blood was established before the development of the heart. Its flow is further augmented by the spiral contraction of the heart. Each bolus of blood that comes from the contraction maintains its spiral shape in an electrically charged circulatory system. That is the difference between what is happening in our blood vessels and what is happening in the water pipes at home. There is no charge associated with the dynamic of your plumbing at home.

The charge in the blood vessels is important and imperative in terms of maintaining the vortical flow and other qualities within the blood. If the charge dynamic in the vessel is disrupted by trauma, the whole thing collapses. Turbulence results and we have dysfunction from that point in the system and continuing downstream.

The point emphasised here is the necessity to understand that the bioelectric dynamic is a significant part of the lesion complex that needs to be addressed, if, in our osteopathic treatment, we are going to successfully recruit the vascular system and resolve the trauma.

Doppler imaging has shown that because of the charge dynamic in the vortical spiralling of the blood, there is an organisation to the componentry of the blood as it passes through the vessels.[15,16] So, there is a ring of plasma around the heavier part, the red blood cells and the platelets, which are organised more centrally within the blood vessel. As a result, a cross-section of the blood passing through the vessel is not a homogeneous fluid; instead, it is organised in response to charge and particle weight in the charge field. Again, once turbulence develops and that charge dynamic is disrupted, the organisation of the elements within the blood is also disorganised.

Blechschmidt repeatedly emphasised the morphogenic functions of the vasculature. Viktor Schauberger described the helical and the spiral vortical flow as a function of nature (Figure 10.11). When you see this vortical flow from the side, what you are seeing in the way these eddies come back is part of the vortical flow. This is palpable as the pulse of the vortical flow. That is the end result of the lateral expression of that vortex functioning in the vasculature.

We saw in the first chapter where the spiralling

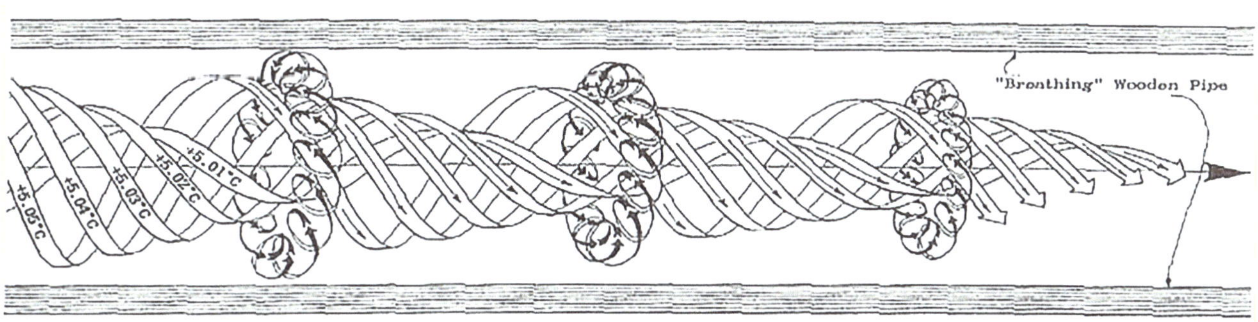


**Figure 10.11 – The Double-Spiral Longitudinal Vortex.** Reprinted from Coats.[17]

of the blood continues into the chambers and spirals back out of the chambers to sculpt the outflow tracts in a spiral configuration.

It is important to remember the aorta is a fulcrum of function but also that the function of the aorta directly relates to venous return. Cardiac output to the cerebrum is directly proportional to venous return. The function of the inferior vena cava (IVC) and the superior vena cava (SVC) coalescing the flows from the rest of the body help to organise the flows into the lungs, an important example of how the arterial functions serve as a vascular fulcrum.[18] As we have worked to optimise flow in patients, either in the IVC or the SVC, we became aware that successfully optimising flow may result in turbulence of flow as venous return increases following removal of any upstream obstruction to flow (the liver being a common site of sluggish return).

We discovered that there are two carenae that prevent chaotic flow and enable vortical flow to continue. The first is the **crista terminalis** (Figure 10.12), which is found at the entrance to the right atrium and facilitates flow coming from above (SVC) and below (IVC).

The second carena is nowhere named, but we have detected what we presume is a carena in multiple patients. It is located in the pulmonary trunk directly above the pulmonary valve. It looks very similar to the carina at the bifurcation of the trachea shown in Figure 10.13.

Next we consider pressure waves; every time the heart coils and uncoils there is a pressure wave that is expressed through the arteries into the tissues. Sound is propagated through water faster than it is through air. Having a redundant communication system with phonons (sound waves first discussed in Chapter 1) from cardiac contraction and reflected waves is another way for the heart to communicate with every cell. So, we have communication by neurotransmitters, communication by light, and communication by sound. All of these pathways

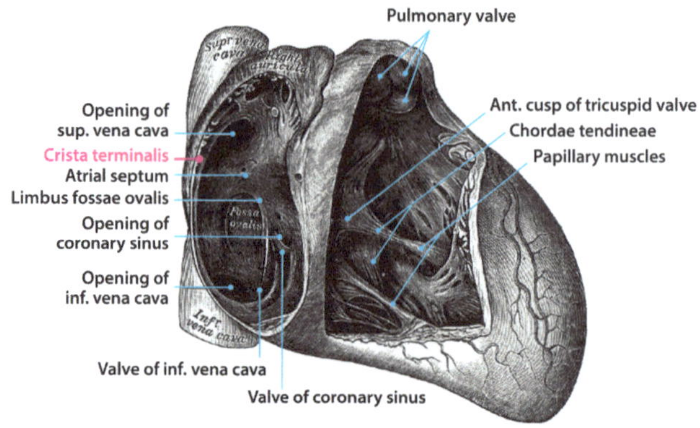


**Figure 10.12 – Crista Terminalis.** Reprinted from Gray.[18]

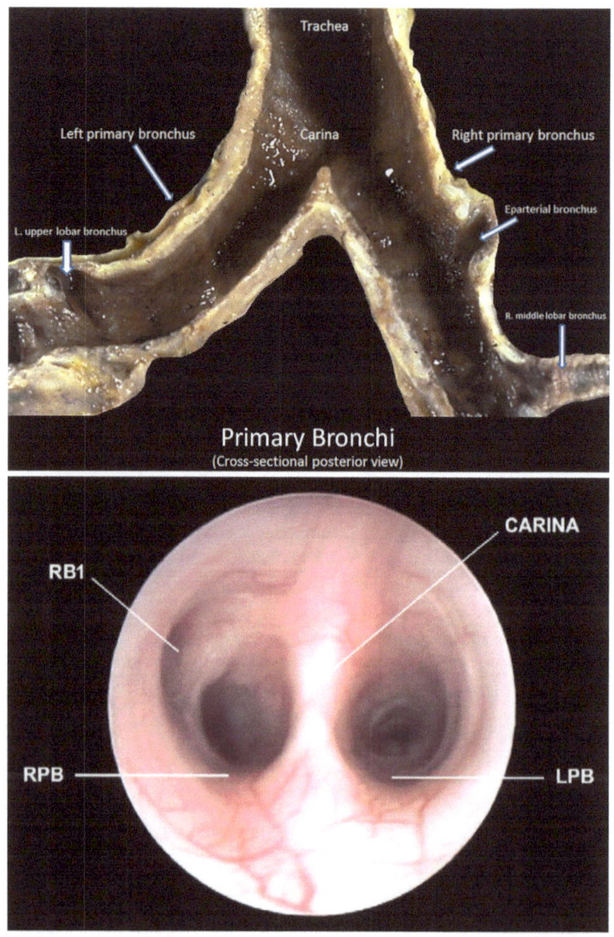


**Figure 10.13 – Carina at the Bifurcation of the Trachea.**[19,20] Carina and right and left principal bronchi (RPB, LPB). It is possible to see the origin of the right cranial lobar bronchus (RB1).

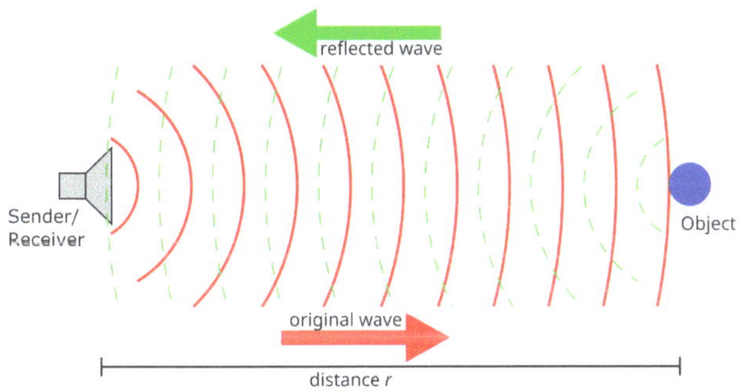


**Figure 10.14 – Continuous Wave Radar.** [41]

form an electromagnetic spectrum communicating with every cell.

Radar works similarly. It sends out a wave and then it gets information from the object via the reflected wave (Figure 10.14). The heart sends out a wave and it gets information back, for example, that there is under-perfusion around our liver and diaphragm and it will vasodilate in relation to that hypo-perfusion. One of the returning signals might be increased levels of nitric oxide that is produced during hypoxia.

Whales and submarines perform the same function under water: they send out signals and receive reflected waves. Bats similarly perform echolocation. The speed that information travels through water and blood is 1,500 m/sec. So within a fraction of a second after the heart's contraction, the heart is communicating with all the tissues.

Anywhere blood flow meets resistance, a reflected wave is created. That reflected wave is the sum of all the resistances. Thus, the bifurcation of the aorta is one of the most important points of resistance below the aortic arch.

In *Gray's Anatomy*,[21] researchers describe how pressure waves, which descend down the aorta with each contraction of the heart, can give rise to reflected waves with pressure oscillations and possible turbulence where it meets the bifurcation which leads into the common iliac arteries (Figures 10.15 through 10.17). This may also be due to the

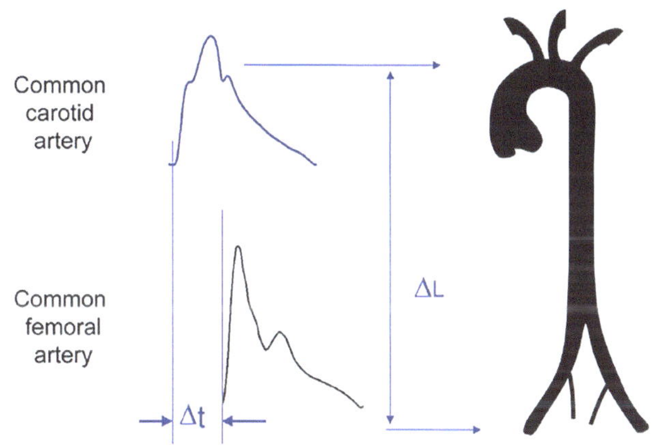


**Figure 10.15 – Measurement of Carotid-Femoral Pulse Wave.** Measurement of carotid-femoral pulse wave velocity (PWV) with the foot-to-foot method. The waveforms are usually obtained transcutaneously at the right common carotid artery and the right femoral artery. The time delay (Δt, or transit time) is measured between the feet of the two waveforms. The distance (ΔL) covered by the waves is usually assimilated to the surface distance between the two recording sites, ie., the common carotid artery and the common femoral artery. PWV is calculated as $PWV = 0.8 \times \Delta L$ (metres)/$\Delta t$ (seconds). Reprinted from Laurent and Boutouyrie with permission.[23]

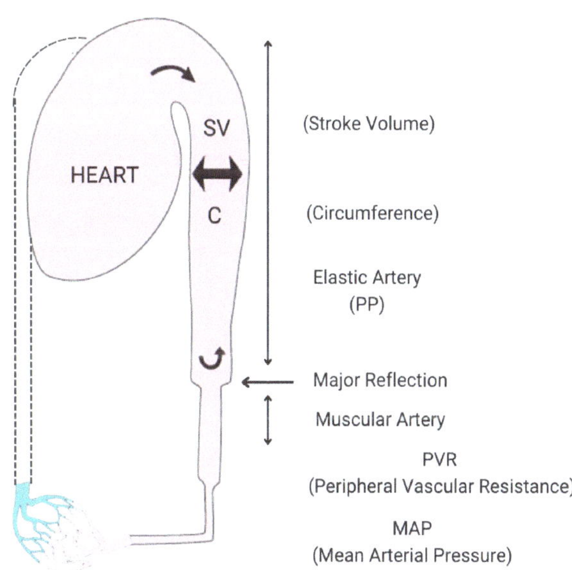


**Figure 10.16 – Aortic Pressure Wave.** Reprinted with permission from Prue Eddie, DO.

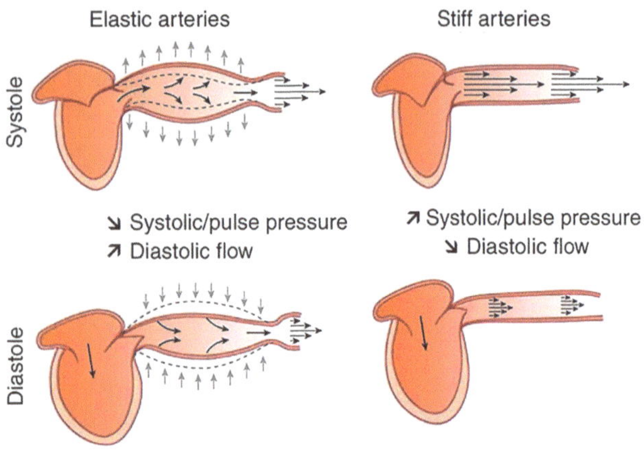


**Figure 10.17 – Elastic and Stiff Arteries in Systole and Diastole.** Schematic representation of the role of arterial compliance (ie., the inverse of arterial stiffness) in dampening blood pressure pulsatility and assuring adapted blood flow through the peripheral circulation. Reprinted from permission from Elsevier and Briet et al.[24]

different luminal sizes. These reflected waves are thought to have the ability to damage the intima of the distal aorta and therefore predispose this area to inflammation and degeneration.[22]

This suggests the importance of blood flow into the common iliac arteries and, for that matter, into any junction between blood vessels where the flow is smooth and without turbulence. Because we are able to palpate the blood flow, osteopathic practitioners can take preventive measures against cardiovascular disease. The vessels develop in an organised coherent flow state. Any reflection or turbulence will result in dysfunction.

It is also important to consider the flow of blood as different from the pressure created by the arterial wall. In *The Dynamic Heart and Circulation*,[25] attention is drawn to the fact that when the heart contracts and blood enters the ascending aorta, the pressure wave created by this can be measured at the big toe about 0.2 seconds after the blood enters the aorta. However, the flow of blood in that time has only reached the abdominal aorta.

The **healthy** arterial system slows down blood flow. It also maintains the pressure wave from the heart, which has a resonance much like a musical instrument. The arterial system is a pressure wave resonator. In the case of atherosclerosis, where plaque forms on the walls of the arterial system in response to damage, the arterial system cannot resonate and therefore cannot perform the function of maintaining the pulsatile pressure wave or allow the communication of information that this resonance carries to the rest of the body.

In addition, in *Stalking the Wild Pendulum*,[26] Ishtak Bentov describes the length of the aorta as half of one wavelength of the sound wave created by the beat of the heart (Figure 10.18). Considering this in the embryo, the length of the embryo is constantly changing as the embryo grows. However, the length of the aorta remains one half of a wavelength of the sound wave created by the heart. The sound wave and the transmission of sound is communicating something to the tissues of the embryo and is related to its growth, in particular the length of the aorta. This function of the heart remains throughout life.

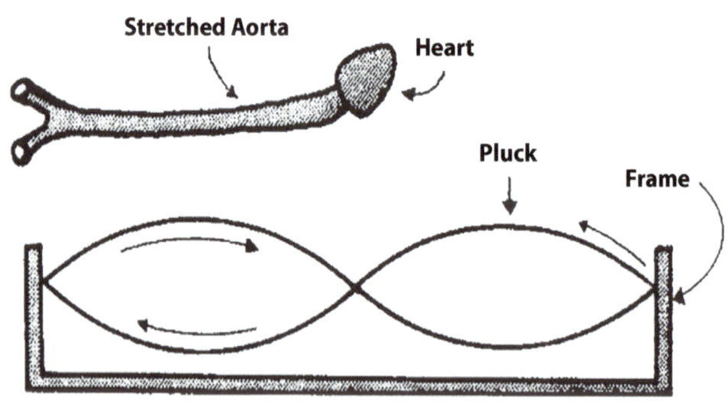


**Figure 10.18 – Length of the Aorta vs Wavelength of Sound From Heartbeat.** *Stalking the Wild Pendulum* by Itzhak Bentov published by Inner Traditions International and Bear & Company, ©1988.[27] All rights reserved. http://www.Innertraditions.com. Reprinted with permission of publisher.

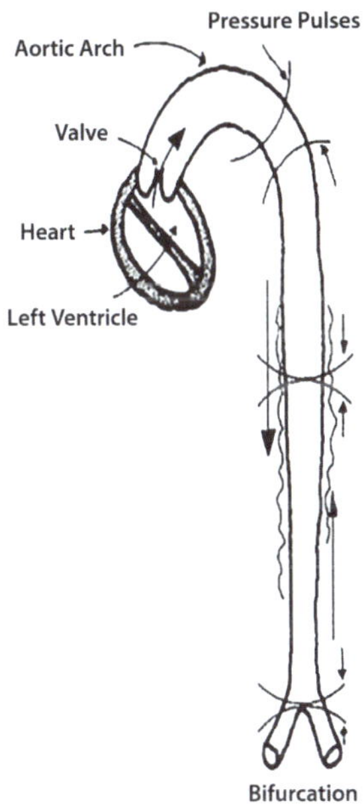


**Figure 10.19 – Showing the Half-way Point With Interference Patterns.** *Stalking the Wild Pendulum* by Itzhak Bentov published by Inner Traditions International and Bear & Company, ©1988.[28] All rights reserved. http://www.Innertraditions.com. Reprinted with permission of publisher.

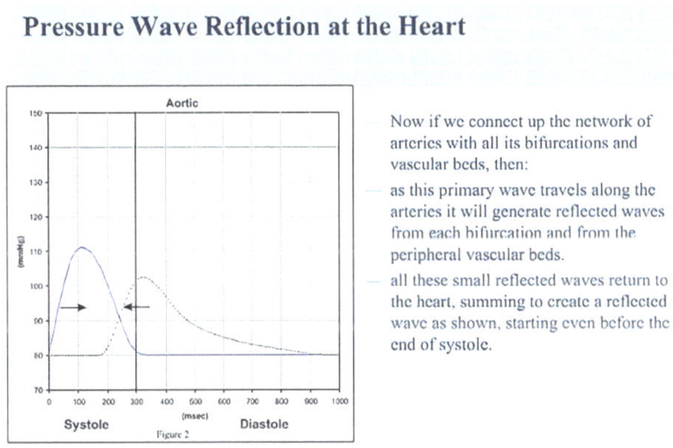


**Figure 10.20 – AtCor Pressure Waves: The Primary Wave.** Image courtesy of AtCor Medical.

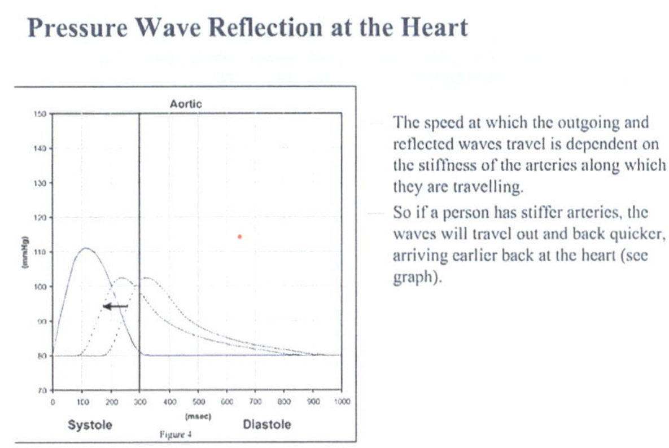


**Figure 10.21 – AtCor Pressure Waves: Arterial Stiffness Alters the Speed and Nature of the Wave.** Image courtesy of AtCor Medical.

If pressure waves cause interference patterns, the vessel walls will vibrate (Figure 10.19).

The Sphygmocor® (made by Core Medical) measures the heart's reflected pressure wave.

Results from using the Sphygmocor®, a vascular biosensing technology which is now used internationally in over 4,000 medical and research institutions, have been published following many clinical trials. The AtCor diagrams above in the series of charts in Figures 10.20 through 10.24 provide an overview of the waves propagated.

These waves are the result of elastic function of the wall of the aorta from its first reflection at that bifurcation of the aorta. The pressure wave is different from blood flow and travels almost as fast as the speed of sound. Blood flow is much slower.

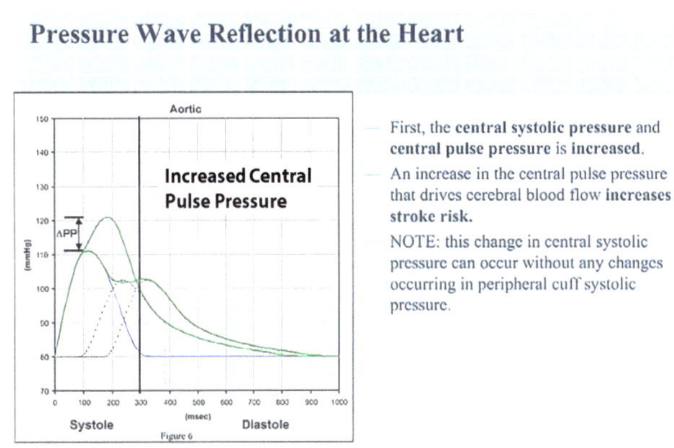


**Figure 10.22 – AtCor Pressure Waves: Increased Central Pressure & Stroke.** Image courtesy of AtCor Medical.

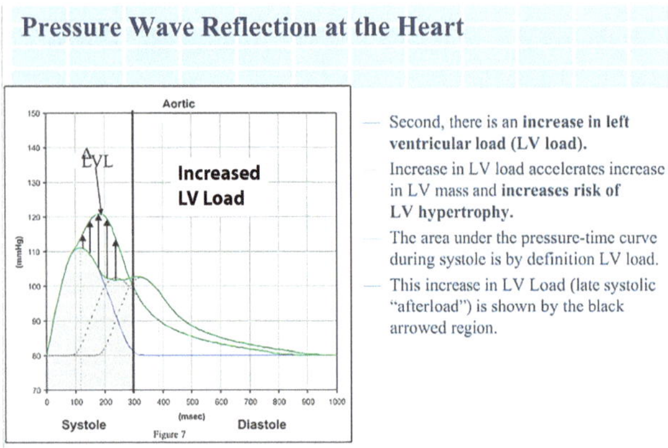


**Figure 10.23 – AtCor Pressure Waves: Increased Load & Ventricular Hypertrophy.** Image courtesy of AtCor Medical.

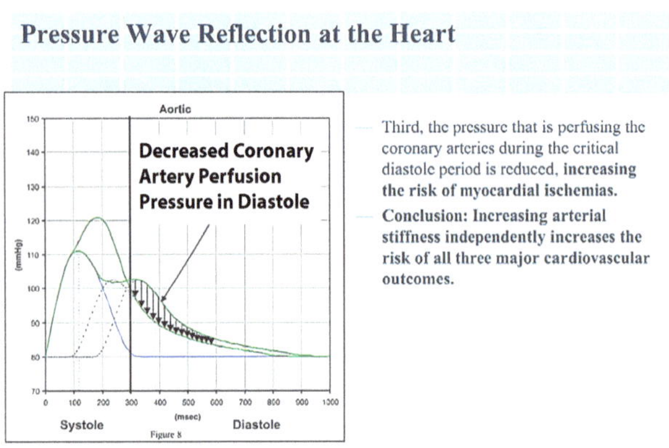


**Figure 10.24 – AtCor Pressure Waves: Myocardial Ischemia.** Image courtesy of AtCor Medical.

The downward arrows in Figure 10.24 represent the decreased volume of blood. Think of the blood as having a hydraulic quality within an open system. Blood flow is much, much slower than the reflected wave. The reflected wave informs the heart about what to do next. These flow graphs demonstrate the compliance of the vascular wall absorbing some of the forces of blood flow and then accentuating it for the function of the heart so that every recoil of the vasculature is accentuating the sound of the heart, just like a beautiful harmonised musical instrument.

The literature confirms how elastic recoil augments flow during diastole.[29–31] When you have an increasing resistance of the stiff arteries,[32] they don't allow ease of flow,[33] resulting in hypertension. The two areas that have the most significant branches from the aorta are going to be most affected by this: the brain and the kidneys.[34,35] In the kidneys, it is the renal arteries affected by hypertension that damage the parenchyma of the kidneys; this same process occurs in the vasculature to the brain.[36]

Developing an understanding of the continuity of tissue between artery and vein helps the osteopathic practitioner to perceive what the tissues feel like. Figure 10.25 emphasises how the tissue between the artery and the vein is continuous and also blends with all of the lymphatics. Take one really important example: the carotid sheath. The function of the artery, the vein, and the vagus in the carotid sheath are all interrelated. However, as Tsamis et al found, "It is the connective fibres within this microstructure, elastin and collagen, which impart elastic properties and strength respectively."[37]

There is evidence to show that a healthy rate in the carotid artery acts like a pacemaker for the function of the parasympathetics. For example, anxiety is mediated by vagal receptors,[39,40] which serve as little pacemakers on the vagus, to restore

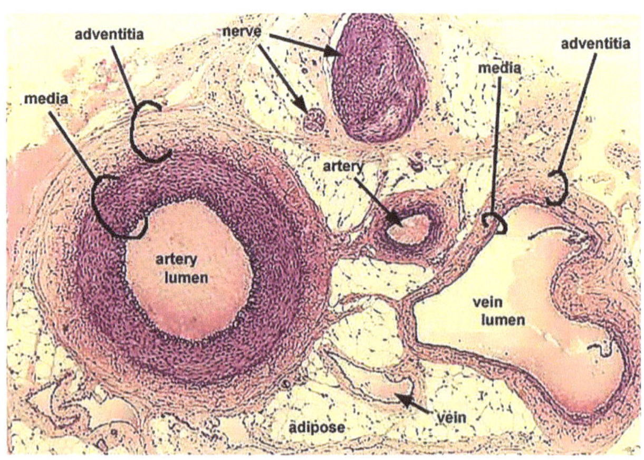


**Figure 10.25 – Continuity of the Tissues.** Image copyright David G. King, 2024, used with permission.[38]

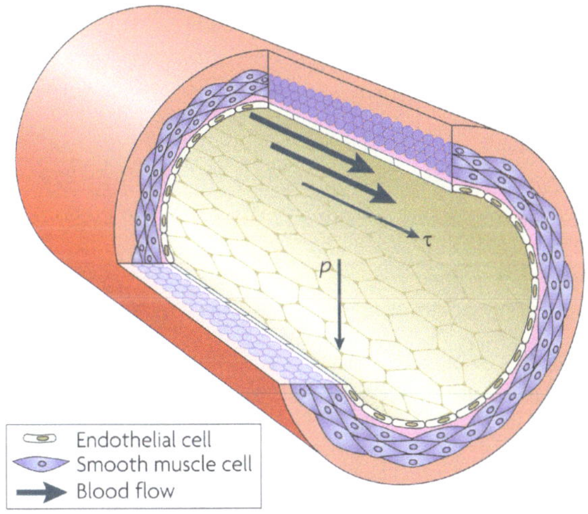


**Figure 10.26 – Blood Flow Through Lumen.** Reprinted from Hahn and Schwartz.[43]

blood flow that may have been affected by stress.

Flow performs a function. Endothelial cells experience high shear stress from blood flow. Within the endothelial cells of vessels, integrins project into the vascular lumen. Information from integrins signal that flow is normal and that parmeation of nutrients is satisfying tissue need. However, bad posture, and other biophysical influences may result in one side of the aortic bifurcation becoming turbulent, thereby affecting integrin function. That turbulent flow may result in permeation and endothelial stress. This may cause inflammation and protective plaque formation. So, the primary event in atherosclerotic formation is turbulence of the endothelial cell wall interfering with those integrins.

Hahn and Swartz found that "in a healthy, atheroresistant artery with high, laminar shear stress, endothelial cells are aligned in the direction of flow and remain in a quiescent state with low rates of both proliferation and death." In addition, Hahn and Swartz found that they express low levels of adhesion receptors and cytokines that attract leukocytes. So, vortical flow maintains a healthy endothelium (atheroprotective). Figure 10.26 demonstrates fluid shear stress (τ), or frictional force from flowing blood, acting on the endothelial cells that line the vessels.[42]

This diagram shows a healthy atheroresistant artery that has high shear stress along the endothelial cells. The cells are aligned in the direction of flow, as function and flow demand. Epithelial cells remain quiescent with low rates of proliferation and death. They express low levels of adhesion receptors and inflammatory chemicals that attract immune cells and low sympathetic signalling.

Forces associated with blood flow are major determinants of vascular morphogenesis. Blood flow is crucial for vascular development and mechanotransduction, a mechanical signal that a cell recognises as an electrical signal, sound signal or light signal, carried by things like the calcium wave and the means by which mechanical stimulus is converted into chemical activity.

In the *Nature Reviews* article, "Mechanotransduction in Vascular Physiology and Atherogenesis",[44] Hahn and Schwartz determined that **at every bifurcation there is turbulence**. According to their article, "An inevitable consequence of the branched structure of the arterial tree is the appearance of irregularities in flow at places where arteries branch or turn sharply."[45]

Bifurcations relate to chronic inflammation. In Figure 10.27, disturbed shear and turbulence develop where the red appears. There is high endothelial cell turnover, poor alignment, activated inflammatory genes, hyper-atherogenic flow and a lot of oxidative stress.

Where there is healthy vortical high shear stress, there is low endothelial cell turnover, good alignment, low permeability and an anti-inflammatory effect. Flow performs a function and it relates directly to how it developed embryologically. Remember that early in the life of the embryo, endothelial cells experienced parmeation of nutrients, which made them quiescent early on.

Mild inflammation is generally benign, however in older people, where other risk factors are present such as diabetes, hyperlipidaemia and smoking, circulating inflammatory mediators are present and it can become more severe and progress to atherosclerotic plaques. So, it is not just the turbulence alone, but turbulence combined with other factors, that results in the most deleterious effects.

If disturbed flow resolves after a short while, the fluid can revert back to normal laminar flow. However, when a person has all the other factors that are contributing to disturbed flow, as mentioned in the previous paragraph, the possibility of atherogenesis increases. This is summarised in Figure 10.28.

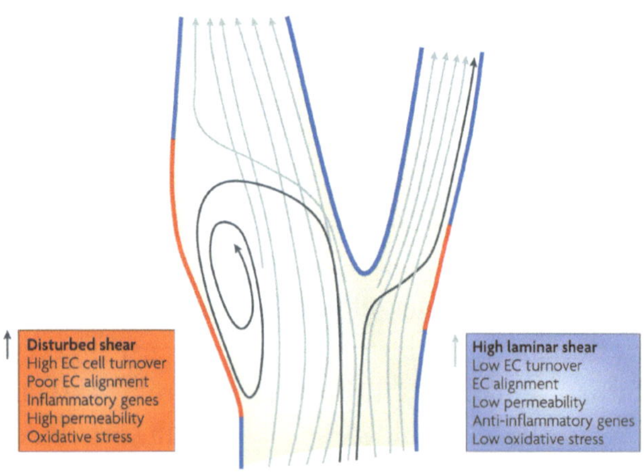


**Figure 10.27 – Disturbed Shear.** Reprinted from Hahn and Schwartz.[46]

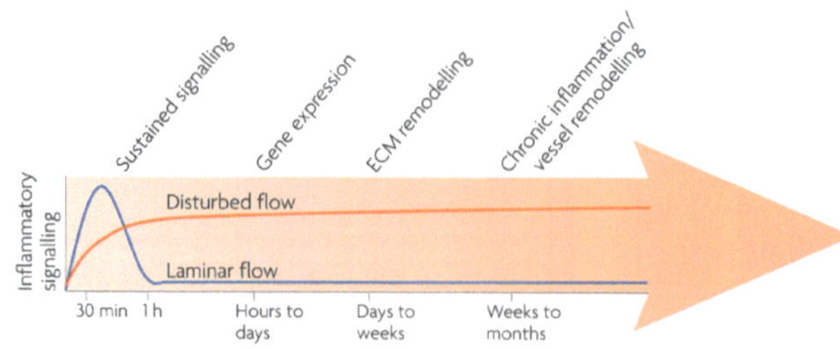


**Figure 10.28 – Inflammatory Signaling.**[47]

Cells in laminar flow, illustrated with the blue line, transiently occurring over 1 hour, activate a variety of inflammatory signalling pathways and then stop those signalling pathways when the combination of all the other factors don't exist. Disturbed healthy shear forces will activate the same pathways in a sustained manner. Changes in gene expression that occur over hours to days from such disturbed healthy flow sustains oxidative stress and the activated phenotype.

## Applications to Osteopathic Practice

Alterations in the extracellular matrix, which occur over days to weeks, lead to engagement of integrins that enhance inflammatory pathways. These changes give rise to a persistently activated phenotype that leads to chronic inflammation and vessel remodeling.

Blood vessel wall stiffness is an early risk factor for cardiovascular disease, coronary events, stroke and mortality that are often seen as age-related changes. The elastic recoil of the arteries can be seen in the elderly, but it requires a certain lifestyle. As we age, there is a decrease in the concentration

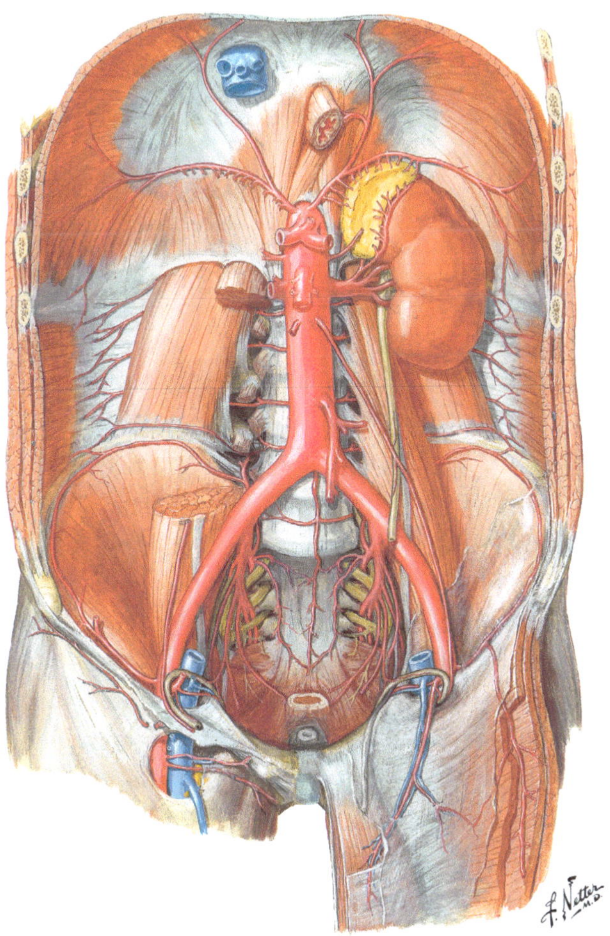

**Figure 10.29 – Ventral Branches of the Aorta.** Reprinted from Netter Images.

and quality of elastin as well as an increase in collagen and less response to the calcium wave/flux and the primary respiratory mechanism.

Figure 10.29 shows the ventral branches of the aorta: the celiac trunk (which supplies the foregut that lies below the respiratory diaphragm at the level of the junction between the 12th thoracic vertebra and first lumbar vertebra); the superior mesenteric artery that arises at the level of the intervertebral disc between the first and second lumbar vertebrae (which supplies the distal one-third of the duodenum, all of the small intestine, the ascending colon and the right half of the transverse colon); and the inferior mesenteric trunk that arises at the level of the third lumbar vertebra (which supplies the hindgut that differentiates into the left part of the transverse colon, the descending colon and the rectum). Those three arterial fulcra relate to the functions of the whole gut; the paraspinal tissues (the erector spinae), the vertebrae, the intervertebral discs, and the spinal canal all relate to the vascular fulcra.

Figure 10.30 depicts T4 that provides the fulcrum for the vasculature and respiration. This is the point where the parts of the cardiovascular system that develop ventrally (ie., the endocardial tube and the aortic arch arteries), meet the parts of the cardiovascular system that develop dorsally, (ie., the dorsal aortae).

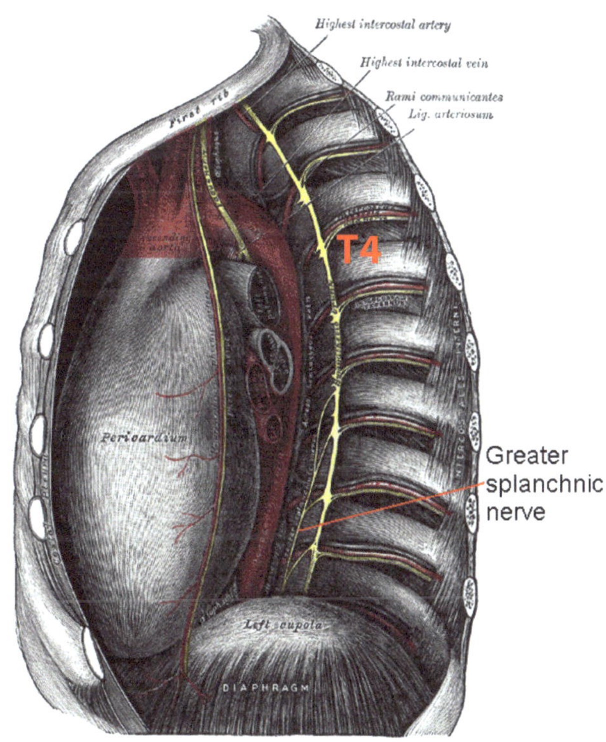


**Figure 10.30 – T4: Fulcrum for vasculature and respiration.** Reprinted from Gray.[48]

The bifurcation of the trachea (Figure 10.31) provides a fulcrum and a function; it works asymmetrically because there are three lobes in the right lung and two lobes in the left lung, providing a wringing movement. The function of that fulcrum is very similar to the function of the bifurcation of the aorta.

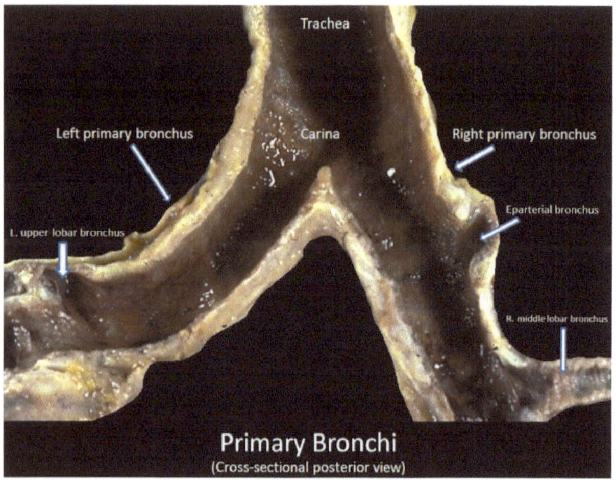


**Figure 10.31 – Bifurcation of the Trachea.**[49]

In *An Osteopathic Approach to Children*, Dr Jane Carreiro discovered a functional fulcrum at the area just to the right of T4 in her treatment of 1,600 neonates. She noted she could palpate a winding up in the meninges starting at the bregma and the coccyx **simultaneously** and moving in a spiral motion to the centre of the thorax around T4. When it reached T4, a fulcrum was created—a still point around which energy organises—and then a gradual expansion spread along the midline axis, between the head and the pelvis, the bregma and the coccyx. When it got there, a long flexion phase occurred, after which the following five phenomena were distinguishable:

- The inherent motility of the brain and spinal cord
- The fluctuation of the cerebrospinal fluid
- The reciprocal tension of the intracranial and intraspinal membrane
- The articular mobility of the cranial bones
- The involuntary motion of the sacrum between the ilia

She noted that she felt this fulcrum was somehow related to the change at birth to breathing air because this observation didn't seem to occur in neonates who did not attempt spontaneous breathing. Thus, Carreiro concluded that T4 is a point of organisation of the primary respiratory mechanism, thoracic respiration and the cardiovascular functions.[50]

When the first breath is taken, the watery fluids that have hitherto created a lot of resistance in the lungs are suddenly expelled from the lungs, which expand under the influence of atmospheric pressure. Because of the asymmetry of the lungs the right side expands more. That expansion is what produces a reciprocal back pressure in the ductus arteriosus and closes it, also causing the foramen ovale to close.

Finally, we see the landmark for gait (the pivot for how we walk) to be the bifurcation of the aorta and not the intervertebral disc between L4/5. The bifurcation of the aorta is at the level of the disc of L4/5. Our true walking fulcrum is the bifurcation of the aorta. The asymmetry in the bifurcation explains the underlying principle for the osteopathic muscle energy technique for the left-on-left sacral pattern described by Dr Gordon Zink; that slight asymmetry creates an efficiency in the way we walk. The asymmetry of our vasculature is part of the slight functional entropy that creates a pivot for more ease in walking.[51]

## Chapter 10 Endnotes

1. Erich Blechschmidt, *The Ontogenetic Basis of Human Anatomy: A Biodynamic Approach to Development From Conception to Birth* (Berkeley, CA North Atlantic Books, 2004), 158.

2. Erich Blechschmidt and Raymond F. Gasser, *Biokinetics and Biodynamics of Human Differentiation: Principles and Applications* (Springfield, IL: Charles Thomas Publishing, 1978).

3. Blechschmidt, *The Ontogenetic Basis of Human Anatomy.*

4. Gary C. Schoenwolf et al., *Larsen's Human Embryology,* 5th ed. (Philadelphia, PA: Churchill Livingstone, 2015).

5. Schoenwolf et al., *Larsen's Human Embryology.*

6. Schoenwolf et al., *Larsen's Human Embryology.*

7. Blechschmidt, *The Ontogenetic Basis of Human Anatomy.*

8. Schoenwolf et al., *Larsen's Human Embryology.*

9. Schoenwolf et al., *Larsen's Human Embryology.*

10. James Bell Pettigrew, *Design in Nature* (London, New York [etc.]: Longman, Green, and co, 1908).

11. Peter A. Stonebridge, "Three-Dimensional Blood Flow Dynamics: Spiral/Helical Laminar Flow," *Methodist Debakey Cardiovascular Journal* 7, no. 1 (January-March 2011): 21–6, https://doi.org/10.14797/mdcj-7-1-21.

12. Stonebridge, "Three-Dimensional Blood Flow Dynamics."

13. Stonebridge, "Three-Dimensional Blood Flow Dynamics."

14. Alick Bartholomew, *Hidden Nature: The Startling Insights of Viktor Schauberger* (Edinburgh: Floris Books, 2003).

15. Alexandru G. Fredriksson et al., "4-D Blood Flow in the Human Right Ventricle," *American Journal of Physiology-Heart and Circulatory Physiology* 301, no. 6 (December 2011): H2344-50.

16. Trung Bao Le et al., "Vortex Formation and Instability in the Left Ventricle," Physics of Fluids 24, no. 9 (September 2012): 91110.17. Callum Coats, *Living Energies: An Exposition of the Concepts Related to the Theories of Viktor Schauberge*r (Dublin: MH Gill & Co., 2001).

18. Henry Gray, *Anatomy of the Human Body* (Lea & Febiger, 1918), plate 493, https://en.wikipedia.org/wiki/Crista_terminalis.

19. Primary bronchi cross-sectional posterior view, https://commons.wikimedia.org/wiki/File:Primary_bronchi_cross-sectional_posterior_view.png.

20. Roberta Caccamo et al., "Endoscopic Bronchial Anatomy in the Cat," *Journal of Feline Medicine and Surgery* 9, no. 2 (April 2007): 140-9, https://doi.org/10.1016/j.jfms.2006.10.003.

21. *Gray's Anatomy: The Anatomical Basis of Clinical Practice*, 41st ed., edited by Susan Standring (Elsevier, October 2015).

22. Marie Briet et al., "Arterial Stiffness and Pulse Pressure in CKD and ESRD," *Kidney International* 82, no. 4 (August 2012): 388–400, https://www.doi.org/10.1038/ki.2012.131.

23. Stéphane Laurent and Pierre Boutouyrie, "Arterial Stiffness and Hypertension in the Elderly," *Frontiers in Cardiovascular Medicine* 7 (October 2020): 544302, https://doi.org/10.3389/fcvm.2020.544302.

24. Briet et al., "Arterial Stiffness and pulse pressure in CKD and ESRD."

25. Craig Holdrege, *The Dynamic Heart and Circulation* (Fair Oaks, CA: AWSNA Publications, 2002).

26. Ishtak Bentov, *Stalking the Wild Pendulum* (Rochester, VT: Destiny Books/Inner Traditions; Bear & Company, February 1988).

27. Ishtak Bentov, *Stalking the Wild Pendulum* (Rochester, VT: Destiny Books/Inner Traditions; Bear & Company, February 1988).

28. Ishtak Bentov, *Stalking the Wild Pendulum.*

29. M. Turzyniecka et al., "Diastolic Function Is Strongly and Independently Associated With Cardiorespiratory Fitness in Central Obesity," *Journal of Applied Physiology* 108, no. 6 (June 2010): 1568–74.

30. Walter P. Abhayaratna, Wichat Srikusalanukul, and Marc M. Budge, "Aortic Stiffness for the Detection of Preclinical Left Ventricular Diastolic Dysfunction: Pulse Wave Velocity Versus Pulse Pressure," *Journal of Hypertension* 26, no. 4 (April 2008): 758–64.

31. Yacine Aggoun et al., "Impaired Endothelial and Smooth Muscle Functions and Arterial Stiffness Appear Before Puberty in Obese Children and Are Associated With Elevated Ambulatory Blood Pressure," *European Heart Journal* 29, no. 6 (March 2008):792–799.

32. Eric J. Brunner et al., "Arterial Stiffness, Physical Function, and Functional Limitation: The Whitehall II Study," *Hypertension*, 57, no. 5 (May 2011): 1003–1009.

33. Arturo Figueroa, Florence Vicil, and Marcos A. Sanchez-Gonzalez, "Acute Exercise With Whole-Body Vibration Decreases Wave Reflection and Leg Arterial Stiffness," *American Journal of Cardiovascular Disease* 1, no. 1 (2011): 60–67.

34. Su-Yan Bian et al., "Association of Glomerular Filtration Rate With Arterial Stiffness in Chinese Women With Normal to Mildly Impaired Renal Function," *Journal of Geriatric Cardiology* 9, no. 2 (June 2012): 158–165.

35. Jun Sugawara, Koichiro Hayashi, and Hirofumi Tanaka, "Distal Shift of Arterial Pressure Wave Reflection Sites With Aging," *Hypertension* 56, no. 5 (September 2010): 920–925.

36. Alma Cypiene et al., "The Impact of Systemic Sclerosis on Arterial Wall Stiffness Parameters and Endothelial Function," *Clinical Rheumatology* 27, no. 12, (December 2008): 1517–1522.

37. Alkiviadis Tsamis, Jeffrey T. Krawiec, and David A. Vorp, "Elastin and Collagen Fibre Microstructure of the Human Aorta in Ageing and Disease: A Review," *Journal of the Royal Society Interface* 10, no. 83 (June 2013): 20121004, https://doi.org/10.1098/rsif.2012.1004.

38. David King. "Artery, vein, nerve," Histology at Southern Illinois University, https://histology.siu.edu/crr/CR025b.htm.

39. Michael S. Fanselow, "Fear and Anxiety Take a Double Hit From Vagal Nerve Stimulation," *Biological Psychiatry* 73, no. 11 (June 2013): 1043–1044, https://doi.org/10.1016/j.biopsych.2013.03.025.

40. Brandon G. Scott and Carl F. Weems, "Resting Vagal Tone and Vagal Response to Stress: Associations With Anxiety, Aggression, and Perceived Anxiety Control Among Youths," 51, no. 8 (August 2014): 718–727, https://doi.org/10.1111/psyp.12218.

41. Georg Wiora. Principle of a sonar or radar distance measurement. https://commons.wikimedia.org/wiki/File:Sonar_Principle_EN.svg#mw-jump-to-license

42. Cornelia Hahn and Martin A. Schwartz, "Mechanotransduction in Vascular Physiology and Atherogenesis," 10, no.1 (January 2009): 53-62, https://doi.org/10.1038/nrm2596.

43. Hahn and Schwartz, "Mechanotransduction in Vascular Physiology and Atherogenesis."

44. Hahn and Schwartz, "Mechanotransduction in Vascular Physiology and Atherogenesis."

45. Hahn and Schwartz, "Mechanotransduction in Vascular Physiology and Atherogenesis."

46. Hahn and Schwartz, "Mechanotransduction in Vascular Physiology and Atherogenesis."

47. Hahn and Schwartz, "Mechanotransduction in Vascular Physiology and Atherogenesis."

48. Henry Gray, (Lea & Febiger, 1918), https://commons.m.wikimedia.org/wiki/File:Greater_splanchnic_nerve.png.

49. Primary bronchi cross-sectional posterior view, https://commons.wikimedia.org/wiki/File:Primary_bronchi_cross-sectional_posterior_view.png.

50. Jane Carreiro, *An Osteopathic Approach to Children* (London: Churchill Livingston, March 2009).

51. J. Gordon Zink and William B. Lawson, "An Osteopathic Structural Examination and Functional Interpretation of the Soma," *Osteopathic Annals* 7, no. 12 (December 1979): 12-19.

# Chapter Eleven

# The Lymphatics

*"We strike at the source of life and death when we go to the lymphatics."*[1]

– Andrew Taylor Still, 1902

Since the time of Hippocrates, human anatomy and physiology have described two major aspects of circulatory function—the circulation of the blood and the drainage of lymph. In the same way that the understanding of venous drainage was less developed than that of arterial circulation, the understanding of the lymphatics has similarly been left wanting. The traditional concept of two areas of function, both separate from cerebrospinal fluid (CSF) dynamics, persisted until very recently. The revelation that lymphatic and venous drainage is inextricably woven into a single and integrated circulatory function was, at first, obscured to scientists who were still staggering from the discoveries of the arterial aspect of function.

In hindsight, the dominant arterial view of circulation was myopic and has served to highlight the deep insight of Dr Still, who accurately described the relationship of the CSF and the lymphatics in his writings more than 120 years ago. As Still wrote back then, "The lymphatics consume more of the finer fluid of the brain than the whole viscera combined."[2]

## Lymphatics – A Cornerstone of Health

Still saw the lymphatics as central to health. In 1902, he compared them to a "fire company with nozzles in all windows ready to flush the burning house."[3] The lymphatics preserve fluid homeostasis; defend against harmful bacteria, fungi, viruses, cancer cells and parasites; collect and transport digestive fat, fat-soluble vitamins and amino acids; transport white blood cells and return excess interstitial fluid to the blood. Their functions are intimately tied to the homeostasis of the interstitial spaces of the extracellular matrix (ECM).

Approximately 4,000 litres of plasma flow through a person's capillary beds each day. From that, about 40 litres of plasma leak through the vessel walls into the interstitium. Substances are then transferred from the plasma to the interstitial fluid via diffusion. This capillary ultrafiltrate combines with excess protein lying within the interstitium. The ultrafiltrate includes water, electrolytes, oxygen, glucose, amino acids, hormones, vitamins and micronutrients. It also combines with excess protein lying within the interstitium.

Ninety percent of the fluid that enters an extranodal extension or extracapsular spread returns at the venular end of the capillary bed, due mostly to osmosis. The remaining 10%—4 to 8 litres per day—includes large proteins and large particulate matter that can't be removed by absorption into the capillaries. This complex enters the lymphatic capillaries and is called lymph (Figures 11.1 and 11.2).

This return of proteins to the blood from the interstitial spaces is an essential function without which edema or pulmonary edema occurs, which can be life threatening.[4] Dr Still's observation that "We strike at the source of life and death when we go to the lymphatics"[5] emphasises how well he understood this system.

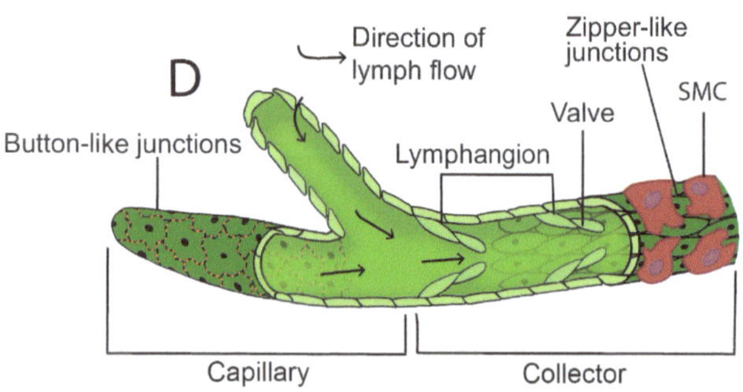


**Figure 11.1 – Terminal Lymph Capillary.** This image of a terminal lymph capillary is shown in relation to a blood capillary passing through it. Image courtesy of SGUL Lymres.[6]

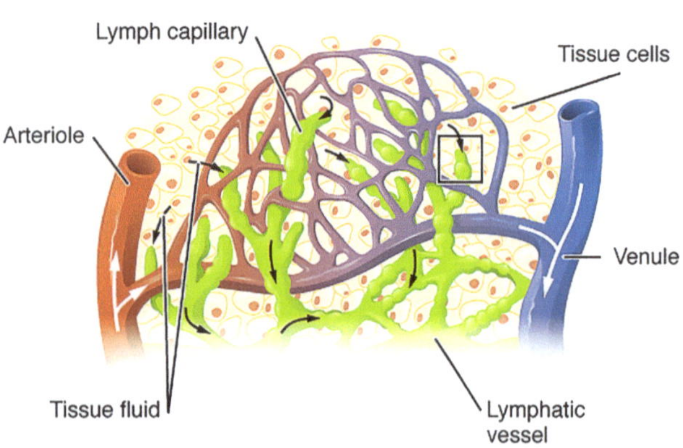


**Figure 11.2 – Lymphatic Capillary Interwoven With Blood Capillary.** Image depicting the interwoven relationships of tissue, vascular capillaries and lymphatic capillaries. Reprinted from https://commons.wikimedia.org/wiki/File:Illu_lymph_capillary.png.[7]

## Drainage From Lymph Node to Vein – An Important Interface

Fifty percent of the water, but none of the proteins, is reabsorbed by lymphatic tissues and passes into the adjacent venous system. This is an opportunity for the blood to interface with the returning lymph; to obtain and return more information to the heart from the water that has diffused back into the vein.

Moving up the lymphatic tree, the lymph becomes increasingly more concentrated so that the volume of lymph that is returned to the thoracic region is about 2 to 4 litres per day. This volume is really important on a palpatory level because the fluid is significantly more viscous and has a different quality to it than either the arterial or the venous fluid.

Ross and Pawlina assert that the lymph node directly returns 35% of the afferent lymph fluid into the venous drainage through the high endothelial venules within the deep cortex of the node.[8] Referring to Ross and Pawlina, Frank Willard has highlighted that, collectively, the lymph nodes return more lymph back to the venous system than the thoracic duct and lymphatic duct, both of which empty their contents into the left and right subclavian veins, respectively[9] (Figure 11.3).

Descriptions of the lymphatics state that they perfuse all tissues except the epidermis, cornea, bone marrow, cartilage and endomysium of muscles. Until recently it was considered that the central nervous system had no lymphatics, but recent studies confirm that lymph vessels exist in the meninges, especially next to the venous sinuses.[10–12] Furthermore, the CSF carries out the functions of

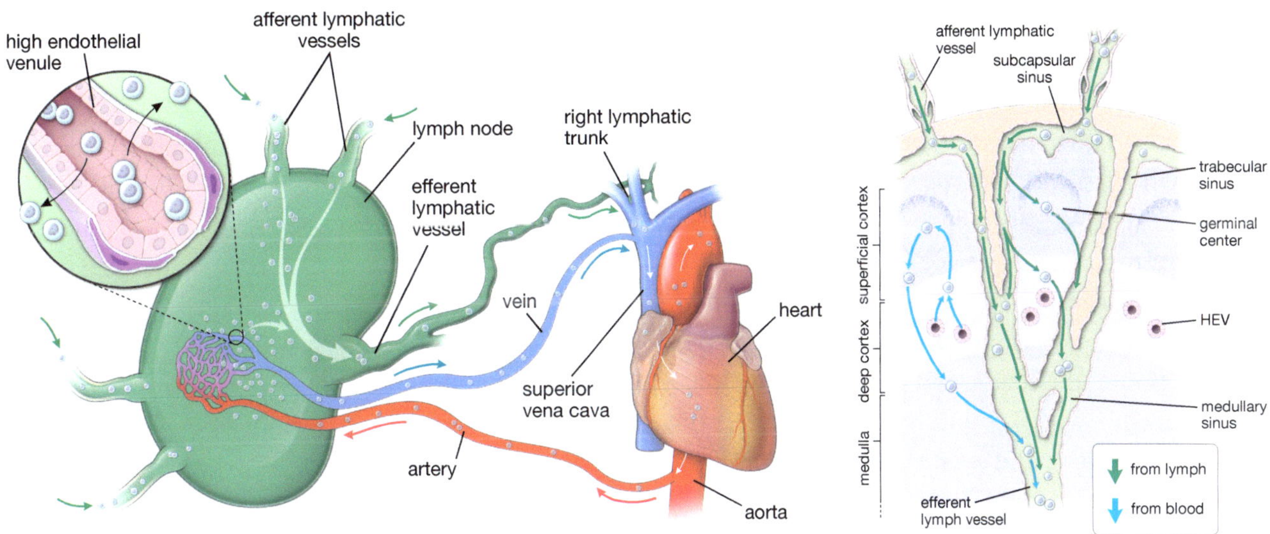


**Figure 11.3 – Drainage of Lymph Via the Veins and Right and Left Lymphatic Duct.** Here lymphocytes are seen draining into both efferent lymphatics and direct into the veins via the high endothelial venules ending in the right lymphatic duct shown here (which drains the right thorax, upper limb, head and neck) and the thoracic duct not shown (which drains the rest of the body). In the inset image, the green arrows show lymphocytes arriving at a lymph node from surrounding tissue. The blue arrows show lymphocytes arriving at the deep cortex of the node via the high endothelial venule and also ending in the superior vena cava.

the lymphatic system for the central nervous system. For the other structures, there are minute interstitial channels called *pre-lymphatics* that drain into the lymphatics directly or via diffusion, but the identification of blood vessels in the margins of the articular cartilage in knee menisci is suggestive that these pre-lymphatic channels are an integral, if modified, part of the system.[13] It is conceivable that the descriptions of lymphatic-free tissues may not be an enduring anatomic truth.

## Lymphatics – An Embryological Perspective

The development of the lymphatics had been poorly researched until recently, and there has been contention between differing theories about its development. Very early in the 20th century, Sabin demonstrated that the lymphatics were derived from the venous system.[14] More recent research has identified separate endothelial cell regulatory proteins—one for each of the arteries, veins and lymphatics—which have been shown to cross regulate each other.[15,16] These findings demonstrate the genesis of the lymphatic system to be an integral part of the circulation as a whole, with neither function separate from the other. Any understanding of the physiology of lymphatic development must always be within the context of the biomechanical forces consequent to the growth movements of the embryo.

The lymphatics may be said to exist because, in the process of embryological folding, fluid accumulates in the folds. The first place this pooling is found is in the area that will become the cervicothoracic junction in the paired jugular sacs at the junction of the subclavian and internal jugular (precardinal) veins. This occurs during week 5 of development. Soon thereafter extensions are seen in the upper limbs.

Pooling also occurs in the subdiaphragmatic space and is associated with the development of the diaphragm and the liver, becoming the unpaired retroperitoneal sac, located at the mesenteric root in the retroperitoneal space. Next, the unpaired cisterna chyli develops dorsal to the mesenteric sac. Finally, the paired posterior iliac sacs appear at the junction of the sciatic and femoral veins.

As the embryo flexes and torsions, it affects the shape, metabolism and even viability of some cells. As a consequence, fluids coalesce in some parts of the mesenchyme, notably the flexion folds; around accumulations of proteins; and other structures too big to return to the cells or circulation through the usual metabolic process of diffusion (Figure 11.4). Paul Lee refers to this as the processes of life occurring at the interstitial level.[17]

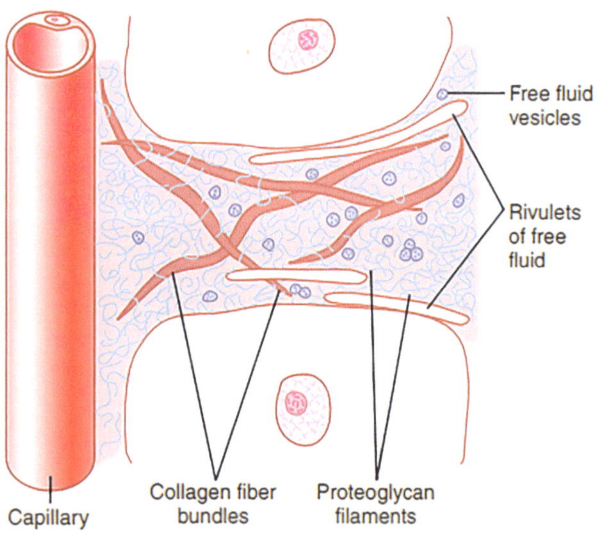


**Figure 11.4 – Structure of Interstitium.** Proteoglycan filaments are everywhere in the spaces between the collagen fibre bundles. Free fluid vesicles and small amounts of free fluid in the form of rivulets occasionally also occur.[18]

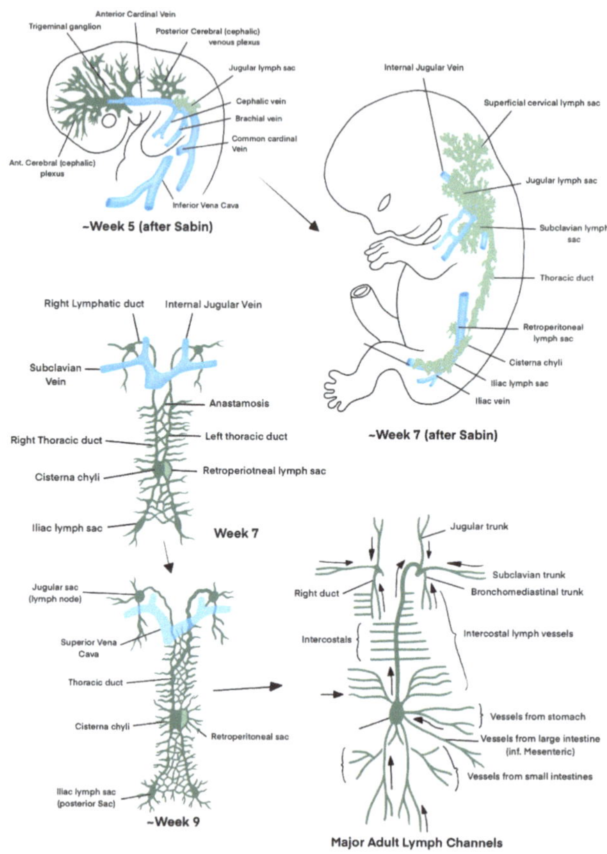


**Figure 11.5 – Weeks 5 Through 8: Paired Jugular Sacs.** Illustration by Hugh France.

One consequence of the pooling in these areas is an inherent tendency for stasis in the fluids, resulting in a change of the mechanical forces in these areas. As the pools increase in size, they exert a hydraulic pressure on the surrounding mesenchyme. The accumulating fluids in the extracellular matrix compress the endothelial cell into a long, thin, spindle-shaped cell. This cell coalesces with other nearby stretched endothelial cells to form the initial lymphatic capillary, which collect lymph.

As the cells flatten into an epithelial form in response to the pressure, they define the shape of the fluid pool. Stretch gaps also appear in the mesenchyme consequent to the mechanical pressure on the cells around the fluid. These become intercon-

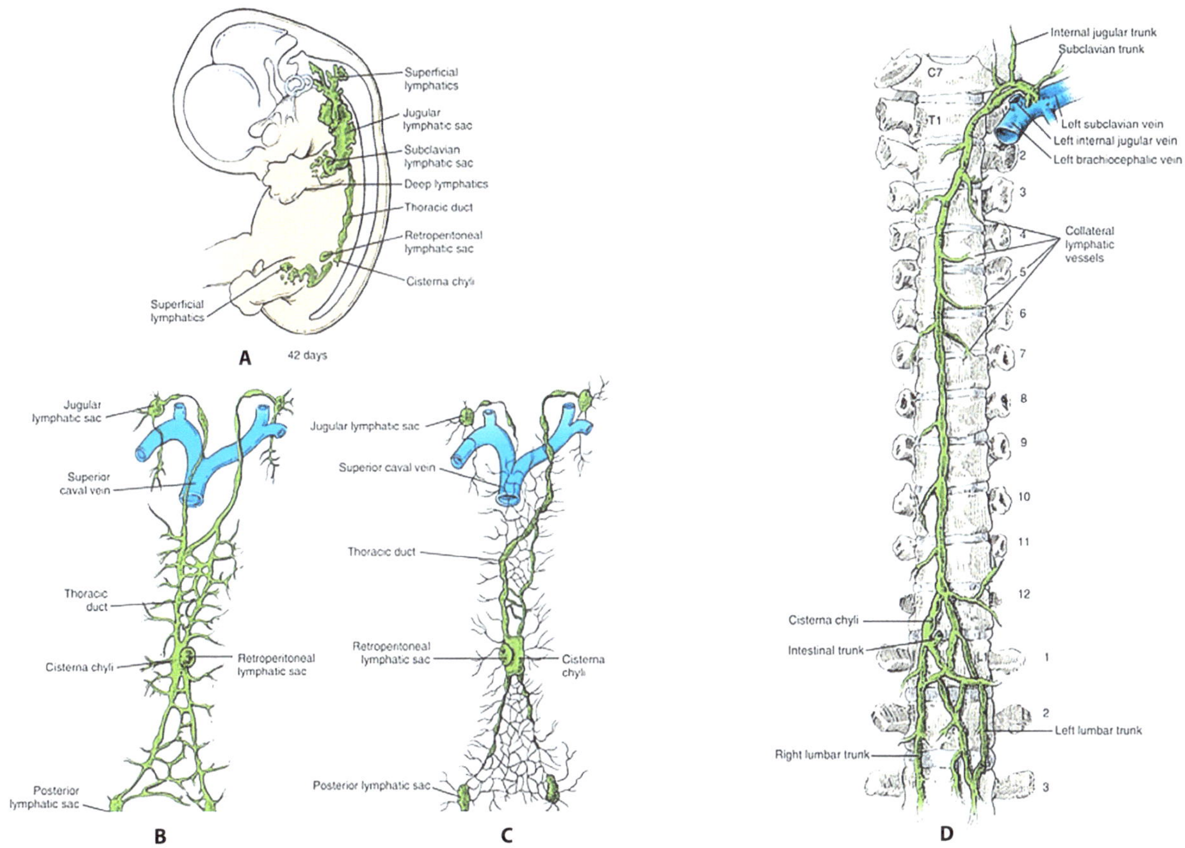


**Figure 11.6 – Lymphatic Network and Development of the Lymphatic System.** A, Several lymphatic sacs and ducts develop by lymphangiogenesis and eventually drain fluid from tissue spaces throughout the entire body. B-D, The single thoracic duct that drains the cisterna chyli and the posterior thoracic wall is derived from parts of the right and left thoracic ducts and their anastomoses. Reprinted from Schoenwolf et al.[19]

necting rivulets and exert the same hydraulic pressure that flatten adjacent cells into the epithelial cells that define the lymphatic vessels, thus allowing the fluid pools to return to circulation.

Blechschmidt described changes in fluid dynamics with the accumulation of interstitial fluid altering the shape and therefore the function of cells. Metabolic gradients form, and where accumulated extracellular fluid stretches cells, gap junctions open. As fluid pressure increases, it shapes the lymphatic endothelial cells to the necessary form and function for a foetus to an infant to a child.

During the fifth week of development, two paired and two unpaired endothelial sacs arise as outgrowths of the venous channels. These sacs form the primordia of the lymphatic system. From weeks 5 through 8, the paired jugular sacs appear first at the junction of the subclavian and internal jugular (precardinal) veins (Figure 11.5). Soon thereafter extensions are seen in the upper limbs.

In Figure 11.5, at 7 weeks (upper right), the embryo is forming primitive lymph sacs and developing vessels. At 9 weeks, the first stage of the formation of the single thoracic duct is seen from the primitive paired lymphatic plexus. The lymphatics at week 7 depict the right and left thoracic ducts connecting the right and left jugular lymph sacs with the cisterna chyli.

Next to develop is the unpaired retroperitoneal sac, located at the mesenteric root in the retroperitoneal space. Soon thereafter, the unpaired cisterna chyli develops dorsal to the mesenteric sac. Finally, the paired posterior iliac sacs appear at the junction of the sciatic and femoral veins.

By the end of the ninth week, these 6 lymphatic sacs are linked together by multiple endothelial channels to form a complicated network of lymphatic vessels (Figure 11.6).

The cisterna chyli also connects to the lower intercostal trunks, the intestinal trunk and the lumbar trunks.

By the end of the ninth week, these 6 lymphatic sacs are linked together by multiple endothelial channels to form a complicated network of lymphatic vessels.

An important point to remember is that while lymphatic vessel formation and repair slows after puberty, it continues developing throughout life.

From the periphery, the lymphatic tree starts in the matrix with the blind-ended lymphatic terminal, leading into the lymphatic capillaries, then to the collecting ducts. These flow through to a set of regional lymph nodes and then into collecting lymphatic trunks before returning to the blood at the left and right thoracic ducts.

Figure 11.5 provides a schematic of the adult form of the lymphatic tree. Notice how early the development of the adult form is evident; it forms that way because it functions that way.

Development into the adult form drives remodelling. Anteriorly, large inguinal accumulations feed into the cisterna chyli. The thoracic ducts differentiate in favour of a significantly greater flow on the right compared to the left, consequent upon a variable transfer, anywhere between T5 and T9, across the midline of the lymphatic return from the lower limbs and pelvis. The result is the drainage of the lower limb, the abdomen and the left side of the chest into that left thoracic duct. These changes in form are consequent to the whole embryo growth, with differentiation occurring within the context of its dynamic growth motion patterns. The functions of the embryo drive the structures to support itself.

As a functioning network, the lymph flows from lymphatic terminals to lymphatic capillaries and then to collecting ducts through a series of regional lymph nodes and, finally, to collecting ducts before returning at the thoracic duct (on the left) or via the right lymphatic duct.

The lymphatic terminals (Figure 11.1) arise in the capillary bed. They are embedded within the extracellular space as a network system of blind-ended, thin-walled vessels. While lymphatic cap-

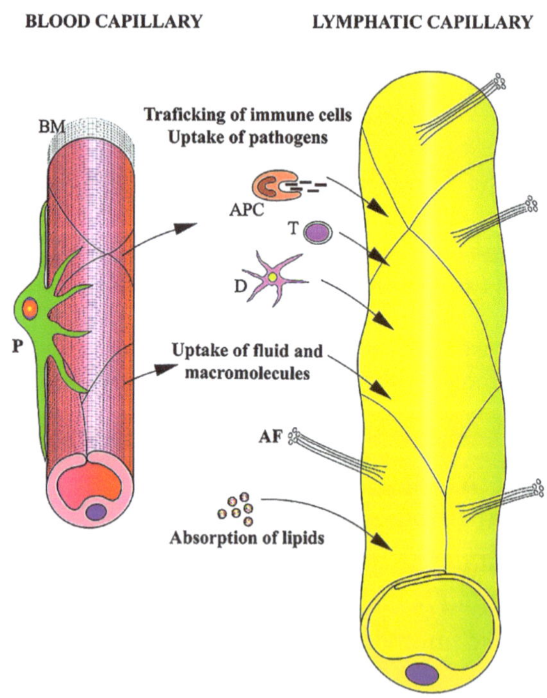


**Figure 11.7 – Blood Capillary Compared With Lymphatic Capillary.** In contrast to the blood capillary, the lymphatic capillary has poorly developed basal lamina (BM) and is devoid of pericytes (P). Lymphatic endothelium is highly attenuated, and cells are connected directly to the interstitial collagen via anchoring filaments (AF). Additional abbreviations in image: T = T cell; D = dendritic cell; APC = antigen presenting cell. Reprinted from Pepper and Skobe.[21]

illaries share the same defining endothelial cell layer as blood capillaries, they lack both a basement membrane and the presence of pericytes—the smooth muscle cells that surround the outer surface of the endothelial cells of blood vessels. Rather than having the smooth, round form of the blood vessels, lymphatic capillaries can be quite irregular; they are also two to three times larger than blood capillaries.[20] These adaptations in their form allow a lymphatic capillary to perform its functions in the uptake of macromolecules, lipids and cells from the interstitium. In Figure 11.7, a lymphatic capillary is compared to a blood capillary.

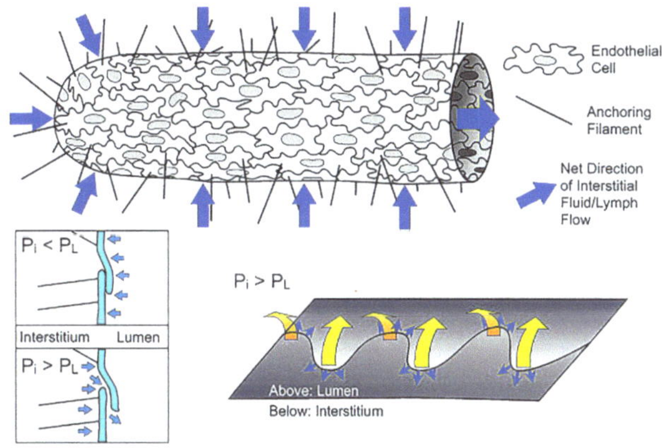


**Figure 11.8 – Valves Formed Between Endothelial Overlaps.** Initial lymphatics and lymph formation. The initial lymphatics are composed of a single layer of oak-leaf-shaped endothelial cells with discontinuous basement membrane and anchoring filaments that project into the interstitium and are the site of interstitial fluid entry (blue arrows). Fluid can pass through leaflets of cell membrane at adjacent endothelial cells when the interstitial pressure (Pi) exceeds luminal pressure (PL). The leaflets are closed when PL > Pi (bottom left; light blue arrows represent net pressure gradient) and open when PL < Pi. The sites where these leaflets are thought to open are along the far edges of the "oak leaf" junction lobes (bottom right). The yellow arrows show the direction of the leaflet movement when PL < Pi, and the small blue arrows show where fluid is thought to pass across these specialised lymphatic endothelial junctions. Reprinted from Breslin.[22,23]

## Function to Form – Initial Lymphatic Vessels

At the junction of the endothelial cells, the edge of one endothelial cell overlaps the edge of the adjacent cell in such a way that the overlapping edge is allowed to flap inwards (Figure 11.8). This forms a minute valve that opens to the interior of the capillary and gives rise to intercellular clefts. The epithelial cells are bound together with a discontinuous series of tight button junctions that support the valve structure. All the epithelial cells have a series of fine strands that serve as anchoring filaments that support the thin-walled lymphatic vessel. These disperse throughout the ECM.

The filaments are fine strands of retinaculum, extending from their insertion on the external surface of the endothelial cell membranes to imbed in the connective tissue matrix of the extracellular space. They bind the endothelial cell to the interstitium. The terminal lymphatic capillary is therefore an extension of the extracellular matrix rather than a separate entity. Terminal lymphatics may be in a state of collapse depending on the amount of fluid in the ECM.

The extracellular space or interstitial space in which the lymphatics are found is a mucopolysaccharide matrix. It is a mat of collagen fibres, and the interstices of this space are filled with a mucopolysaccharide gel-ground substance.

Collagen fibres extend long distances in the interstitial space and bind about 20% of the fluid in the space by charge. These fibres are very strong and provide most of the tensional strength of the tissue. The mucopolysaccharide gel is made up of proteoglycan filaments, which are very thin, coiled molecules composed of mostly hyaluronic acid and a little protein. They form a mat of very fine reticular filaments. The interstitial fluid, which becomes the lymph, is trapped mainly in the minute spaces among the proteoglycan filaments by charge.

The combination of the hydrophilic proteoglycan filaments and the fluid has the characteristics of a gel. Due to the high number of charged proteoglycan filaments, it is difficult for the fluid to flow easily through the tissue gel. Instead, it mainly diffuses through the gel mediated by changes in the charge gradient.

Both the mucopolysaccharide gel and the elastin fibres within the collagen matrix have elastic characteristics that allow them to expand and contract. When expanded, as more fluid enters the extracellular space, the collagen fibres are pushed apart and pockets of free fluid develop within the gel substance. When contracted, the elastic recoil of the compression of the collagen fibres and the gel reticular fibrillae seem to generate suction within the tissue spaces, thus creating the negative tissue pressure noted by Guyton.[24]

The matrix expands and contracts in response to multiple stimuli. It may be from the disruption of the calcium ion flux or from piezoelectric shifts due to altered mechanical, chemical or temperature effects. These stimuli cause pockets of free fluid to develop and be resorbed, either completely or partially, depending on what is happening. Bulk movement of fluid in the interstitial space occurs as areas of free fluid coalesce to form little rivulets that have developed due to changes in the rhythmically expanded and contracted state of the space. Fluid otherwise flows only with great resistance through the charged mucopolysaccharide matrix.

In optimal physiology, the hydrostatic pressure in the vessel is negative and the terminal vessel collapses.[25] Fluid and high molecular weight substances like protein are able to enter the terminal lymphatics due to the overlapping arrangement of the oak-leaf-shaped endothelial cells (Figure 11.9).

As interstitial fluid volume increases, it causes the tissue to swell. Rather than exaggerating the collapse of the terminal, the swelling creates a radial tension on the anchoring filaments embedded in the interstitial space (Figure 11.10). This increases the luminal space of the vessel and opens the intercellular clefts, thus enabling fluid and molecules to move into the lymphangion. With movement of fluid into the vessel, the pressure in the interstitial space decreases and the tissue decongests. The internal pressure within the terminal lymphatic vessel becomes relatively balanced to the extracellular matrix and the valves close, stopping any backflow. The dynamic of the ECM physiology therefore pumps the fluid into the vessel rather than the fluid passively draining (Figure 11.10).

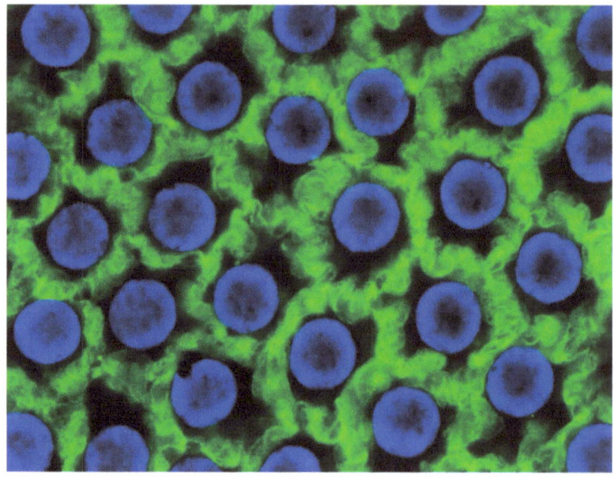

**Figure 11.9 – Endothelial Cells' Overlapping Arrangement.**[26]

With mechanical pressure on the ECM, an injection of fluid from the terminal vessel to the next part of the vessel occurs until the fluid reaches the collecting vessels in the system. At this point the epithelial cells, now involved in transport rather than collection, connect with zipper-like tight junctions and close the valves connecting the lumen to the ECM. A basement membrane now appears, as

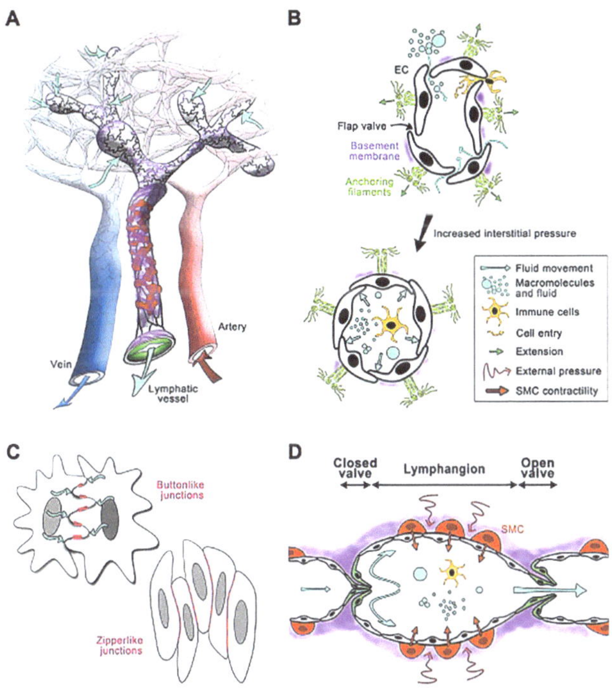


**Figure 11.10 – Organisation of Lymphatic Vasculature.** (A) The lymphatic vasculature resorbs fluid, macromolecules, and cells from the interstitium. (B) Mechanism of lymph formation in capillaries. Interstitial components penetrate lymphatic capillaries via openings between the lymphatic endothelial cells (LECs). The specialised structure of such openings prevents the return of lymph back to the interstitium. Anchoring filaments attach LECs to the extracellular matrix and prevent vessel collapse under conditions of increased interstitial pressure (black arrow). (C) Junctional organisation of LECs in lymphatic capillaries and collecting vessels. Both "buttons" and "zippers" share a repertoire of adherens and tight junction–associated proteins (eg., VE-cadherin, zonula occludens-1, occludin, and claudin-5). The main difference between them resides in their organisation (Baluk et al., 2007).[27] (D) Mechanism of lymph propulsion in collecting vessels. Coordinated opening and closure of lymphatic valves is important for efficient lymph transport. Smooth muscle cells (SMCs) covering each lymphangion possess intrinsic contractile activity. Reprinted from Schulte-Merker et al.[28]

do smooth muscle cells involved in propelling the lymph fluid back to general circulation.

Contractile actomyosin filaments have also been found attached to the endothelial cells in the terminal lymphatics, and these rhythmically push the lymph into the lymphangion. Calcium waves, described in Chapter 13, may also play a role in contracting these actomyosin filaments to perform this function.[29]

## Lymphangion Function – An Expression of the PRM

Lymphangions are the morphological functional unit of the lymphatic vessel. This includes the vessel and an internal valve, and the adjacent portion of the lymphatic vessel extending to the next valve. The lymphangion has been referred to as the "little heart" of the lymphatic system, a moniker given because of the peristaltic movement and the role T-type $Ca^{2+}$ channels play in lymphatic pacemaking.[30] Once fluid moves out of the terminal lymphatic into the collecting lymphatics, two to three layers of spiralling smooth muscle are found within the vessel. These smooth muscle cells spontaneously depolarise and generate action potentials that result in the contraction of the lymphangion.

Distension of the lymphangion wall stimulates the depolarisation of the smooth muscle cells that contract and push the fluid, opening the internal valve. As the smooth muscle relaxes, the valve closes, and this stimulates the contraction in the next lymphangion. The result is a series of contractions all the way to the lymphatic duct and along the thoracic duct until the lymph reaches the venous structures. The lymph is essentially pushed along from one collecting vessel to the next until it reaches the thoracic ducts, where the movement of venous blood back to the heart generates a degree of suction, pulling the lymph fluid into the venous stream.

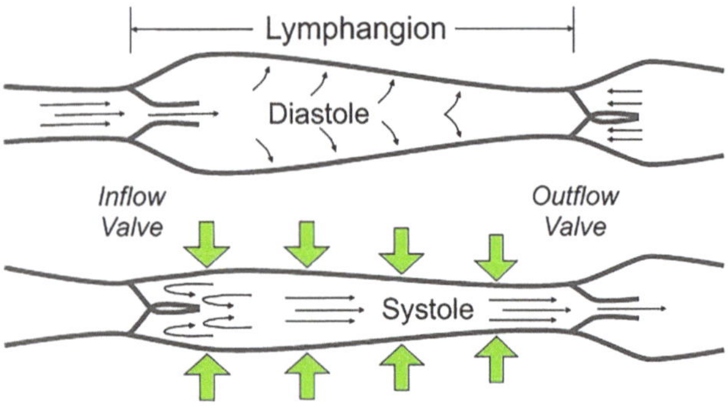


**Figure 11.11 – Lymphangion Diastole and Systole.** Like the heart, collecting lymphatics have a period of brisk contraction (systole) and relaxation (diastole) between each phasic contraction. During diastole, the inflow value of the lymphangion opens for filling. During systole, the inflow valve closes and the phasic contraction forces the lymph forward through the outflow valve. Phasic contraction frequency and force depend on the outflow pressure (afterload), the inflow pressure (preload), and the flow of lymph (shear stress).[31]

The peristaltic wave of contraction in the lymphatic vessels (Figure 11.11) is mediated by the autonomic nervous system. This rate of contraction does not occur at the same rate as the heart. Sources vary as to the rate of contraction, with some citing a rate of **5 to 8 times per minute** and others 5 to 20 times per minute. Regardless of the cited rates, the variable rate reflects the ability of the system to respond to the differing requirements of the extracellular space metabolism in different conditions.

Both external and internal mechanical stimuli can increase the rate of contractions; the presence of oedema is an example of increased internal mechanical pressure. Increases in temperature increase the rate of contractions whereas decreases in temperature decrease the rate. For example, in a situation where someone is fighting an infection, there is an associated rise in temperature. The need for the lymphatic system to function more rapidly as a part of an integrated, general immune response demands this.

The movement of fluid is a prime function of the lymphatic system, but it is also involved in the immune response. The vessels are a conduit for lymphocytes and antigen-presenting cells to regional nodes. It is at these nodes that the immune system interfaces with the lymph fluid and all it contains. During inflammation, macrophages, B cells and dendritic cells at the nodes regulate the node function via the chemokine and cytokines they secrete. Additionally, rather than being a passive vessel delivering material to immune cells, Choi and colleagues found that the lymphatic epithelial cells have the ability to modulate an inflammatory response directly by suppressing dendritic cell maturation. The process of ongoing lymphangiogenesis has also been linked to the suppression of chronic skin and joint inflammation.[32]

The increase in lymphangion contraction in the inflammatory state is indicative of the intrinsic relationship of the lymphatic system to the immune system. Hormones like epinephrine and norepinephrine and pharmacological agents like caffeine and acetylcholine have also been shown to affect lymphangion function.

When tracking the vessels from caudal to cranium, it is observed that as they coalesce and increase in size, the vessel wall becomes larger. As their size increases, they acquire more layers, with the larger collecting lymphatic trunks and vessels having three—subtly differentiated—layers.

The tunica intima, which is the innermost layer, consists of endothelium. It has an irregular appearance with a thin subendothelial layer of fibrous tissue. The tunica media contains smooth muscle cells arranged in a circular form. The tunica adventitia is mainly fibrous connective tissue with collagen, elastin and nerve fibres.

Larger lymphatic vessels and collecting ducts, like the thoracic duct, are also fortified with a plexiform vasa vasorum and nerve fibres.

In the abdomen, the drainage from the small intestine is extensive. The lymph from the intestinal field is a milky fluid containing emulsified fats and free fatty acids. Hippocrates described this as being "white blood" and called it *chyle*. The fluid is taken up by specialised terminal vessels, called lacteals, and drains into the cisterna chyli—a sac-like structure formed at the confluence of several lymphatic trunks. The cisterna chyli was one of the original lymphatic sacs, and part of it can remain as a saccular dilation or it may present as a mesh of lymphatic vessels. All lymphatic drainage from the lower extremities and pelvis pass through the cistern. Its function is intimately related to diaphragmatic function. The thoracic duct, ranging from 38 to 45 cm in length, starts at the cisterna chyli, passes through the aortic aperture and ascends to the right of the midline with the vertebral column posterior to it. The duct travels up the right side to approximately the T5 level of the spine and then crosses to the left side.

The vessel then runs up as high as the C7 transverse process, passing 3-4 cm above the level of the clavicular arches, medial to the jugular vein. It then enters into the junction of the left subclavian and internal jugular veins, though its position can vary. The junction includes a bicuspid valve that prevents retrograde flow into the lymphatic vessel.

The right lymphatic duct does not course as high as the left before entering the subclavian vein. The right duct drains the right side of the head and neck, the upper extremity, the right side of the chest and most of the lymph from the heart. As with the left lymphatic duct, the position and structure of the right duct may vary.[34]

## Lymphatic Drainage of the Heart

The lymph from the heart itself is drained outwards in atypical, valveless channels (Figure 11.12). The movement of fluid is continuous as a result of the heart's uninterrupted spiral wringing motion. Lymph passes through the valveless channels that develop around the continuous flow of the lymphatic fluid from the myocardium. The vessels organise into the subendocardial plexus and myocardial plexus. The illustration in Figure 11.13 shows the drainage of the left side of the heart.

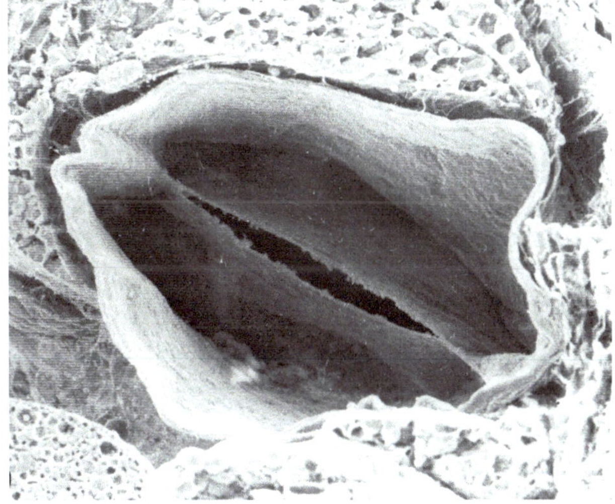

**Figure 11.12 – A Cross-sectional View of a Secondary Valve in a Pulomonary Lymphatic Vessel.** The pair of leaflets originates along the circumference of the inner lymphatic wall, projecting to the lumen of the vessel.[33]

The lymphatics are most plentiful in the left ventricle, and it is this pathway that makes up the majority of drainage from the heart. The left anterior coronary lymphatic trunk is joined by an anterior lymphatic trunk, which continues on to meet the right coronary lymphatic trunk, which lies on the anterior aspect of the pulmonary trunk.

The combined vessel then passes to the pretracheal node found between the pulmonary trunk and the arch of the aorta. From there a single vessel runs to what is called the *cardiac lymph node*. This lymph node is consistently located between the superior vena cava and the right brachiocephalic artery, and it drains to the right lymphatic duct.

The drainage of the right-hand side of the heart is more variable than that of the left with the two coronary lymphatic vessels sometimes merging where they cross before continuing up the left lym-

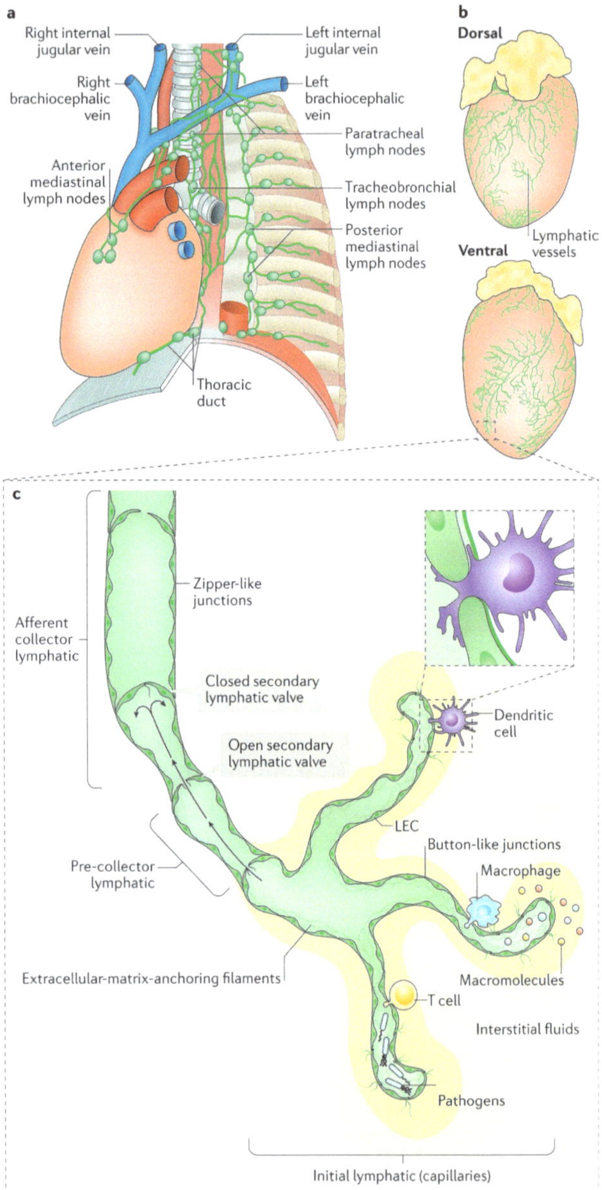


**Figure 11.13 – Structure and Function of Cardiac Lymphatic Vessels.** This image shows adult mouse cardiac lymphatics. The lymphatic endothelial cells (LEC) that are connected to the button-like junctions are collection points for fluids, pathogens and macromolecules in the interstitium. Lymph then moves through pre-collector vessels into the afferent collectors 'C' where zipper-like junctions connect to mediastinal lymph nodes.[35]

phatic duct. The contralateral drainage of the sides of the heart reflects the twisting motion of the embryologic development in the heart and displays the myocardium's spiral pattern, which facilitates the "wringing out" of the lymphatic fluids from the myocardium.[36]

The lymphatics follow the neural conducting pathways within the heart, again, following the embryological growth pattern. It has been shown[37] that an infarction of the right interventricular area will impact drainage up to the bundle of His and the atrioventricular (AV) node. The AV node drains into the left thoracic duct, and lymphedema in that area may cause delays in AV conduction. The sinoatrial node drains into the right lymphatic duct. In working with patients after myocardial infarction, consideration of the lymphatics is going to be significant (Figure 11.14).

The pericardium drains via a number of channels. Vessels from the pericardium follow the phrenic vessels, and while some of it returns to the right lymphatic duct, most is returned to the left thoracic duct.

The lymphatics of the heart valves are sparse, with the mitral valve having the greatest representation. They are thought to drain following their respective ventricles: mitral draining to the left, tricuspid to the right. It has been suggested that it is highly probable that the AV valves lymphatics are connected to that of their corresponding aortic and pulmonary valves.

We began this chapter by recalling Dr Still's assertion that the cerebral spinal fluid (CSF) and the lymphatics were connected. Tracer studies have demonstrated that a significant proportion (14%-47%) of CSF drains into deep cervical lymph nodes within a short time (Figure 11.15). When Indian ink is injected into the cisterna magna, it reaches the deep cervical lymph nodes within 1 min in a rabbit[39] and 30 min in a rat.[40]

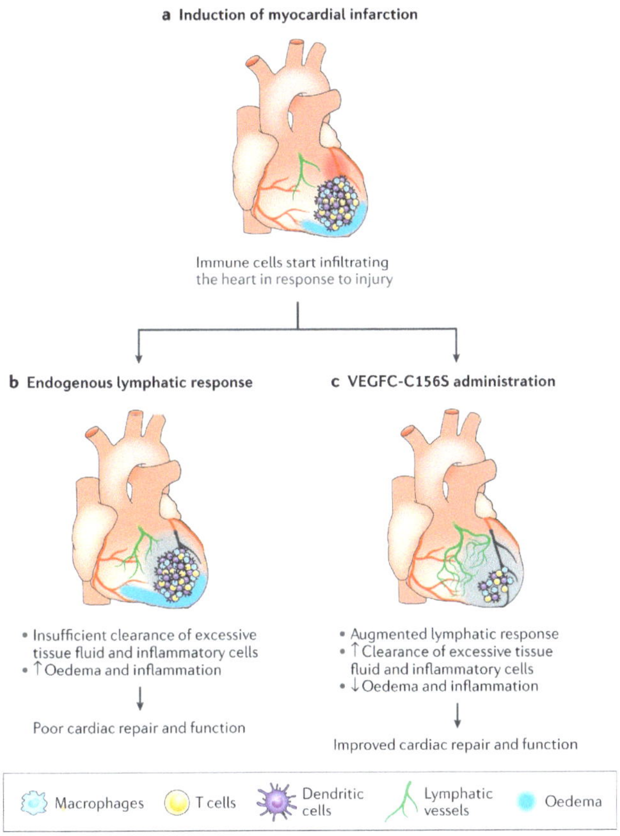


**Figure 11.14 – Cardiac Lymphatic Response to Myocardial Infarction.** Endogenous and VEGFC-C156S-augmented cardiac lymphatic response to myocardial infarction. Schematic illustration of the endogenous response of the lymphatic vessels to myocardial infarction and the augmented response induced by administration of vascular endothelial growth factor C (VEGFC)-C156S. a | After induction of myocardial infarction through surgical ligation of the left anterior descending coronary artery, accumulation of fluids leads to oedema and infiltration of immune cells, such as macrophages, dendritic cells and T cells, into the myocardium. b | In response to myocardial infarction, cardiac lymphatic vessels undergo lymphangiogenesis in an attempt to clear the excessive tissue fluid and the inflammatory cells. However, this response is insufficient and the heart is repaired through fibrotic scar formation. c | Augmentation of the lymphangiogenic response through administration of VEGFC-C156S leads to decreased oedema and increased immune cell clearance and subsequently to improved cardiac healing and function.[38]

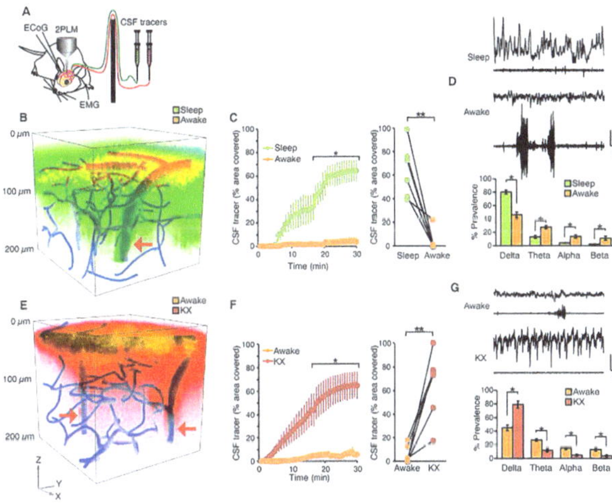


**Figure 11.15 – Wakefulness Suppresses Influx of CSF Tracers.** (A) Shows the experimental setup used for two-photon imaging of cerebral spinal fluid (CSF) tracer movement in real time. (B) Shows the distribution of CSF tracers injected in a sleeping mouse and then again after the mouse was awakened. (E) Three-dimensional reconstruction of CSF tracer influx into the mouse cortex. Arrows point to penetrating arteries. (F) Comparison of time-dependent CSF influx in awake versus anesthesia. (Right) The tracer intensity during the two arousal states at the 30-min time point was compared. $^{**}P < 0.01$, *t* test. (G) Electrocochleography and electromyography recordings in the awake mouse and after administration of ketamine/xylazine. Power spectrum analysis of all the animals analysed in the two arousal states. Reprinted from Xie et al.[41]

## Glymphatics

The routes the fluid takes are yet to be fully understood but current research has given some insight. In 2013, Maiken Nedergaard and her team at Rochester Medical Center discovered a previously unknown brain cleansing system, a "shadow plumbing system", more formally referred to as the *glymphatic system*. This highly-organised system of "piggybacking pipes" utilises glial cells to clear waste from the brain, functioning in a similar way to the lymphatic system throughout the rest of the body. What they found was a system that travels along the outside of the blood vessels, forcefully pumping CSF through a dense web of aquaporins (channels created by projections from glial astrocytes) that deliver nutrients and clear waste.[42] Xie et al found a pathway through the subarachnoid space surrounding the olfactory bulbs, through the cribriform plate, and into the lymphatics of the nasal mucosa.[43] Dr Sutherland was aware of this fact and mentioned that sneezing resulted in a sudden increase in CSF draining from the cribriform plate.[44]

In 2015, Louveau et al published an article in *Nature* on the structural and functional features of the lymphatics of the central nervous system lining the dural sinuses, which they discovered while researching T-cell gateways in the meninges. Louveau and his team found the following:

> "These structures express all of the molecular hallmarks of lymphatic endothelial cells, are able to carry both fluid and immune cells from the cerebrospinal fluid, and are connected to the deep cervical lymph nodes. The unique location of these vessels may have impeded their discovery to date, thereby contributing to the long-held concept of the absence of lymphatic vasculature in the [central nervous system]."[45]

That same year, Aspelund and his team published similar results in *The Journal of Experimental Medicine,* as well as some images captured using the newly developed immunofluorescence, a staining technique that uses fluorophores to visualise various cellular characteristics.[46] Figure 11.16 shows a dural lymphatic vascular system that drains brain interstitial fluid and macromolecules within mouse meninges; lymphatic vessels (red) are shown alongside the blood vasculature (green).

Aspelund and colleagues stated,

> "Here we report the surprising finding of a lymphatic vessel network in the dura mater of the mouse brain. We show that dural lymphatic vessels absorb CSF from the adjacent subarachnoid space and brain interstitial fluid (ISF) via the glymphatic system. Dural lymphatic vessels transport fluid into deep cervical [lymph nodes] via foramina at the base of the skull."[48]

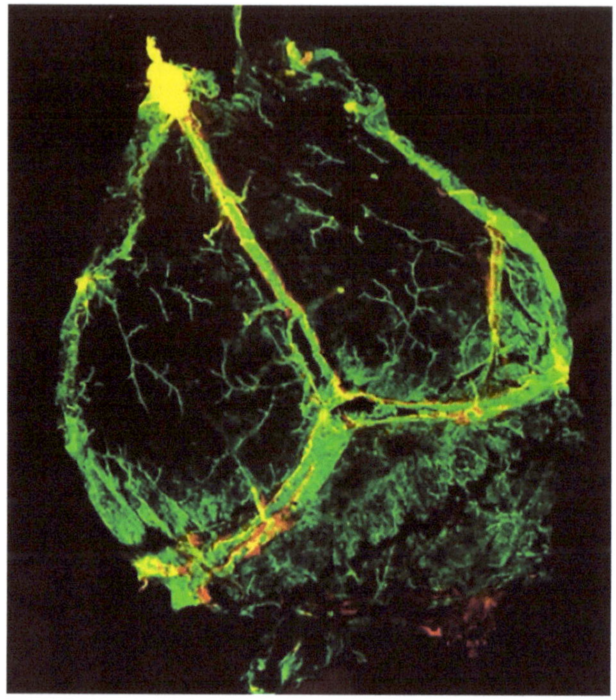

**Figure 11.16 – Dural Lymphatic Vascular System Within Mouse Meninges.**[47]

Still's insight, as recorded in his writings, was that the lymphatics can "consume more of the finer fluid of the brain than the whole of the viscera combined".[49] The recent description of the whole lymphatic system has been a validation of his insight and vindication of osteopathic approaches that have been in use for many years.

Just recently in 2022,[50] meningeal lymphatic vessels have been shown to have dural lymphatic structures along the dural venous sinus (Figure 11.16).

Glymphatic drainage in the human brain is via the cribriform plate anteriorly, via the cranial and spinal epidural spaces to cervical lymph nodes, and along cranial nerves ventrally.

Additionally, direct connections were detected between glymphatic channels along the cranial

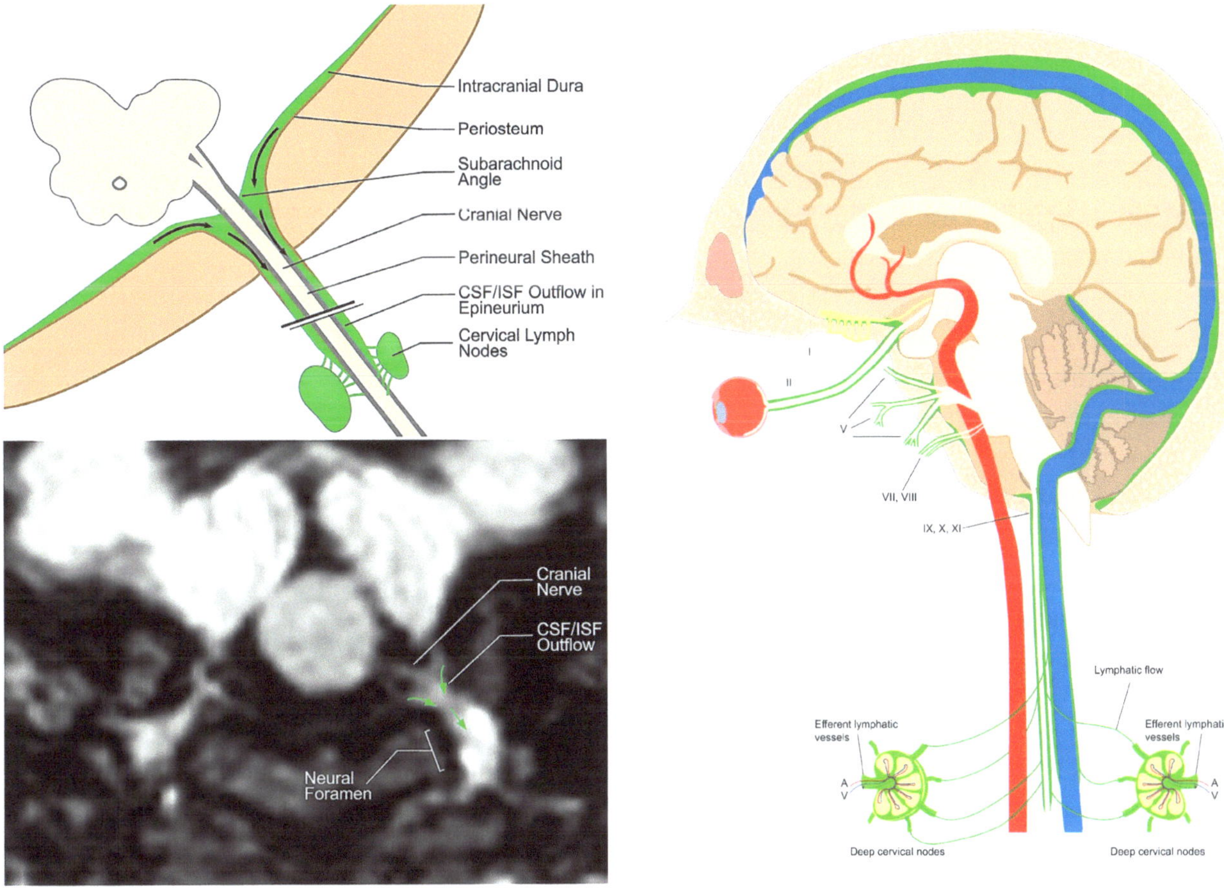


**Figure 11.17 – Extensive connections between the glymphatics and cranial and spinal nerves.**

nerves, adjacent blood vessels and cervical lymph nodes. Still wrote, "Finer nerves dwell with the lymphatics than even with the eye…. No atom can leave the lymphatics in an imperfect state and get a union with any part of the body. There the atom obtains form and knowledge of how and what to do."[51] How insightful he was!

Figure 11.17 shows a transverse section of a terminal lymphangion, which has these long, flattened epithelial cells in its wall; the cells overlay each other and the overlapping is the mechanism of a valve presentation. Although the lymphatic vessel has no associated basement membrane, it does have a series of little strands that are the anchoring filaments that support the thin-walled lymphatic vessel.

These filaments are fine strands of retinaculum that extend from their insertion on the external surface of the endothelial cell membranes and imbed themselves in the connective tissue matrix of the extracellular space. They blend the endothelial cell to the interstitium. The terminal lymphatic capillary is therefore an extension of the ECM rather than a separate entity.

There is a cycling accumulation of fluid, including molecules, in the ECM. This creates a swelling of the associated cells, and the pressure facilitates an opening of the overlap between the epithelial cells. This enables fluid and molecules to move into the lymphangion. As the extracellular pressure around the lymphangion reduces with the inward movement of fluid, the flaps and the internal pressure become relatively balanced to the ECM. As a result, the flaps close. As mechanical pressure in the ECM is expressed, there is an injection of fluid from one part of the lymphangion to the next.

## Formation of Lymph Vessels – Evidence for Blechschmidt's Principles

In 2012, Paz et al validated Blechschmidt principles by demonstrating how lymph vessels form.[52] The accumulating fluids in the ECM compress the endothelial cell into a long, thin, spindle-shaped cell (Figures 11.18 and 11.19). This cell coalesces with other nearby stretched endothelial cells to form the initial lymphatic capillary, collecting the lymph.

This understanding supports the notion of the differentiation of tissues forming from the outside in that it is not a gene-driven event—it is under biodynamic and fluid mechanical influences.

So, a function, *used* in embryological development, prepares the function *needed* in adulthood. It is also important to remember that lymphatic vessel formation and repair continues in adult life.

Typically, we talk about the lymph draining, but it does not really do this. The hydrostatic pressure is negative, but it is broken by valves and nodes. So how does the lymph enter into the terminal lymphatic and end up back in the venous system?

When we are treating someone with a conduction problem, it is important to bear in mind that the AV node drains to the left to the thoracic duct, and that the SA node drains to the right lymphatic duct.

When considering valve problems (although they are lightly lymphatic, the mitral has the most), recall that they are thought to drain following their respective ventricles; mitral draining to the right, tricuspid to the left.

The routes the fluid takes is yet to be fully understood. The current research into the glymphatic system may shed some more light.

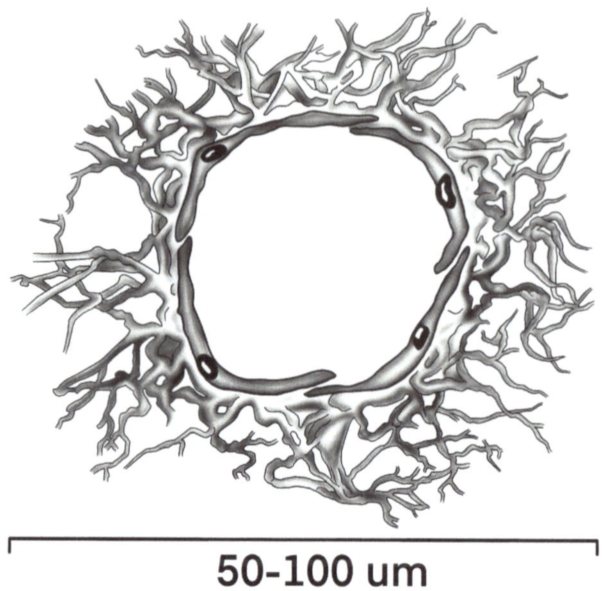


**Figure 11.18 – Transverse Section of a Terminal Lymphangion.** Illustration by Hugh France.

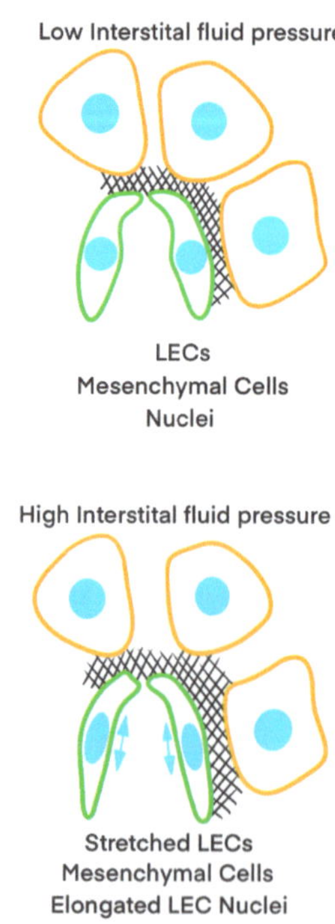


**Figure 11.19 – Nuclear LEC Elongation - Function Shapes Form.** LEC = lymphatic endothelial cell. Illustrations by Hugh France.

## Applications to Osteopathic Practice

The lymphatic system performs essential physiological functions for protein homeostasis and immune surveillance. Eighty-five percent of blood that returns to the heart is drained by the venous system. Fifteen percent leaves the circulation and enters interstitial spaces that are drained by the lymphatic system.

Lymphatic drainage into the thoracic ducts is purposeful and organised by the syphoning forces in the subclavian veins. Tissue respiration helps to guide excess fluids into terminal lymphangions. Osteopaths recognise this as an effect of primary respiration in the extracellular matrix (ECM). The importance of somatic dysfunction and lymphatic drainage is emphasised when the response of the ECM is altered by trauma or disease.

Understanding the function of the liver and gastrointestinal tract to produce approximately 70% of lymph emphasises the importance of these organs in the momentum of lymph and their roles in immunity. Recognising that 30% of lymph is reabsorbed in the lymph glands once again underscores the importance and relevance of tissue respiration.

The biomechanics of lymphatic flow provides a guide to Osteopaths in how to sequence their treatment. This will optimise treatment outcomes and prevent adverse reactions.

An analysis is made of the lower extremities and the syphoning strength of the lymph nodes at the groin.

Next, the mesenteric stem can be assessed via the umbilicus, which in a slender patient overlies the body of L3. The root of the mesentery contains the superior mesenteric vein, lymphatics and lymph nodes as well as autonomic nerves. From the umbilicus the mesenteric stem is followed from above-right (patient's left) to below-left (patient's right). Points of pain, often associated with inflammation and congestion, are noted. A gentle compression is applied and then lifting to enhance lymphatic syphoning.

Below the lowest point of the mesenteric stem, the caecum area is found. The iliocaecal valve frequently requires attention. Find the point of balanced tension in the mesenteric tissue and maintain that point of tension as the inherent forces are engaged. Observe a release or softening, or an improvement in fluid function.

Repeat the same process with the mesentery related to the ascending, descending and sigmoid colon.

Next assess the function of the cisterna chyli, that may have a varied configuration of nodes converging on the cisterna. There is a cluster of nodes around the entrance to the Cisterna Chyli which is variable (Figure 11.20).

Gather the tissue around the cisterna, observing any congestion or points of pain, match the tension and find the balance point. As the release occurs an increase in suction occurs.

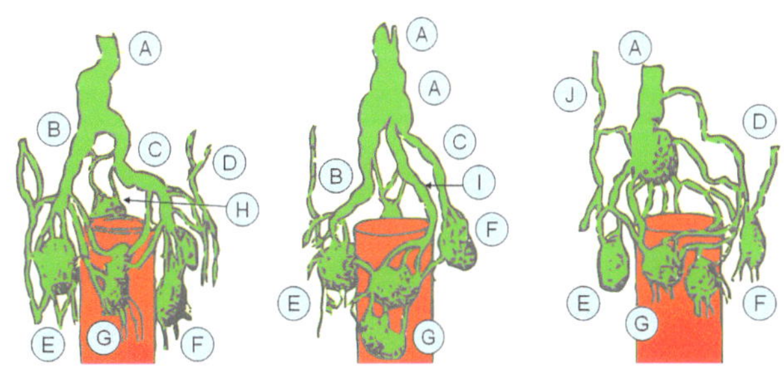


**Figure 11.20 – Cisterna Chyli.**[53]

The crossover of the lymphatic duct is particularly important and should always receive attention.

The lymphatic channels from the heart's left ventricle empty into the junction of the internal jugular and subclavian veins. The left clavicle and first rib are important in that they can influence the function at the junction. Achieving a balance of the fascia and articulatory tissues will improve the suction of lymph at the junction.

In the cranium, the function/tension of the anterior dural girdle is assessed and its functional link to the free border of the tentorium is observed. The drainage of the superior and inferior sagittal sinus, the cavernous, petrosal and basilar sinuses is assessed in relation to the reciprocal tension membrane. The inherent motion and function of the ethmoid (and particularly the cribriform plate) is observed. All the above information is considered in relation to glymphatic cranial function.

## Before Moving On

The following links provide visual examples of some of the topics discussed in this chapter. For those reading the print version, a QR code is included for each video for your convenience.

A video in real time of lymphatic drainage can be seen at https://www.youtube.com/watch?app=desktop&v=cPirnvc5x9o. This video shows the rhythmic collapse of the lymphatic wall as lymphatic fluid is passed from one lymphangion to another.

A beautiful film in black and white recorded by Dr Klabunde in 1991 can be viewed at https://m.youtube.com/watch?v=eIThhKUTBeg. It shows spontaneously contracting lymphatic vessels found in the mesentery of an anesthetised rat.

The video at https://www.youtube.com/watch?v=Rqs0yC9Ei_8 shows our lymphangion in action.

These YouTube videos are shown in real time and give a sense of how slow the pulsatile movement of lymph is. The videos also show the movement of blood running along these vessels accompanying the lymphatics and the pulsatile movement in them as well. It also shows an ebb and flow of particles within the lymphangion.

## Chapter 11 Endnotes

1. A.T. Still, *Philosophy and Mechanical Principles of Osteopathy* (Kansas City, MO: Hudson-Kimberly Pub Co., 1902).

2. Still, *Philosophy and Mechanical Principles of Osteopathy*.

3. Still, *Philosophy and Mechanical Principles of Osteopathy*.

4. Achilles J. Pappano and Withrow Gil Wier, "The Microcirculation and Lymphatics," in *Cardiovascular Physiology* (10th Ed.), (Elsevier, 2013), 153–170, https://doi.org/10.1016/B978-0-323-08697-4.00008-3.

5. Still, *Philosophy and Mechanical Principles of Osteopathy*.

6. SGUL Lymres, Lymphatic capillary and collector.tif, Wiki Commons Images, accessed September 22, 2023, https://commons.wikimedia.org/wiki/File:Lymphatic_capillary_and_collector.tif.

7. Lymph capillaries in the tissue spaces, Wiki Commons Images, accessed September 22, 2023, https://commons.wikimedia.org/wiki/File:Illu_lymph_capillary.png.

8. Michael H. Ross and Wojciech Pawlina, *Histology: A Text and Atlas* (Philadelphia: Wolters Kluwer/Lippincott Williams & Wilkins Health, 2011), 509.

9. Michael H. Ross and Wojciech Pawlina, *Histology: A Text and Atlas* (Philadelphia: Wolters Kluwer/Lippincott Williams & Wilkins Health, 2011), 469.

10. Sandro Da Mesquita et al., "Functional Aspects of Meningeal Lymphatics in Ageing and Alzheimer's Disease," *Nature* 560 (2018): 185-91.

11. Aleksanteri Aspelund et al., "A Dural Lymphatic Vascular System That Drains Brain Interstitial Fluid and Macromolecules," *Journal of Experimental Medicine* 212, no. 7 (June 2015): 991-9.

12. Martina Absinta et al., "Human and Nonhuman Primate Meninges Harbor Lymphatic Vessels That Can Be Visualized Noninvasively by MRI," *Elife* 6 (October 2017): e29738.

13 Van Schie, P., van der Lelij, T.J.N., Gerritsen, M. *et al.* Intraoperative assessment of the vascularisation of a cross section of the meniscus using near-infrared fluorescence imaging. *Knee Surg Sports Traumatol Arthrosc* 30, (2022): 1629–1638, https://doi.org/10.1007/s00167-021-06690-w.

14. Florence R. Sabin, "On the Origin of the Lymphatic System From the Veins and the Development of the Lymph Hearts and Thoracic Duct in the Pig," *American Journal of Anatomy* 1, no. 3 (May 1902): 367-89, https://onlinelibrary.wiley.com/doi/10.1002/aja.1000010310.

15. Inho Choi, Sunju Lee, and Young-Kwon Hong, "The New Era of the Lymphatic System: No Longer Secondary to the Blood Vascular System," *Cold Spring Harbor Perspectives in Medicine* 2, no. 4 (April 2012): a006445.

16. Yulia A. Komarova et al., "Protein Interactions at Endothelial Junctions and Signaling Mechanisms Regulating Endothelial Permeability," *Circulation Research* 120, no. 1 (January 2017): 179-206, https://doi.org/ 10.1161/CIRCRESAHA.116.306534.

17. R. Paul Lee, "The Living Matrix: A Model for the Primary Respiratory Mechanism," *Explore* 4, no. 6 (November-December 2008): 374-8.

18. Arthur Guyton and John Hall, "Chapter 16: The Microcirculation and Lymphatic System: Capillary Fluid Exchange, Interstitial Fluid, and Lymph Flow," *Guyton and Hall Medical Textbook of Physiology,* 12th ed. (Philadelphia: Saunders-Elsevier, 2011), 180.

19. Gary C. Schoenwolf et al., *Larsen's Human Embryology* (Philadelphia: Elsevier, 2015).

20. Michael S. Pepper and Mihaela Skobe, "Lymphatic Endothelium: Morphological, Molecular and Functional Properties, *Journal of Cell Biology 163*, no. 2 (October 2003): 209-13.

21. Pepper and Skobe, "Lymphatic Endothelium."

22. Jerome W. Breslin, "Mechanical forces and lymphatic transport," *Microvascular Research* 96 (November 2014): 46-54, https://doi.org/10.1016/j.mvr.2014.07.013.

23. "Lymph Channels of the Body," BrainKart, accessed February 24, 2023, https://www.brainkart.com/article/Lymph-Channels-of-the-Body_19286/

24. Arthur C. Guyton, Malcolm Frank and Berry Abernathy. "A Concept of Negative Interstitial Pressure Based on Pressures in Implanted Perforated Capsules," *Circulation Research*. April 1963;12:399–414.

25. Robert P. Weenik and Thijs T. Wingelaar, "The Circulatory Effects of Increased Hydrostatic Pressure Due to Immersion and Submersion," *Frontiers in Physiology* 12 (July 2021): 699493.

26. "Cell Flower," Wikimedia Commons, accessed September 22, 2023, https://commons.wikimedia.org/wiki/File:Cell_flower-1.jpg.

27. Peter Baluk et al., "Functionally Specialized Junctions Between Endothelial Cells of Lymphatic Vessels," *Journal of Experimental Medicine* 204, no. 10 (September 2007): 2349–62.

28. Stefan Schulte-Merker, Amélie Sabine, and Tatiana V. Petrova, "Lymphatic Vascular Morphogenesis in Development, Physiology, and Disease," *Journal of Cellular Biology* 193, no. 4 (May 2011): 607–18. https://doi.org/10.1083/jcb.201012094

29. Lee, R Paul, "The Living Matrix: A Model for the Primary Respiratory Mechanism," *Explore (New York, N.Y.)* vol. 4, no. 6 (2008): 374-8. https://doi.org/10.1016/j.explore.2008.08.003.

30. Dirk F. van Helden, "The Lymphangion: A Not so 'Primitive' Heart," *Journal of Physiology* 592, no. 24 (December 2014): 5353-4, https://doi.org/10.1113/jphysiol.2014.286039.

31. Jerome W. Breslin, "Mechanical Forces and Lymphatic Transport," *Microvascular Research* 96 (2014): 46-54, https://doi.org/10.1016/j.mvr.2014.07.013.

32. Inho Choi, Sunju Lee, and Young-Kwon Hong, "The New Era of the Lymphatic System: No Longer Secondary to the Blood Vascular System," *Cold Spring Harbor Perspectives in Medicine* 2, no. 4 (April 2012): a006445.

33. Jerome W. Breslin et al., "Lymphatic Vessel Network Structure and Physiology," *Comprehensive Physiology* 9, no. 1 (January 2019): 207-299.

34. "Variations of the Entry of the Thoracic Duct into the Venous System," in *Vascular Surgery*, eds. G. Heberer and R.J.A.M. van Dongen (Berlin, Heidelberg: Springer-Verlag, 1989).

35. Konstantinos Klaourakis, Joaquim M. Vieira, and Paul R. Riley, "The Evolving Cardiac Lymphatic Vasculature in Development, Repair and Regeneration," *Nature Reviews Cardiology* 18 (January 2021): 368–79.

36. Marios Loukas et al., "A General Outline of the Cardiac Lymphatic System," in *The Cardiac Lymphatic System: An Overview*, ed. Ganga Karunamuni (New York: Springer, 2013).

37. Loukas, *The Cardiac Lymphatic System,* 11.

38. Konstantinos Klaourakis, Joaquim M. Vieira, and Paul R. Riley, "The Evolving Cardiac Lymphatic Vascualture in Development, Repair and Regeneration," *Nature Reviews Cardiology* 18, no. 5 (January 2021): 368-79, https://doi-org.fortlewis.idm.oclc.org/10.1038/s41569-020-00489-x.

39. R. Deane, A. Sagare and B. V. Zlokovic, "The Role of the Cell Surface LRP and Soluble LRP in Blood-Brain Barrier Abeta Clearance in Alzheimer's Disease," *Current Pharmaceutical Design* 14, no. 16 (2008): 1601-5.

40. Kevin Hellman et al., "Genetic Evidence for a Role for Protein Kinase A in the Maintenance of Sleep and Thalamocortical Oscillations," *Sleep* 33, no. 1 (January 2010): 19-28.

41. Lulu Xie et al., "Sleep Drives Metabolite Clearance from the Adult Brain," *Science* 342, no. 6156 (October 2103), https://doi.org/

42. Scientists Discover Previously IUnknown Cleansing System in the Brain," University of Rochester, published August 15, 2012, https://www.urmc.rochester.edu/news/story/scientists-discover-previously-unknown-cleansing-system-in-brain.

43. Xie et al., "Sleep Drives Metabolite Clearance."

44. William G. Sutherland, *Teachings in the Science of Osteopathy* (Rudra Press, 1990), 82.

45. Antoine Louveau et al., "Structural and functional features of central nervous system lymphatics," Author manuscript, PubMed Central (January 16, 2016), published in final form in *Nature* 523, no. 7560 (July 2015): 337–41.

46. Lekan Oyejide, Odete R. Mendes and Igor Mikaelian, "Molecular Pathology," *A Comprehensive Guide to Toxicology in Preclinical Drug Development* (Academic Press, 2013), 237-76, https://doi.org/10.1016/B978-0-12-387815-1.00010-1.

47. Antoine Louveau et al., "Structural and Functional Features of Central Nervous System Lymphatic Vessels," *Nature* 523, no. 7560 (July 2015): 337-341, https://doi.org/10.1038/nature14432.

48. Aleksanteri Aspelund et al., "A Dural Lymphatic Vascular System That Drains Brain Interstitial Fluid and Macromolecules," *Journal of Experimental Medicine* 212, no. 7 (June 2015): 991-9. https://doi.org/10.1084/jem.20142290.

49. A.T. Still, *The Philosophy of Osteopathy* (Kansas City: Hudson-Kimberly Pub. Co., 1899), 104.

50. Mehmet Sait Albayram et al., "Non-invasive MR Imaging of Human Brain Lymphatic Networks With Connections to Cerivical Lymph Nodes," *Nature Communications* 13, no. 1 (January 2022): 203, https://doi.org/10.1038/s41467-021-27887-0.

51. Still, *Philosophy and Mechanical Principles of Osteopathy*, 66.

52. Lara Planas-Paz et al., "Mechanoinduction of Lymph Vessel Expansion," *The EMBO Journal* 31, no. 4 (February 2012): 788-804.

53. Henry Gray, *Anatomy of the Human Body* (Lea & Febiger, 1918), https://en.wikipedia.org/wiki/Cisterna_chyli.

# Chapter Twelve

# The Circle of Willis

*"A disturbed artery mark[s] the period to an hour and minute, when disease begins to sow its seeds of destruction in the human body."*[1]

– Andrew Taylor Still, 1901

The circle of Willis is an anastomosis of several arteries located at the base of the brain, winding around the optic chiasm and the stalk of the pituitary gland. It supplies important communications between the blood supply of the forebrain and hindbrain (ie, between the internal carotid and vertebrobasilar systems following obliteration of primitive embryonic connections).

## The Circle of Willis – A Harmonising of Anterior and Posterior Flow

The structure of the circle of Willis (Figure 12.1) includes the left and right internal carotid arteries, the middle and anterior cerebral arteries, the posterior cerebral arteries and the rostral branches of the basilar artery.

Both the nervous and vascular systems comprise highly branched and complex networks. Both networks also exhibit a certain degree of plasticity and undergo dynamic remodeling postnatally. The concept of activity-induced vascular plasticity during postnatal development has gained support.[3,4] Lacoste et al[5] found that vascular density and

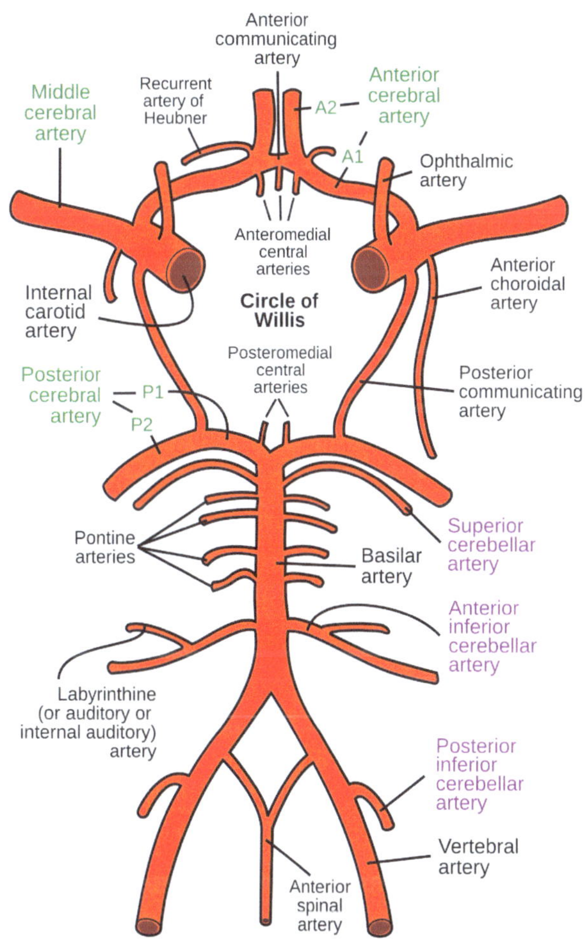


**Figure 12.1 – Schematic of the Circle of Willis**[2]

branching, as well as endothelial cell proliferation, were decreased in layer IV of the primary somatosensory cortex when sensory input was reduced by either a complete deafferentation, by a genetic impairment of neurotransmitter release at thalamocortical synapses, or by a selective reduction of sensory-related neural activity.

The way in which this developing denseness dramatically increases continues to be studied, and it appears that the neuronal structure is not necessarily involved in vascular patterning, but rather neural activity may play a role.[6]

We know from Moskalenko's studies[7–11] that osteopathic treatment can actually encourage the growth of dendrites between the front and the back, which was what he was looking at—expanding frontal occipital connections.

## Anterior Dural Girdle – Flow in the Middle Cerebral Artery

Building an osteopathic palpatory perception is a slow process. After working with several hundred children with learning difficulties over the course of 20 years, we became aware of the importance of the anterior dural girdle (Figure 12.2) in relation to the middle cerebral artery and its branches into the prefrontal cortex. The anterior dural girdle attaches to the anterior clinoid process (Figure 12.3) and then to the lesser wing of the sphenoid. Changes in tension of the girdle can influence flow in the middle cerebral artery.

With the advent of the general availability of specialised positron emission tomography scans, it became evident that certain areas of the brain were routinely found to be hypoperfused. As can be seen in Figure 12.4, which shows the number of imaging studies referenced in the U.S. National Library of Medicine, the frontal cortex was most frequently involved.[12]

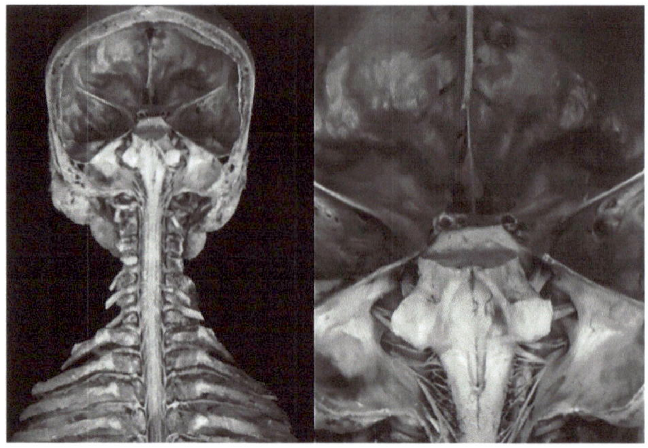

**Figure 12.2 – Anterior Dural Girdle.** Posteroanterior view of the anterior dural girdle: its attachment at the anterior clinoid process and the start of the middle cerebral artery. Image reprinted with permission from Frank Willard at the University of New England.

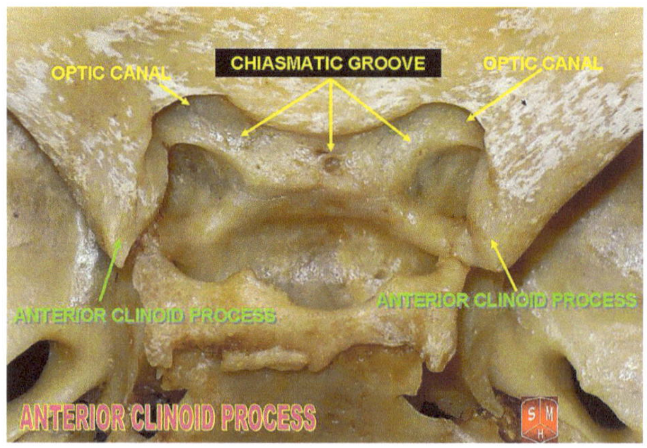


**Figure 12.3 – Anterior Clinoid Process.**

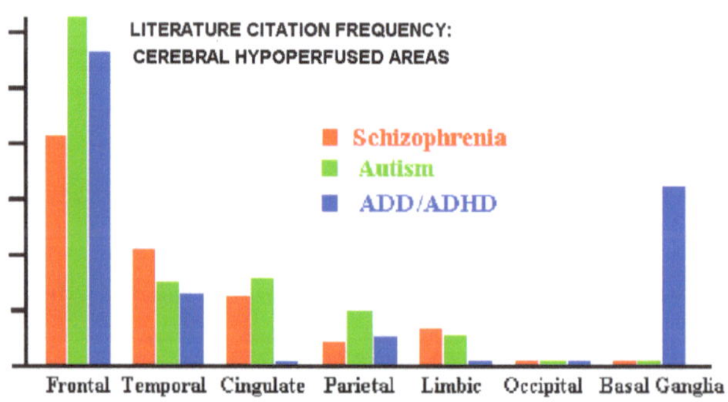


**Figure 12.4 – Cerebral Hypoperfusion by Diagnosis.**[13] Areas of hypoperfusion reported for three groups of patients. Abbreviation: ADD/ADHD = attention deficit disorder/attention deficit/hyperactivity disorder.

In 2001, Surgeef et al demonstrated that cranial manipulation favourably affects the Traube-Hering wave.[14] This explained a change in the Traube-Hering wave we had been experiencing with our patients for the previous 15 years. Repeatedly, we perceived an increase in suction and a shift in the rate, smoothness and amplitude of blood flow—changes that happen when there is a shift in the hypoperfusion of the prefrontal cortex during osteopathic treatment. A vasodilation is perceived by the treating osteopath, and the patient often reports a sensation of warmth.

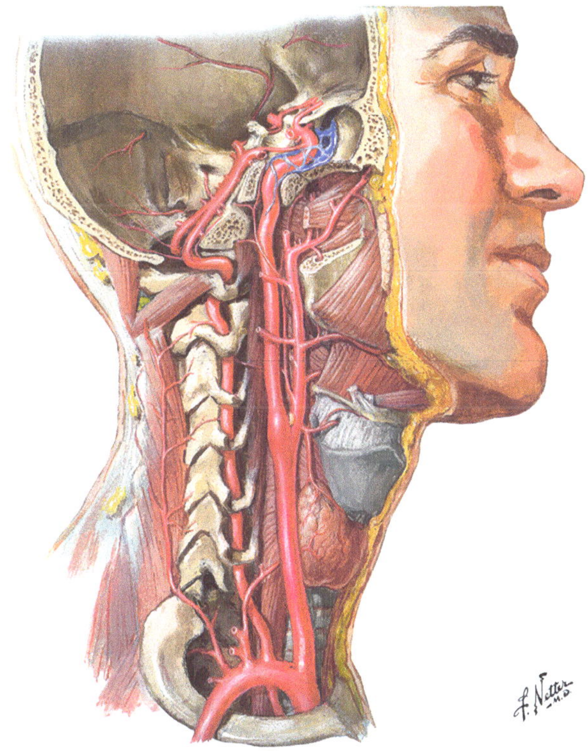

Figure 12.5 – The Flip. The arrows show the sharp turn of the vertebral and internal carotid arteries. Reprinted from Netter.[15]

## Internal Carotid and Vertebral Arteries' "Flip" on Entry

Another two areas that we progressively became aware of in terms of our osteopathic experience were the "flips" that occur both in the vertebral and the internal carotid arteries. This is seen in Figure 12.5. The flip results in a heightened vibrational quality to the blood as it moves into the cranium.

In health, it appears that both these areas have a particularly important harmonising role in terms of what Pienta and Coffey[16] saw as a continuous vibratory and resonant interaction between the capillary bed, the matrix and the cellular cytoplasm and cytoskeleton.

From our observations, we believe the flip induces a particular spin, frequency or waveform into the blood and that part of the circle of Willis provides the opportunity for the system to check how we are doing: Are the front and the back of the head "matching up?" It ensures that resonance and coherence persist.

This appears to be in part borne out by the information presented by Schubert et al, whose 2011 study concluded the following:

> "Arterial flow patterns [in the internal carotid artery] showed a significant reduction in [the pulsatility index and the peak acceleration of blood] when compared distal to proximal to the carotid siphon. The observed attenuation of flow pulsatility is most likely related to the contorted shape of the distal [internal carotid artery] and may bear a protective effect for downstream cerebral vasculature."[17]

In the case of the vertebrobasilar system, the vertebral arteries come up through the foramen magnum and then become the basilar artery. There are numerous small branches out of the basilar artery above the foramen magnum, and they supply the brainstem and cerebellum. The posterior inferior cerebellar artery is one that supplies the cerebellum and can be subject to compromise in later life (eg. degeneration of the vessel wall as a cause for unsteadiness).

The internal carotid artery becomes the middle

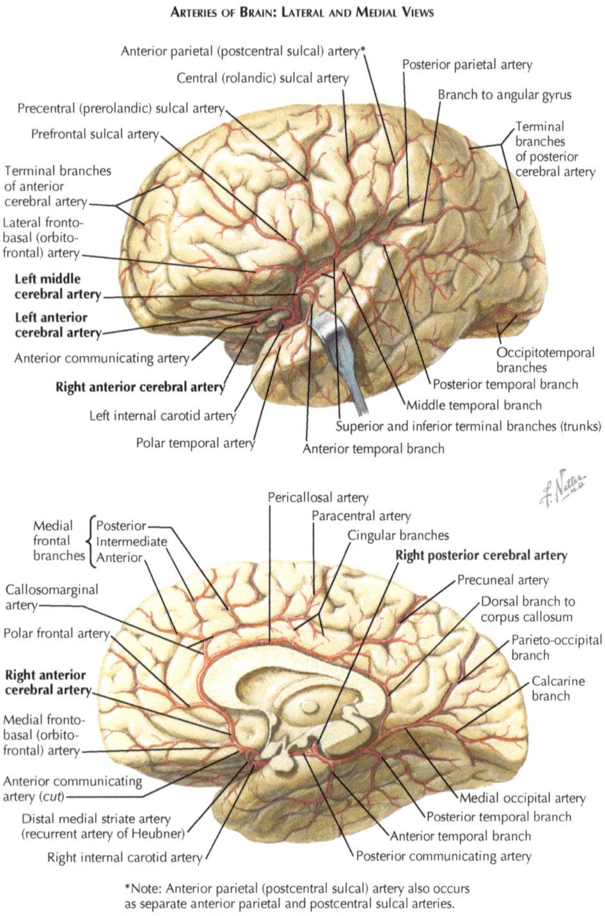


**Figure 12.6 – Wide Area of Supply of the Middle Cerebral Artery.**[18]

cerebral artery. The part of the internal carotid that lies in the carotid canal in the petrous temporal bone is surrounded by venous and sympathetic plexuses. Then the internal carotid runs in the cavernous sinus to emerge through the dural roof of the sinus, sending out petrosal branches as well as branches to the trigeminal ganglion and to the walls of the cavernous sinus. It also supplies the hypophysis and is dependent on good return through the venous system that is in the adjacent diaphragma sellae. Figure 12.6 shows the supply from the anterior and middle cerebral arteries.

Note the medial surface of the temporal lobe being supplied. The extensive supplier to the prefrontal cortex can also be seen. In clinical practice, the anterior dural girdle, anterior cerebral artery and the middle cerebral artery and its branches should be routinely observed. Crucial structures that are supplied by the middle cerebral artery include the limbic system, the hippocampus and the insula, lying opposite. More posteriorly lies Wernicke's area for speech. All these areas are particularly important for children with learning difficulties.

More centrally, the ophthalmic artery, posterior communicating arteries and the anterior choroidal artery all branch off the internal carotid artery. The anterior choroidal artery arises just distal to the ophthalmic artery but just below the circle of Willis. The anterior choroidal artery is important in terms of the production of cerebrospinal fluid (CSF) as a super filtrate. It is in close proximity to the anterior clinoid, as can be seen in Figure 12.7.

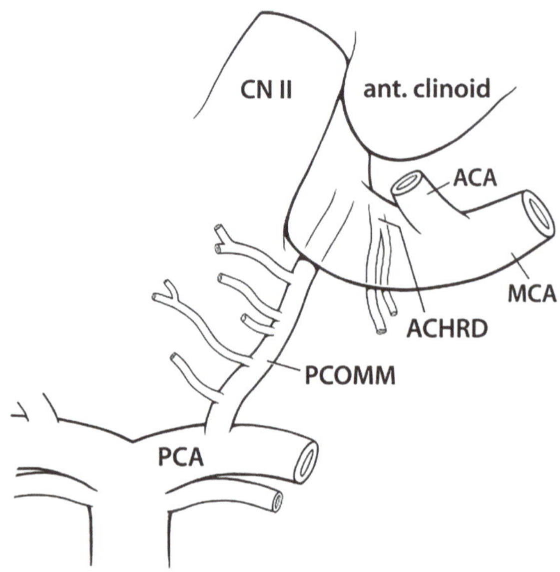


**Figure 12.7 – Proximity of the Anterior Cerebral Artery to the Anterior Clinoid Process.** ACA = anterior cerebral artery; ACHRD = anterior choroidal artery; CN = cranial nerve; MCA = middle cerebral artery; PCA = posterior cerebral artery; PCOMM = posterior communicating artery. Reprinted from Neupsy Key.[19]

## CSF and Cognition

Research shows that the CSF is very important for cognition[20] because there are peptides secreted into the CSF that progress from the lateral ventricles to the third ventricle and from the third ventricle down to the fourth ventricle. The CSF passing out through the foramen of Magendie tends to move or fluctuate caudad, whereas the CSF coming out of the foramina of Luschka tends to go cephalad so that it has to go over the free border of the tentorium and then around the brain within the anterior fossa. It is suggested that roughly 30%–40% of the CSF is going out through the cribriform plate.[21,22]

So the CSF, which is carrying peptides, bathes the brain and establishes a **mood** that can persist for some time. Vreening found that vasopressin influences behaviour and emotional states like aggression, fear, and anxiety whereas cortico trophin-releasing factor (CRF) led to depression states.

Candace Pert described molecules of emotion, a kind of neuropeptide, that change the chemistry and electricity of every cell in the body and mind. Jiang and co-workers suggest three monoamine neurotransmitters play the following roles in emotions: dopamine—joy, norepinephrine—fear (anger), serotonins—disgust (sadness).[23]

You can get CSF produced in response to a particular situation that will set the mood within a minute of being exposed to that situation and lasting up to an hour thereafter. So, paying attention to the choroidal artery, the anterior clinoid process and the anterior dural girdle or where it touches the lesser wing of the sphenoid are all important in terms of the production of CSF and its carriage of peptides.

The anterior cerebral artery supplies the orbital and medial surfaces of the frontal and parietal lobes. The anterior cerebral artery lies immediately adjacent to the falx cerebri and thus will be influenced by any alterations in the tension of the falx. The anterior cerebral artery supplies the cingulate gyrus, which is critical to the management of emotion. The cingulate is like the gear stick between the frontal and limbic system. If you have a child that just gets stuck on a particular problem and cannot move on to anything else, usually there is a problem in the area of the cingulate and the anterior falx.

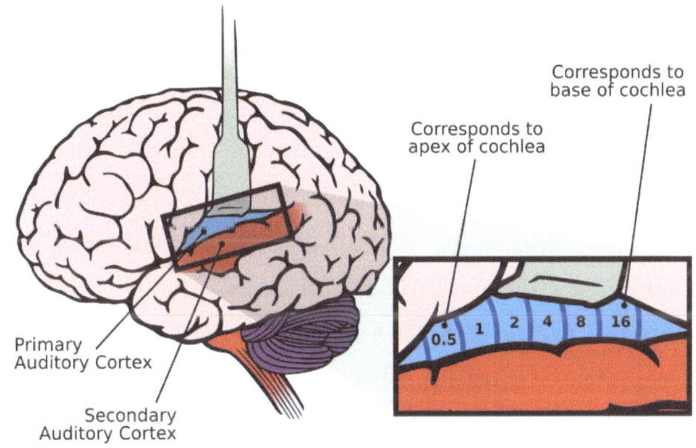


**Figure 12.8 – Auditory Dominance Columns.** Reprinted from Brockmann.[25]

The cortical branches of the middle cerebral artery supply the entire lateral surface of the brain. This includes the primary motor cortex, Broca's area, Heschl's gyrus and Wernicke's area, which is the primary auditory cortex (Figure 12.8).

We now know that just as there are ocular dominance columns that are established within the first year of life, so too are there auditory dominance columns.[24]

The auditory dominance columns are specialised for certain frequencies. In relation to children with learning difficulties, we know that there will be some frequencies that they cannot respond to; either at all or very well. According to Dr Alfred Tomatis, the otolaryngologist pioneer of the sound therapy, the Tomatis method, if they cannot hear it, they cannot spell it. If they cannot spell it, they have difficulty reading it.[26] The Tomatis method can speed up the process when osteopathically treating children with learning difficulties. So being aware of the branching of the middle cerebral artery into this area is really important osteopathically.

Now turning to the branches of the middle cerebral artery that supply the basal ganglia, the medial lenticulostriate branch supplies the head of caudate, the lateral lenticulostriate arteries supply the putamen and the anterior choroidal artery supplies the tail of the caudate and the globus pallidus. (Note that it is the penetrating branches of the posterior cerebral arteries coming off the basilar artery that supply the substantia nigra and the subthalamic nuclei.)

The bar graph in Figure 12.4 highlights the hypoperfusion of the basal ganglia in children with learning difficulties and the need for augmenting flow in the branches of the middle cerebral artery. Dr Viola Frymann stressed that the birth process can induce strains that remain and subsequently affect function, which is expressed in many children as learning difficulties.[27] Because there are common patterns, there are also common strains observed. The left occiput anterior presentation of an infant is the most common strain at birth and results in a right frontal-left occipital strain pattern with concomitant hypoperfusion in those two areas.

Jeremy Schmahmann, a Harvard University professor of Neurology and considered a world thought leader on the cerebellum, has changed the way in which the function of the cerebellum is viewed.[28] According to Schmahmann, "just as the motor portions of the cerebellum regulate the speed, capacity, and appropriateness of movements, the posterior cerebellum regulates these same features of thought."[29] The cerebellum does not just regulate the fluency of movement, its timing and its rhythm, but it performs a similar role in cognition. Theoretically, it transitions early-stage learning, taking things from where one might be struggling to learn, to automating the process so that you no longer have to think about it. It is the cerebellum that achieves the automation of learning.

So in a child who, as an infant, had a left occiput anterior presentation, the left cerebellar hemisphere is less well-perfused. Then, if there is also a hypoperfusion in the prefrontal cortex and in the basal ganglia (where learned patterns of movement or higher order thinking are stored), there is commonly a history of a parent who says, "I taught John this yesterday, I taught John this the day before, and the day before that and it is like pouring water into sand." This experience is typical for a child who has a cerebellum that is not working for him or her. In addition to that, if the child is hypoperfused in the basal ganglia area, they will show a difficulty in expressing those patterns.

It is therefore important to keep in mind the function of the anterior dural girdle and its relation with the internal carotid artery as it becomes the middle cerebral artery. It is the area where there is the most immediate contact with the middle cerebral artery. In the newborn, the attachment of the anterior dural girdle to the anterior clinoid process, which is also the attachment of the free border of the tentorium, highlights how much these structures work hand in glove. So, if there are strains in the reciprocal tension membrane, they will frequently express themselves around the anterior clinoid and as a result, the middle cerebral artery will be compromised. This is where the harmonising function of the temporal bone at the petrosphenoidal ligament plays an important balancing role.

## Importance of the Petrosphenoid Ligament

As the temporal bone moves into external rotation, it winds up the petrosphenoid ligament. When it reaches the limit within its elastic modulus, it prompts the unwinding process that occurs in internal rotation.

At the point at which there is a shift in function and an augmentation in blood flow, these children may feel an improvement in blood flow—so much so that the more dysfunctional they are, the more sensitive they are to it. When that happens and a change in perfusion is felt by the osteopath and reported by the child being treated, the osteopath can be confident that things will start to change for the child. Paraphrasing the words of Dr Still, "Show me the moment when the blood flow was altered and I will show you the start of disease." The converse is also true: Show me the moment the blood flow was altered for the better and I will show you the moment when health started to return.

## Applications to Osteopathic Practice

The circle of Willis acts to provide collateral blood flow between the anterior-posterior blood supply to the brain, protecting against ischaemia in the event of vessel disease or damage.

Moreover, it can assist in ensuring that adequate blood flow occurs when persistent patterns of hypoperfusion have developed. It is important to remember that the arteries that complete the circle sometimes are not fully formed or are absent. For example, it is commonly understood that the posterior communicating artery (Figure 12.9) may have multiple structural variations, have hypoplasias, or even have one or both completely absent.[30] This can also occur in other arteries of the circle, including, though more rare, the anterior communicating arteries and the anterior cerebral arteries. A completely formed circle of Willis is only seen in 20-25% of individuals.[31,32,33]

So, if malformations of the circle of Willis occur, the adaptability of the area will be compromised. As a result, in treatment it is necessary to assess the flow in the arteries between front and back and to ensure that the blood flow of the vertebral arteries and the internal carotid are harmonised.

As mentioned earlier in this chapter, positron emission computed tomography studies have made it possible to understand how these patterns of hypoperfusion can influence cognitive function.

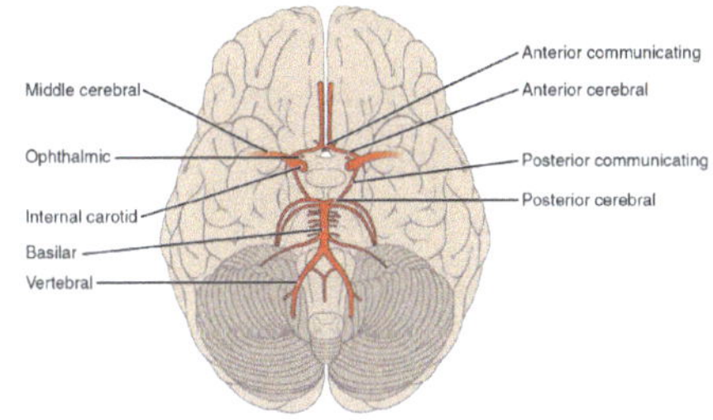


**Figure 12.9 – The Circle of Willis.** Reprinted from Betts et al.[34]

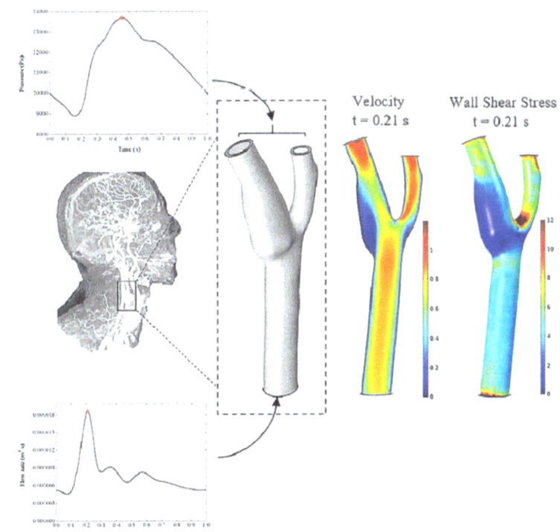


**Figure 12.10 – Turbulence in the Common Carotid Artery.** There is reduced flow on the left due to increased shear. On the right, the shear is low and blood flow is unimpeded. Reprinted from Lopes et al.[42]

Attention to the anterior dural girdle and its connection to the free border of the tentorium cerebelli can influence arterial supply. It is not uncommon for there to be an imbalance in blood flow between the basilar and internal carotid arteries. The circle of Willis provides a way in which to rebalance arterial supply to the infra- and supratentorial areas of the brain. However, it is impossible, at this time, to show that cerebral perfusion has been improved following osteopathic treatment.[35, 36]

Turbulence can also have similar adverse effects on cognitive function. Any such turbulence usually occurs at the point where an artery branches or where two arteries join to become one. Figure 12.10 shows a haemodynamic study of the bifurcation of the common carotid artery.[37]

In the past decade, osteopathic studies have shown that turbulence can be reduced by osteopathic treatment, which then has the effect of reducing the elevated tone in the sympathetic nervous system. It also has the effect of positively influencing heart rate variability.[38–,41]

Wherever there is turbulence, the resulting forces affect the epithelial cells in the wall of the artery, and atherosclerosis can start to develop.

In terms of the venous part of the system, the superior sagittal sinus and inferior sagittal sinus both relate to the straight sinus.

One of the defining aspects of the reciprocal tension membrane (the falx cerebri, the falx cerebelli and the tentorium cerebelli) is that they all have sinuses in them; so too does the anterior dural girdle, which carries the sphenoparietal sinus (Figure 12.11). All of the dural sinuses meet in the confluence of sinuses, which eventually empty into the internal jugular vein and all are subject to mechanical insult.

In the straight sinus where Dr Sutherland's fulcrum is located, there is a shift in the fulcrum: anteriorly in the flexion phase and posteriorly in the extension phase. During this shift, as the tentorium spreads, there is an increased patency in flexion (the point where the great vein of Galen joins the straight sinus) with greater ease of drainage. The converse occurs in the extension phase.

The distance between the anterior and posterior clinoid processes has been observed to be different from one side to the other. A 3- to 5-mm difference between the anterior and posterior clinoids can occur depending on whether the cranial base is hyperflexed or hyperextended. When the cranial base is hyperextended, the anterior clinoid is pulled back and there is a much narrower gap between the anterior and the posterior clinoid processes.

With a hyperextended pattern at the cranial base, the drainage into the great vein of Galen is less than optimal, and the draining of all the core structures (including the lateral ventricles, the striatum and the limbic system) are affected. Note too that the middle cerebral vein (draining a correspondingly extensive area to that supplied by the middle cerebral artery) drains back into the great vein and the same principles of biomechanics influencing drainage apply.

There is a very fine plexus of veins that forms the cavernous sinus area. The superior middle cerebral vein and superior and inferior ophthalmic veins drain into the cavernous sinus, which can flow in either direction. The pterygoid venous plexus is connected with the cavernous sinus through veins that pass through the sphenoidal emissary foramen (foramen of Vesalius), the foramen ovale and the foramen lacerum; it is also connected with the orbit via the inferior ophthalmic vein(s). Flexion and extension of the cranial base assist drainage of the

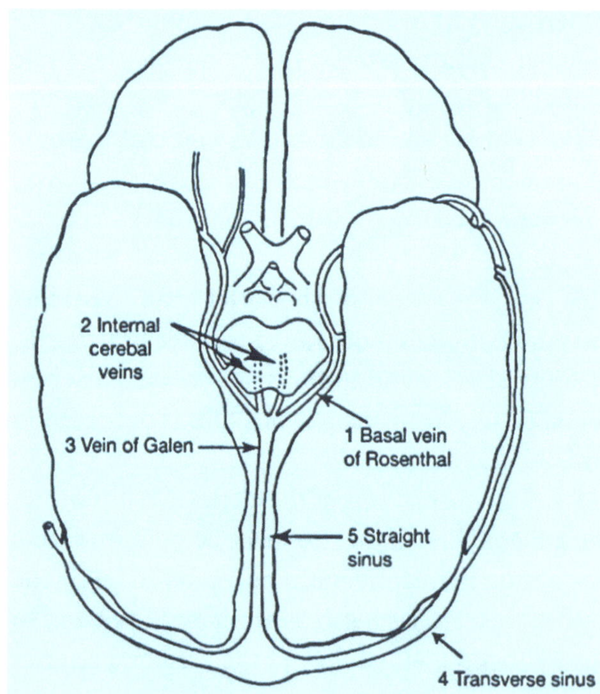


**Figure 12.11 – Cerebral Veins and Sinuses.** Illustration of the flow of venous blood that drains into the great cerebral vein of Galen and straight sinus. Reprinted from Kilic and Akakin, 2008, with permission.[43]

sinus, which can be compromised by either a compression of the petrobasilar suture, affecting the inferior petrosal sinus, or tension of the tentorium cerebelli, affecting its attachment along the petrous ridge and thereby altering flow in the superior petrosal sinus.

There is a very dense plexus of interlacing veins that lie between the layers of the dura mater of the clivus (the basilar portion of the occiput) into which the inferior petrosal sinuses and cavernous sinuses flow. Veins drain blood from the pons and medulla into the superior and inferior petrosal sinuses and vertebral venous plexus (Figure 12.12).

So a compression or a lateral or a vertical strain of the sphenobasilar synchondrosis can compromise drainage of the reticular activating system in the medulla, which osteopathic practitioners can facilitate in infants whose parents report prolonged periods of crying following a difficult delivery.

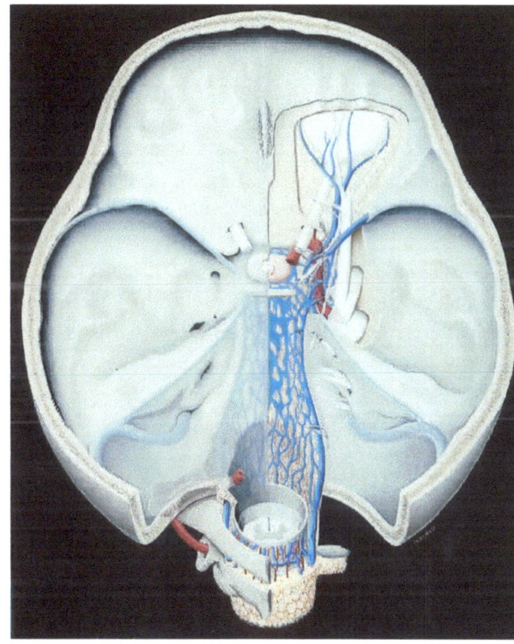

**Figure 12.12 – The Basilar Venous Plexus.** Reprinted from "Extradural Neural Axis Compartment" by Dwight Parkinson.[44]

## Chapter 12 Endnotes


1. A.T. Still, "Dr. A. T. Still's Department," *The Journal of Osteopathy* VII, no. 9 (February 1901): 33, https://www.atsu.edu/museum-of-osteopathic-medicine/wp-content/uploads/2019/04/JournalofOsteopathy1901February.pdf.

2. Schematic representation of the Circle of Willis; arteries of the brain and brain stem, https://commons.wikimedia.org/wiki/File:Circle_of_Willis_en.svg.

3. E.G. Argandoña and J.V. Lafuente, "Effects of Dark-Rearing on the Vascularization of the Developmental Rat Visual Cortex," *Brain Research* 732, no. 1–2 (September 1996): 43–51.

4. E.G. Argandoña and J.V. Lafuente, "Influence of Visual Experience Deprivation on the Postnatal Development of the Microvascular Bed in Layer IV of the Rat Visual Cortex," *Brain Research* 855, no. 1 (February 2000): 137–42.

5. Baptiste Lacoste et al., "Sensory-Related Neural Activity Regulates the Structure of Vascular Networks in the Cerebral Cortex," *Neuron* 83, no. 5 (September 2014): 1117–30.

6. Lacoste et al., "Sensory-related neural activity."

7. Yu E. Moskalenko et al., "Periodic Mobility of Cranial Bones in Humans," *Human Physiology* 25, no. 1 (January-February 1999): 51–8.

8. Yury Moskalenko et al., "Physiological Background of the Cranial Rhythmic Impulse and the Primary Respiratory Mechanism," *American Academy of Osteopathy Journal* 13, no. 2 (Summer 2003): 21–33.

9. Y.E. Moskalenko et al., "Variations in Blood Volume and Oxygen Availability in the Human Brain," *Nature* 202 (April 1964): 159–61.

10. Yu E. Moskalenko et al., "Slow Rhythmic Oscillations Within the Human Cranium: Phenomenology, Origin, and Informational Significance," *Human Physiology* 27 (March 2001): 171–8.

11. Y.E. Moskalenko, V.M. Frymann, and T. Kravchenko, "A Modern Conceptualization of the Functioning of the Primary Respiratory Mechanism," in H.H. King. (Ed.), *Proceedings of International Research Conference: Osteopathy in Pediatrics at the Osteopathic Center for Children in San Diego, CA* (Indianapolis, IN: American Academy of Osteopathy, 2005), 12-31.

12. Hershel Toomim, *Homoencephalography: The Study of Regional Cerebral Blood Flow*, http://216.117.166.12/HEGTALK1-AConceptualIntroductiontoHEG.pdf.

13. Hershel Toomim, *Homoencephalography.*

14. Nicette Surgeef, Kenneth E. Nelson, and Thomas Glonek, "Changes in the Traube-Hering Wave Following Cranial Manipulation," *American Academy of Osteopathy Journal* 11, no. 1 (Spring 2001): 17.

15. Frank H. Netter, *Atlas of Human Anatomy,* 7th ed. (Elsevier, 2018).

16. K.J. Pienta and D.S. Coffey, "Cellular harmonic information through a tissue tensegrity-matrix system," *Medical Hypothses* 34, no. 1 (January 1991): 88–95.

17. T. Schubert et al., "Dampening of Blood-Flow Pulsatility Along the Carotid Siphon: Does Form Follow Function?" *American Journal of Neuroradiology* 32, no. 6 (June-July 2011): 1107–12.

18. Frank Netter, "Arteries of Brain: Lateral and Medial Views Arterial Supply of the Brain-Lateral and Medial Aspects," Netter illustration used with permission of Elsevier Inc. All rights reserved. www.netterimages.com

19. Nepsy Key, "Aneurysms of the Internal Carotid Artery at the Origins of the Posterior Communicating and Anterior Choroidal Arteries," Clinical Tree, https://neupsykey.com/aneurysms-of-the-internal-carotid-artery-at-the-origins-of-the-posterior-communicating-and-anterior-choroidal-arteries/.

20. Jan G. Veening and Henk P. Barendregt, "The Regulation of Brain States by Neuroactive Substances Distributed Via the Cerebrospinal Fluid; A Review," *Cerebrospinal Fluid Research* 7 (January 2010): article 1.

21. Veening and Barendregt, "The Regulation of Brain States."

22. M. Preuss et al., "Updated Physiology and Pathophysiology of CSF Circulation—The Pulsatile Vector Theory," *Child's Nervous System* 29, no. 10 (October 2013): 1811–25.

23. Yao Jiang et al., "Monoamine Neurotransmitters Control Basic Emotions and Affect Major Depressive Disorders," *Pharmaceuticals* 15, no. 10 (September 2022): 1203, https://doi.org/10.3390/ph15101203

24. Anthony J. Castro et al., *Neuroscience: An Outline Approach* (Mosby, 2002).

25. Chittka L. Brockmann, "Perception Space–The Final Frontier," *PLoS Biology* 3, no. 4 (April 2005): e137, https://doi.org/10.1371/journal.pbio.0030137.

26. Deborah Ross-Swain, "The Effects of Auditory Stimulation on Auditory Processing Disorder: A Summary of the Findings," *International Journal of Listening.*

27. Viola M. Frymann, Richard E. Carney, and Peter Springall, "Effect of Osteopathic Medical Management on Neurological Development in Children," *The Journal of the American Osteopathic Association* 92, no. 6 (June 1992): 729–44.

28. Georgios P.D. Argyropoulos et al., "The Cerebellar Cognitive Affective/Schmahmann Syndrome: A Task Force Paper," *Cerebellum* 19, no. 1 (2020): 102–25.

29. Christopher Berglund, "Harvard Research Shows How the Cerebellum Regulates Thoughts: The Cerebellum Is Responsible for Monitoring Both Motor and Non-motor Functions," *Psychology Today,* May 21, 2016. https://www.psychologytoday.com/us/blog/the-athletes-way/201605/harvard-research-shows-how-the-cerebellum-regulates-thoughts.

30. Sandhya Arvind Gunnal, Mujibuddin S. Farooqui, and Rajendra N. Wabale, "Anatomical Variability of the Posterior Communicating Artery," *Asian Journal of Neurosurgery* 13, no. 2 (2018): 363-9.

31. Cagatay Ustun, "NEUROwords Dr. Thomas Willis' Famous Eponym: The Circle of Willis," *Journal of the History of the Neurosciences* 14, no. 1 (2007): 350.

32. H.R. Harnsberger et al., *Diagnostic and Surgical Anatomy* (Lippincott Williams & Wilkins, 2006).

33. P. Butler, A. Mitchell, and J.C. Healy, *Applied Radiological Anatomy*, (Cambridge University Press, 2012).

34. J. Gordon Betts et al., *Anatomy and Physiology*, 2nd ed. (Rice University, 2022), Figure 20.27, https://openstax.org/details/books/anatomy-and-physiology-2e Pulled from wiki commons https://commons.wikimedia.org/wiki/File:2123_Arteries_of_the_Brain.jpg.

35. Frederica Tamburella et al., "Cerebral Perfusion Changes After Osteopathic Manipulative Treatment: A Randomized Manual Placebo-Controlled Trial," *Frontiers in Physiology* 10 (April 2019): 403, https://doi.org/10.3389/fphys.2019.00403.

36. Michelle Dickerson et al., "Osteopathy in the Cranial Field as a Method to Enhance Brain Injury Recovery: A Preliminary Study," *Neurotrauma Reports* 3, no. 1 (October 2022): 456–72, https://doi.org/10.1089/neur.2022.0039.

37. D. Lopes et al., "Influence of Arterial Mechanical Properties on Carotid Blood Flow: Comparison of CFD and FSI Studies," *International Journal of Mechanical Sciences* 160 (September 2019): 209–18.

38. Mauro Fornari, Luca Carnevali, and Andrea Sgoifo, "Single Osteopathic Manipulative Therapy Session Dampens Acute Autonomic and Neuroendocrine Responses to Mental Stress in Healthy Male Participants," *The Journal of the American Osteopathic Association* 117, no. 9 (September 2017): 559–67, https://doi.org/10.7556/jaoa.2017.110.

39. Charles E. Henley et al., "Osteopathic Manipulative Treatment and Its Relationship to Autonomic Nervous System Activity as Demonstrated by Heart Rate Variability: A Repeated Measures Study," *Osteopathic Medicine and Primary Care* 2 (June 2008): 7, https://doi.org/10.1186/1750-4732-2-7.

40. Luca Carnevali et al., "Exploring the Effects of Osteopathic Manipulative Treatment on Autonomic Function Through the Lens of Heart Rate Variability," *Frontiers in Neuroscience* 14 (October 2020): 579365, https://doi.org/10.3389/fnins.2020.579365.

41. Brian Budgell and Barbara Polus, "The Effects of Thoracic Manipulation on Heart Rate Variability: A Controlled Crossover Trial," *Journal of Manipulative and Physiological Therapeutics* 29, no. 8 (October 2006): 603–10, https://doi.org/10.1016/j.jmpt.2006.08.011.

42. D. Lopes et al., "Influence of Arterial Mechanical Properties on Carotid Blood Flow: Comparison of CFD and FSI Studies," *International Journal of Mechanical Sciences* 160 (September 2019): 209–18.

43. Türker Kiliç and Akin Akakin, "Anatomy of Cerebral Veins and Sinuses," *Frontiers of Neurology and Neuroscience* 23 (2008): 4-15, https://doi.org/10.1159/000111256.

44. Dwight Parkinson, "Extradural Neural Axis Compartment," *Journal of Neurosurgery* 92, no. 4 (2000): 585-8.

# Chapter Thirteen

# Ion Waves and Their Electromotive Force

*"As an electrician controls electric currents, so an Osteopath controls life currents and revives suspended forces."*[1]

– Andrew Taylor Still

This chapter reviews the origin and nature of the primary respiratory mechanism: *How* did it start and *how* is it maintained?

At conception, when the sperm enters an egg, it elicits a surge of calcium that triggers the release of zinc from the egg. This is the beginning of the calcium flux and, as cells divide, the calcium flux continues to occur in each of those new cells. The biphasic increase and decrease of calcium results in a swelling and receding pattern of cell function: increasing intracellular $Ca^{2+}$ causes cell volume to shrink, while reducing intracellular $Ca^{2+}$ results in swelling of the cell. Solutes move into and out of cells with these modulations of intracellular $Ca^{2+}$. The $Ca^{2+}$-sensitive potassium channel is activated by cell shrinkage and inhibited by cell swelling.[2,3]

The calcium flux, which acts as a second messenger influenced by intracellular $Ca^{2+}$, continues to occur in every cell as the fertilised egg becomes a zygote in the fallopian tube, then the morula within the uterus, then the blastocyst at implantation (Figure 13.1). The extracellular flux of calcium ions occurs at a rate of 7-10 cycles per minute (CPM),

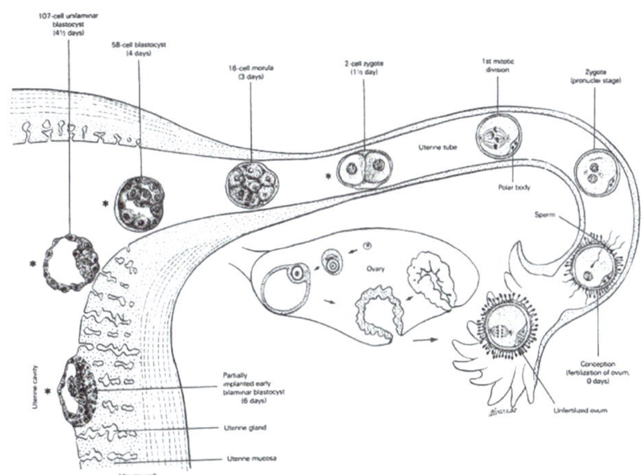


**Figure 13.1 – Cycle of a Fertilised Egg.** The stages of embryonic development during the first week and the general location of each in the uterine tube or uterus. Reprinted with permission from Gasser.[4]

which is consistent with the primary respiratory mechanism as described by Dr William Sutherland.

In the placenta, the placental ionic flux and the maternal Traube-Hering wave (discussed in Chapter 5) meet.

In 1932, John Lewis Bremer, professor of Anatomy and Surgery at Harvard University, filmed the development of a chick embryo heart and made the remarkable observation that circulation is already in motion before the heart and valves have formed. As blood starts to move within the embryo, spiralling is intrinsic to its movement and the gas within the blood is essential to the development and maintenance of vortical flow.[5] When the heart begins to beat, there is no turbulence but instead an amplification and an increased complexity of a process already in motion.

Some years before Bremers work, in 1927, Prof Kurt Bergel of Berlin University recorded automatic pulsations in small blood vessels around the egg sac of a bird's egg a few days after incubation, though no heart had yet been formed. Bergel also rejected the popular theory of the heart as a pump, insisting that "this function was carried out by the millions of highly active capillaries permeating the body, and that health or disease is primarily dependent on the faultless or disturbed activity of the capillaries."[6] Bergel is not alone in his suggestion. Over the generations, other puzzled clinicians and scientists have similarly questioned the pump model and suggested the capillaries as the drivers for circulation.[7–14] In those earlier times, the difficulty has been to adequately explain how, without imposing pressure, flow might be maintained in capillaries.

Bergel theorised that the pulsation of the capillaries initiates the circulation of the blood, augmented by the configuration of the blood vessels themselves. As part of this function, there was an assumption that the viscosity of the blood is reduced in the finer blood vessels so that the blood's ability to flow freely is not compromised.

Much more recently, Pollack and Zheng[15] have again demonstrated peripheral flow, this time in a 3-day-old chick, selected particularly because smooth muscle in the vessel walls are not fully functional.[16–19] In this report, circulation beyond the heart was shown to be augmented, not by imposing pressure, but by using infrared energy to activate/augment flow. Earlier, Pollack had shown the existence of an exclusion zone adjacent to the vessel wall,[20,21] and his associates had already shown[22] that flow can arise from a driving force or energy, such as infrared energy affecting tubular surfaces.[23] The surface activity can bring about longitudinally directed chemical gradients that drive intratubular flow and act as a tiny engine, fuelled by IR energy, within the lumen of capillaries.[24–27] The diagram below shows the experimental set up.

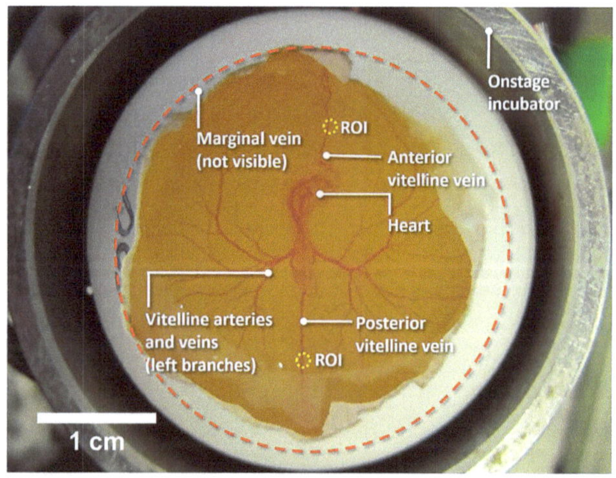


**Figure 13.2 – Three-Day Old Chick Embryo, Showing the Vitelline Vascular Network.**

The egg was held in an incubator. The embryo is just above the middle of the egg with the region of interest (ROI) supplied by the anterior vitelline vein above and the posterior vitelline vein below.

The following image demonstrates the arrangement of the equipment for directing the infrared light at the chick embryo.

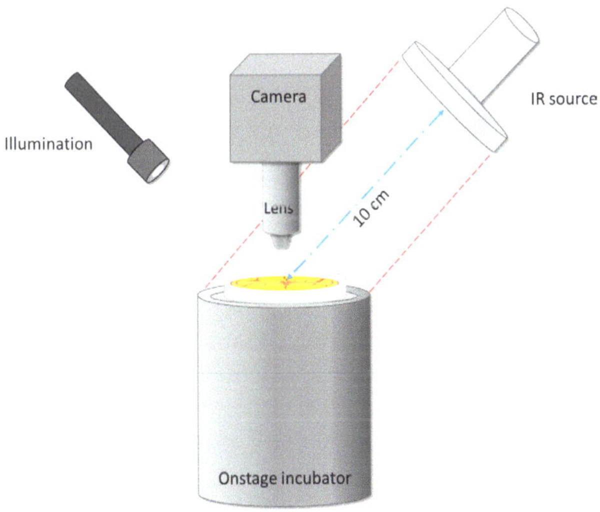


**Figure 13.3 – Experimental Configuration for Applying Infrared Light to the Chick Embryo.**

The authors also showed that the relative difference in diameter of the capillaries compared to the venules with the different surface tensions in the capillaries and venules so that a surface-induced tension promotes flow towards the venules.

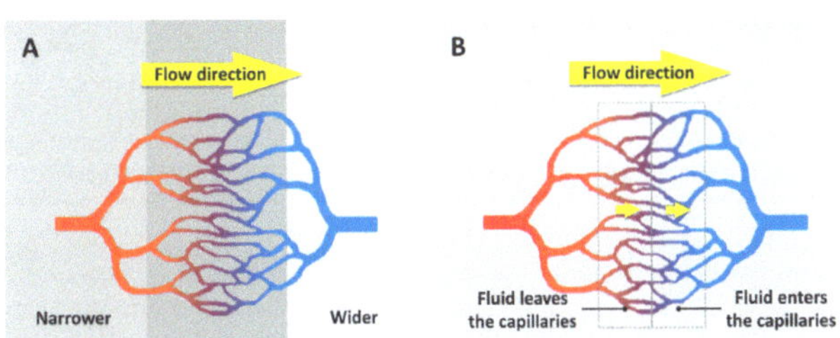


**Figure 13.4 – Surface-Induced Flow in a Capillary Bed.**

(A) Compared to venules (blue), the arterioles (red) are narrower; thus, the water-surface interaction drives capillary flow from arteries to veins. (B) As fluid (mainly water) leaves the capillaries through the capillary wall at the arteriolar end, a surface-induced flow is generated pointing from the arteries to the capillaries. Meanwhile, as fluid enters the capillaries at the venular end, a surface-induced flow is generated, pointing from the capillaries to the venules.[28]

Take a moment to scan the QR codes for the following videos:

**Video 1: Postmortem Venous Blood Flow**

**Video 2: Postmortem Arterial Blood Flow**

When blood flowing in the embryo arrives at the developing choroid plexus of the brain, the blood is spiralling and expressing the ionic calcium flux, which becomes the Traube-Hering wave (discussed more fully in Chapter 5). The cerebrospinal fluid is produced in the choroid plexus in waves that reflect the arriving blood and result in the fluctuation of the cerebral spinal fluid at a rate of 7 to 10 cycles per minute, as reported by osteopaths.

The amplified motion of cerebral tissue can be seen in the video at https://vimeo.com/812217885, or you may scan the QR on the next page.[29] The video demonstrates that every part of the parenchyma of the brain is affected by the circulatory process. When watching the video, observe the strength of the vascular motion at the sphenobasilar synchondrosis, the way in which the cerebrum moves towards the lamina terminalis, the motion of the occipital lobe and the shortening of the frontal lobe on an anteroposterior axis. Try to see where no movement can be detected. If you observe closely, every part of the cranium is in motion as it interfaces with the circulation.

In a series of lectures entitled "Human Embryology from a Biodynamic Perspective," Prof Brian Freeman spoke of the "hunger of the tissues," or oncotic pressure, that provide the suction force that draws blood from the heart to the periphery.[30,31] Blood with high oxygen and nutrient concentration will pass through the capillary vessel wall and be drawn by osmotic pressure towards cells.[32]

Further, the research of Aleksandr and Svetlana Goncharenko[33] (a colleague of Dr Vladimir Voeikov, biophysicist and professor at the Biological Faculty at Lomonosov Moscow State University) suggests that ponderomotive force explains how blood is sucked from the left ventricle towards the periphery. A ponderomotive force occurs where a charged particle is not subject to uniform electrical and magnetic forces within the space it occupies. These variations often take the form of waves. In such a non-uniform environment, the charged particle tends to move towards an area of weaker field strength.

Goncharenko and Goncharenko review how changes in blood volume occur in various clinical settings. For instance, in pregnancy the blood volume can increase by up to 50% when moving from lying to standing. Goncharenko and Goncharenko consider that cavitation may explain this very rapid change in volume.[34]

Cavitation is the process of gas-filled caverns (also called cavities or bubbles) appearing at the points of a flowing liquid where its speed increases and the pressure falls below the critical value of structural stability. As associates of Voeikov,[35] Goncharenko and Goncharenko were clearly working on the assumption that the water in the ventricle is structured and that cavitation is the result of a sheer between layers of structured water that can rupture:

> "At points of the liquid's rupture, if it contains dissolved gases, and in the conditions of alternating pressure, an unlimited growth of cavitation bubbles is observed (with gas diffusing into the bubbles from the liquid). They grow in size, the pressure within them also grows and exceeds the ambient pressure. The energy from the movement of these bubbles and their vibration create new bubbles around them. They grow in numbers and this increased volume creates ponderomotive forces which lead to displacement of the surrounding liquid and its self-motion…
>
> "The study of regurgitation, using a contrast-enhanced Doppler echocardiography, registered the appearance of voids (caverns) in the blood volume of the heart cavities at the moment when the recurrent blood stream leaves the heart. The appearance of caverns in heart cavities coincides in time with the short-term decrease in blood volume and pressure drop. This helps us to understand the mechanism of a 'spontaneous' increase of blood volume in the heart.
>
> "The recurrent stream is released at the speed of 3 to 15 m/s, developing the pressure of up to 800 mm Hg at 30–40 mm distance of its way between the valves, and leaving behind a cavity in the blood volume (vacuum cavern) with negative pressure and exposed ionic bonds. This is an active source of 'pure' physical force.
>
> "The surrounding blood from areas with higher pressure flows into it. But since at this point, the blood is already limited by a hermetically closed cavity of the heart, the movement of its particles towards the cavern is only possible with multiple ruptures of the water layers in blood. Blood gases move into the created microcavities, and bubbles are formed.
>
> "The growing number of bubbles increases the blood volume. This vacuum provocation of the heart instantly releases the gases dissolved in blood and increases the size of gas bubbles within blood. This is the cause of such a significant increase of its volume in the isometric phase (1).
>
> "An instant increase in this volume empowers the

> blood with ponderomotive forces which act rapidly and independently from the heart muscles contractions. Since the power of the heart's muscles contraction takes 1/6 part in the blood transfer, the remaining 5\6 derive from ponderomotive forces of cavitation, which are the 'pushing' forces vis a fronte. ('vis a fronte' = a force operating from in front, as in attraction or suction – Oxford dictionary).
>
> "[So] it can be argued that the heart has one more function: to excite the cavitation in blood.
>
> "This function is the main power source of its circulation in vessels."[36]

This is how negative pressure can be measured by the SphygmoCor (discussed previously in Chapter 10) in the aortic arch and at the bifurcation of the aorta. It is negative pressure/suction that is driving the process.

Goncharenko and Goncharenko also observed that this powerful ponderomotive force is accompanied by sound (phonons), electromagnetic, luminescent (photons), thermal and kinetic effects.

As we observed in Chapter 1, there are at least four ways that the heart communicates with the brain and body: neurologically, biophysically (through pulse waves), biochemically (which includes hormonal communication) and, as Szent-Györgyi suggested, electronically. It is in the plasma layer that the electrons "skip" between ionised molecules in the plasma.

We came to our study of the heart with a neurocentric view of body function derived from the predominating anatomic-physiologic view of our era. We progressively came to understand that Dr Still's insight of a conscious heart that imparts information to the blood had a reality to it that was compelling.

We realised that of the 37,000 billion billion reactions occurring every second within the human body, only 5000 billion nerve impulses occur. Thus, neural activity constitutes less than 1% of all the activity occurring within the human body. Then we became aware of research that showed that slime mould (introduced in Chapter 6), without a nervous system, was able to make conscious decisions in order to escape a maze and was able to adapt based on memory of earlier attempts in the maze. Baluska and Levin reviewed this topic in an article entitled "On Having No Head: Cognition Throughout Biological Systems."[37] In addition to paracrine signalling (chemical into cellular messengers), autocrine signalling (cell targets self), endocrine signalling (via the bloodstream) and signalling by direct contact (cell to cell), there is also the electronic signalling as Szent-Györgyi expected.

Prof Ross Adey, of Loma Linda University, wrote:

> "We have discovered some of the keys to understanding how body cells 'whisper' to one another, and, in so doing we have discovered some of the keys to understanding how electromagnetic fields, so weak that some scientists have regarded them as incapable of biological effects, are detected by living tissues, and we have studied some of the likely consequences for human health…These fields can exert effects even at intensities near zero, in other words, a lower limit or threshold may not exist."[38]

As Grundler and Kaiser have pointed out, "Living cells exhibit a high degree of information processing and communication…It is clearly demonstrated that a fast oscillating, very weak outer field is influencing biological reactions of cells."[39]

Dr Robert O. Becker, renowned for his work in bioelectricity, determined that there are extensive semiconductor networks within the body. A semiconductor has a conductivity between a conductor (such as copper) and an insulator (such as rubber). In his seminal work *The Body Electric*, Becker explains that "Semiconduction can occur in materials that have an orderly molecular structure, such as crystals [or bone], in which electrons can move easily from the electron cloud around one atomic nucleus to the cloud around another."[40] If unobstructed, information can pass along a semiconductor network at light speed. It turns out that we are full of semiconductors!

Semiconductor networks can include bone (as elucidated by Dr Becker, above), the docosahexaenoic acid in our cell membranes, the extracellular matrix, tendons, blood vessel walls, muscles, skin, melatonin, serotonin, dopamine and collagen. One of the qualities of semiconductors is piezoelectricity. This means that pressure (squeezing or stretching) can give rise to electricity and, conversely, electricity can produce a vibration.

The research of Prof Fritz-Albert Popp drew our attention to the importance of light as a part of body physiology. Although sonoluminescence was first discovered by scientists at the University of Cologne in 1934, it was only in the late 1990s that interest in and research related to sonoluminescence began to develop rapidly.[41,42,43] Interestingly, the emission of light by micro bubbles in a liquid were excited by low-pressure sound waves.

In Chapter 3, we discussed the results of the research of Prof Gerald Pollack, who said that water organises into an exclusion zone around hydrophilic surfaces. This water is more stable, constrained and aligned and has an associated electrical potential. As a result of the cleavage of hydrogen ions from the hexagonal ring structure that forms in the exclusion zone, there is a gradient of charge between the central core of fluid and the exclusion zone. The reason that this battery does not run down is because it is maintained by infrared light, which is ubiquitous day and night. The photons present in the blood also have a charging effect.

Gas is essential to the development and maintenance of vortical flow, which starts to occur in the very early stages of embryonic development. The charge and the fluid dynamics hold gases in the stable state so that their behaviour does not match that of gases held under pressure where there is a tendency to expand and dissipate.

These vortices within the circulating blood have been observed using cineradiology[44], Doppler imaging and magnetic resonance velocity mapping.[45, 46]

Cortical flow ensures that substances in the blood are not scattered randomly; instead, in flow it is observed that heavier objects migrate to the centre and lighter objects to the periphery. So the red blood cells are found in the core of the flow and the lighter platelets are peripheral to the red blood cells. A sleeve of plasma is found at the very periphery of the vessel. Plasma within the blood is highly conductive and so, as stated earlier, electrons move freely in the plasma.

The vortical motion in blood flow generates a pulsatile pattern within the moving blood, which occurs beginning early in the embryo's development. Prof Peter Stonebridge has stated that the description of the laminar flow of blood has come from the two-dimensional representations of flow. However, MRI and colour Doppler flow imaging techniques have demonstrated that there is a spiral, helical and rotational property to laminar blood flow.[47]

The pulsatile pattern of flow represents a standing wave in relation to which the fractaline code in the fluid is arranged. As we noted in Chapter 5, this pulsatile pattern of flow was described in the late 1800s by Traube, Hering and Mayer, who observed a moving equilibrium in the average arterial pressure. The pulse pressure (systole minus diastole) remained about the same, but the average pressure of blood in the vessel varied with the cycle occurring at a rate of approximately 7 to 9 times per minute. Mayer discovered a longer wave, about 2 to 3 times per minute.[48]

These "vasomotor" waves or oscillations of pressure reflex control systems were reported to be independent of respiratory activity and have been measured in association with blood pressure and heart rate.[49–55] The origin of this oscillation is regarded as multifactorial, including baroreceptor and chemoreceptor responses as well as the central nervous system ischemic pressure control mechanism relating to cerebrospinal fluid pressure.[56]

The effect of osteopathic treatment and its effect on turbulence and the restoration of vortical flow in relation to sympathetic nervous system activity is briefly reviewed below (see references 56-59).

In a personal communication in 1990, Prof Al Kelso, emeritus professor of physiology at the Midwestern University Chicago College of Osteopathic Medicine, suggested that part of what cranial osteopaths had been palpating, perceiving and reporting was a vascular phenomenon. Not long after that communication, Nelson and Glonek reported that osteopaths were able to accurately palpate and record the Traube-Hering wave.[57] Subsequently, Surgeef et al showed that the Traube-Hering wave was responsive to osteopathic treatment.[58] Thus, we came to see the relationship between the rate of the Traube-Hering wave and the rate of fluctuation of the cerebral spinal fluid.

Varga suggested that the heart and circulation together are a carrier of electrical charge and that a current exists in the blood. He calculated that each red blood cell, when oxygen-rich, carries about 7000 free electrical charges and that there are approximately $5.5 \times 10^9$ erythrocytes/cm$^3$ in the blood.[59] It was reported to us quite recently[60] that the same view of the blood was being taught in the 1930s to osteopathic students at the Kirksville College of Osteopathic Medicine (formerly the American School of Osteopathy, which was founded by Still). We have elsewhere followed the blood flow from the heart to the periphery, in which "a key to healthy circulation is the propelling of the negatively charged red blood cells towards the veins as a consequence of the voltage drop between the arteries and the veins. Because the veins are more acidic, the negatively charged RBCs [red blood cells] naturally migrate in the direction of lower pH (positive charge)."[61] This is illustrated in Figure 13.5.

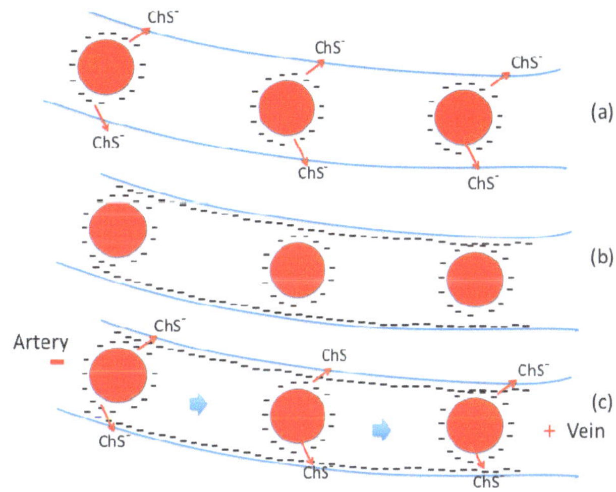


**Figure 13.5 – Red Blood Cell Sheds Negative Charge.** Reprinted from Davidson and Seneff.[62]

Vascular tone, which refers to the degree of constriction or dilation of blood vessels, is primarily regulated by the autonomic nervous system (ANS). The sympathetic branch of the ANS acts to cause vasoconstriction by releasing noradrenaline (ie. it causes blood vessels to constrict). However, sensory nerves also play a crucial role in this regulation. These nerves act not only as sensors but also have an efferent role. Specifically, sensory fibres release a neuropeptide known as calcitonin gene-related peptide, which causes a vasodilation to occur. This then counteracts the constriction usually caused by the sympathetic nervous system. Thus, the balance between these opposing forces helps maintain proper vascular tone and blood flow.[63]

All endothelial vascular structures develop with the flow of nutrients parallel to their membranes. As you'll recall from Chapter 2, this is **parmeation** of nutrients, where the flow is parallel to the blood vessel wall, which allows them to function and grow at a relatively slower metabolic rate. They are metabolically quiescent when experiencing normal and healthy flow.

In a healthy, atheroresistant artery with high,

laminar shear stress, endothelial cells are aligned in the direction of flow and remain in a quiescent state with low rates of both proliferation and death (Figure 13.6). They also express low levels of adhesion receptors and cytokines that attract leukocytes.[64]

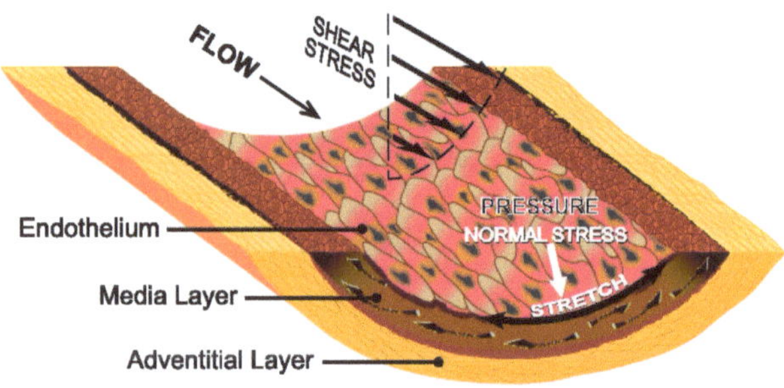


**Figure 13.6 – Shear Stress and Normal Stress.** Schematic diagram showing the generation of shear stress (parallel to the endothelial cell surface) by blood flow and the generation of normal stress (perpendicular to the endothelial cell surface) and circumferential stretch due to the action of pressure. Reprinted from Chiu and Chien.[65]

However, any turbulence of flow will generate an ANS response that leads to a process of increased tone reflected in the musculoskeletal system.

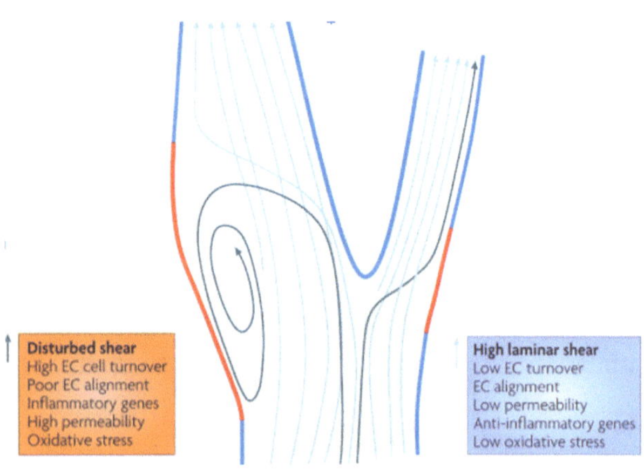


**Figure 13.7 – Laminar Stress.** EC = endothelial cell.

## Vascular Branching and Flow Patterns

In regions where arteries are relatively straight, the rate of blood flow changes during the cardiac cycle but flow is always in the same direction and patterns are laminar (blue segments). In regions where arteries divide, branch or curve sharply, there are regions where complex flow patterns develop (red segments). Flow in these regions is slower and can even reverse direction during the cardiac cycle, and so it is called oscillatory flow, where rippling and swirling occurs.

Endothelial cells (ECs) respond to the mechanical forces exerted by blood flow, particularly shear forces, which significantly influences their function and physical composition. In areas where blood flow is consistent and smooth (ie. high, laminar shear stress), endothelial cells adopt a quiescent, anti-inflammatory pattern of flow. In this state the endothelial cells align themselves with the direction of blood flow and they express or activate genes that protect against inflammation. These cells experience reduced oxidative stress and there is low to minimal cell turnover and low permeability, meaning the blood vessel walls are stable and less likely to allow substances to pass through. These conditions make the endothelial cells less susceptible to atherosclerosis.

In contrast, in areas where blood flow is irregular or disturbed, endothelial cells exhibit an activated, pro-inflammatory pattern. This is marked by poor alignment of cells to blood flow, increased cell turnover, leading to a less stable endothelial layer and higher levels of oxidative stress. The increased turnover and stress result in higher permeability, allowing more substances to penetrate the vessel walls. These conditions increase the risk of developing atherosclerosis in these regions.[66]

These sites show a low level of chronic inflammation not only in healthy individuals but also in newborns and other mammals that are highly resistant to atherosclerosis. Blood flow is a key factor in atherosclerosis; despite the systemic nature of major risk factors, it occurs mainly in regions of arteries that experience disturbances in fluid flow.

Osteopathic treatment can reduce turbulence, thus resulting in a reduction in ANS activity with de-facilitation, a restoration of normal biomechanics and a return to normal blood flow.[67–70]

In Chapter 5 we reviewed the transfer of the code from the capillary bed to the extracellular matrix. Nordenström observed that there were groups of ions on the matrix side of the paravasal mantle or perivascular space. Furthermore, he suggested that these groups of ions must collect in the extracellular matrix because of metabolic activity and local differences in the capillary bed circulation (due to the Traube-Hering wave), matrix properties (primarily the calcium flux) and ionic size and mobility (Figure 13.8).[71] As mentioned in Chapter 5, Lee has hypothesized that within the matrix, a calcium flux drives motion from the capillary bed to the cells at a rate of 7 to 8 cycles per minute (see Appendix).

An article in 2018 referred to a previously unrecognised structure named the *interstitium*, yet more than 100 years earlier, in 1902, Still emphasised the importance of the fascia, and since that time, osteopaths have viewed it as a tissue that holds vital significance in health. Still wrote:

> "In every view we take of the fascia, a wonder appears. The part the fascia takes in **life** and **death** gives us one of the greatest problems to solve. It surrounds each muscle, vein, nerve, and all organs of the body. It has a network of nerves, cells, and tubes running to and from [and through] it; it is crossed and no doubt filled with millions of nerve-centers and fibers which carry on the work of secreting and excreting fluids vital and destructive. By its action we live and by its failure we die."[72]

We also described how calcium is attracted to negative charges in the matrix in Chapter 5. Water also moves from positive to negative charge. Parenchymal cell membranes are negatively charged.

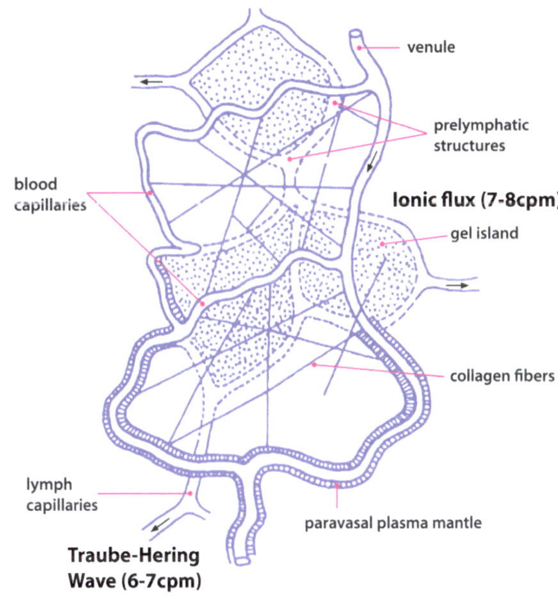


**Figure 13.8 –Traube-Hering Wave and Ionic Flux.** Reprinted from Holdrege.[50]

Calcium ions' positive charge depolymerises the glycose-aminoglycans of the extracellular matrix as it moves from the relative positive to negative domains, simultaneously freeing water that is bound to the negative charge of the sulfates in the polymerised glycose-aminoglycans. Water and calcium ions flow from the more positively charged region of the interface of capillary plasma and interstitial fluid towards the parenchymal cell membrane carrying with them nutrients delivered by the capillaries.

Gases, water, ions and compounds of low molecular weight pass over the capillary membrane by diffusion, filtration and osmosis. Transmural hydrostatic pressure differences, colloid osmotic pressure and concentration differences across the membrane play important roles. The endothelial cells themselves are permeable to lipophilic substances but not hydrophilic ones. Hydrophilic substances pass through the capillary walls through interepithelial spaces (called stomata), pores or leaky junctions.

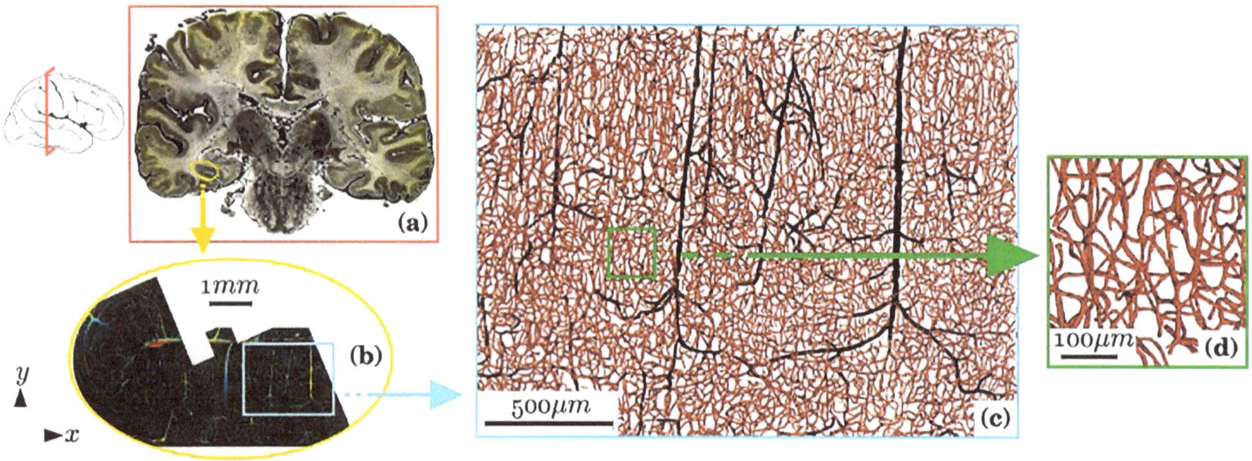


**Figure 13.9 – Multiscale Architecture and Scales of Microvascular Networks in the Human Brain.** Representation of different length scales: (a) Brain scale (*63 cm$^2$ × 300 μm): 300 μm-thick cortical section, where blood vessels have been injected with India ink for contrast enhancement. (b) Macroscopic scale (*18 mm$^2$ × 300 μm): reconstruction of parts of the collateral sulcus by confocal laser microscopy. (c) Mesoscopic scale (*5 mm$^2$ × 300 μm): region of interest in which vessels more than 10 μm in diameter are coloured in black and vessels less than 10 μm in diameter are coloured in red (diameters have been multiplied by 2 for visualisation). In contrast with the capillary bed, the arteriolar and venular trees have a quasi-fractal structure. (d) Microscopic scale (*0.07 mm$^2$ × 300 μm): detailed view of the capillary bed. The capillary bed is dense and space-filling over a cut-off length of * 50 μm. Reprinted from Peyrounette et al.[51]

Electricity drives the process in which these transitions occur, resulting in transient changes of viscosity and a movement of ions and nutrients from the capillary bed to the cells, which cannot be more than 150 μm away. This is because oxygen cannot diffuse beyond 150-200 microns in living tissue at 37° C. Constant adaptation and angiogenesis is therefore required in order for oxygen and nutrients to be adequately supplied (Figure 13.9).

Intracellular activity is also charge driven. In Figure 13.10, found in James Oschman's book *Energy Medicine in Therapeutics and Human Performance,*[75] Oshman noted the receptor on the left, which is the primary locus of electromagnetic field effects. Each of these (sound, pulsed electromagnetic field therapy, laser therapy and osteopathic treatment) can have an effect on the voltage-gated calcium channel so that each can influence this locus.

The calcium flux results in more calcium coming into the cell and then less as it is released into the

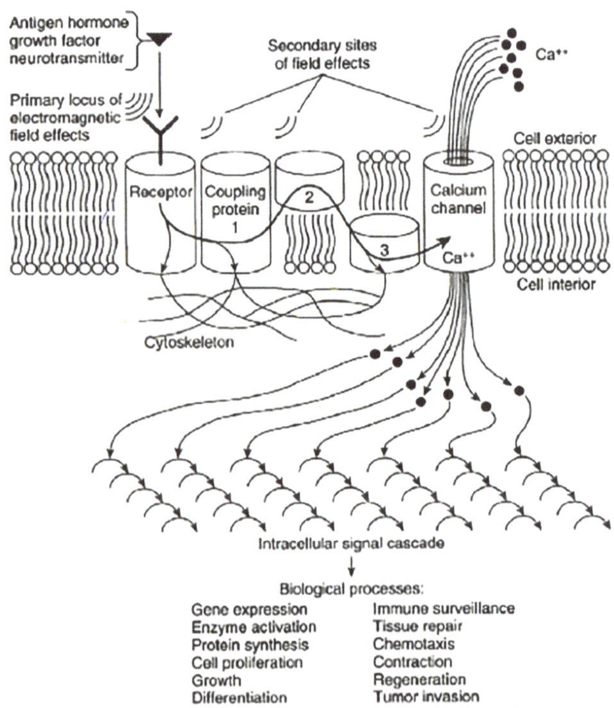


**Figure 13.10 – Charge-Driven Intracellular Activity.** Reprinted from Oschman.[76]

cytoplasm; the cells shrink (extend/expire) as calcium is high and swell (flex/inspire) as calcium is low. Cellular pH shifts between an alkalinity of 7.45 and the slightly lower alkalinity of 7.35 with the charge of the cell membrane oscillating between -90 mV and -70 mV. So, we see the **calcium flux as the interface of Still's celestial and terrestrial**—the physical expression of the **Breath of Life.**[77]

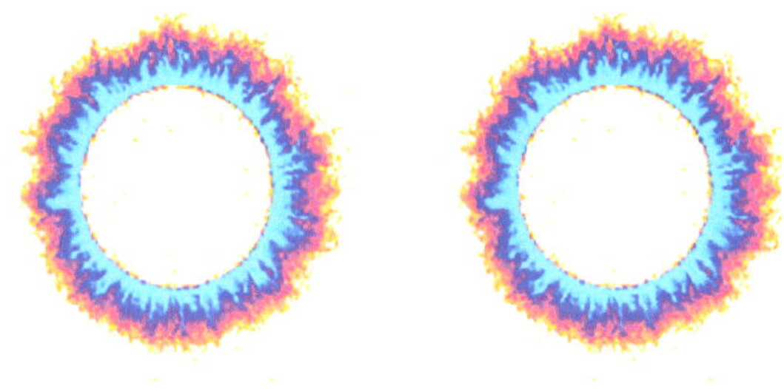

**Figure 13.11 – BioWell Gas Discharge Visualisation Images of Two Digits.**

## Practical Applications to Osteopathic Clinical Practice

There is a link to the calcium flux, the inherent wave of vortical flow of blood that starts its spiral flow before the heart starts breathing. This wave is similar to the Traube-Hering wave which, when supplying the choroid plexus, generates a fluctuant wave of cerebrospinal fluid. When the Traube-Hering wave in the circulation arrives at the capillary bed, it sets up the **ionars**, or ion groups, that cross the paravasal mantle or perivascular space. This is the fascial gateway that allows the heart's code to be transferred to the cells. Goncharenko's experiments[78] (referred to earlier in this chapter as well as in Chapter 7) demonstrated how the blood is "packaged" in the left ventricle and transferred to a specific target area of the body.

Korotkov[79] has developed a device (the BioWell) for measuring the bio-energetic output of the fingers and thumbs and an algorithm to interpret that output (Figure 13.11). Bearing in mind, in the recent research of Li and Pollack, it is possible to envisage the IR emanating from the digits of the osteopath influencing the blood flow of the patient being treated.

It is also possible to observe the synchronisation of waves so that the coherence increases across all areas of the body. At this moment, if there are one or more focal areas of dysfunction, they may become apparent to the osteopathic observer. This is just as Prof Irwin Korr described: one soldier in the regiment out of step becomes immediately apparent.[80]

The presence of a suction force has already been referred to in Chapter 10 where the SphygmoCor measurements of aortic pressure waves are referred to. Seneff describes the suction forces in electrical terms as "a voltage change from artery to vein which propels red blood cells through arteries to capillaries like a magnet."[81] These magnetic/suction forces can be perceived by the trained osteopath.[82,83] This knowledge can then be used to reduce vascular turbulence and restore normal vortical flow, with a downregulation in autonomic nervous system tone resulting in improved musculoskeletal function.[84,85]

## Chapter 13 Endnotes

1. A.T. Still, *Autobiography of Andrew Taylor Still* (Kirksville, MO: A.T. Still, 1908), 224.

2. J.K. Foskett and K.R. Spring, "Involvement of Calcium and Cytoskeleton in Gallbladder Epithelial Cell Volume Regulation," *American Journal of Cell Physiology* 248, no. 1 (January 1985): C27–36.

3. A. Schwab et al., "Migration of Transformed Renal Epithelial Cells Is Regulated by $K^+$ Channel Modulation of Actin Cytoskeleton and Cell Volume," *European Journal of Physiology,* 438, no. 3 (August 1999): 330–7.

4. Raymond F. Gasser, "The First Week of Life: Conception to Implantation Period," Atlas of Human Embryos (R.F. Gasser, 1975), Fig. 1-1, reprinted in The Endowment for Human Development, https://www.ehd.org/classics/gasser_ch1.php.

5. J.L. Bremer, "The Presence and Influence of Two Spiral Streams in the Heart of the Chick Embryo," *American Journal of Anatomy* 49, no. 3 (January 1932): 409–40.

6. Viktor Schauberger, *Our Senseless Toil: The Cause of the World Crisis: Progress Through Transformation of the Atom - Not Its Destruction!,* vol. II (Krystall Verlag Vienna, 1933), 34, https://archive.org/details/Our_Senseless_Toil/mode/2up

7. J.L.W. Thudichum, "On the Cause of the Emptiness of the Arteries After Death," *American Medical Journal* 3, no. 10 (February 1855), 122-7.

8. J. Snow, "On the Circulation in the Capillary Blood Vessels, and on Some of Its Connections With Pathology and Therapeutics," *London Medical Gazette* 31 (1843): 810-6.

9. Leon Manteuffel-Szoege, "Energy Sources of Blood Circulation and the Mechanical Action of the Heart," *Thorax* 15, no. 1 (1960): 47-53, https://thorax.bmj.com/content/15/1/47.

10. Yandell Henderson et al., "The Third Major Mechanical Factor in the Circulation of the Blood," *Science* 79, no 2057 (June 1934): 508-10.

11. C.D. De Langen, "The Vis a Tergo, Capillary Pressure and Capillary Function," *Acta Medica Scandinavica* 140, no. 6 (January/December 1951): 437-45.

12. Branko Furst, *The Heart and Circulation: An Integrative Model,* 2nd ed. (London: Springer International Publishing, 2020).

13. Branko Furst, "The Heart: Pressure-Propulsion or Organ of Impedence?" *Journal of Cardiothoracic and Vascular Anesthesia* 29, no. 6 (December 2015): 1688-1701, https://doi.org/10.1053/j.jvca.2015.02.022.

14. Nuno Koch Esteves, "Regional Thermal Hyperemia in the Human Leg: Evidence of the Importance of Thermosensitive Mechanisms in the Control of the Peripheral Circulation," *Physiological Reports* 9, no. 15 (August 2021): e14953.

15. Zheng Le and Gerald H. Pollack, "On the Driver of Blood Circulation Beyond the Heart," *PLoS One* 18, no. 10 (October 2023): e0289652, https://doi.org/10.1371/journal.pone.0289652.

16. M.E. Murphy and E.C. Carlson, "An Ultrastructural Study of Developing Extracellular Matrix in Vitelline Blood Vessels of the Early Chick Embryo," *American Journal of Anatomy* 151, no. 3 (March 1978): 345-75, https://doi.org/10.1002/aja.1001510304.

17. M.L. Kirby, J.W. McKenzie, and T.A. Weidman, "Developing Innervation of the Chick Heart: A Histofluorescence and Light Microscopic Study of Sympathetic Innervation," *The Anatomical Record* 196, no. 3 (March 1980): 333-340.

18. Margaret Loewy Kirby, *Innervation of the Developing Heart* (New York: Oxford University Press, 2007), 179-97.

19. Jung Yeop Lee and Sang Joon Lee, "Hemodynamics of the Omphalo-Mesenteric Arteries in Stage 18 chicken Embryos and "Flow-Structure" Relations for the Microcirculation," *Microvascular Research* 80 (no. 3), 402-11, https://doi.org/10.1016/j.mvr.2010.08.003.

20. B. Chai, A.G. Mahtani, and G.H. Pollack, "Unexpected Presence of Solute-Free Zones at Metal-Water Interfaces," *Contemporary Materials* 3, no. 1 (2012): 1-12, https://doi.org/10.7251/COM1201001C.

21. Jianming Zheng and Gerald H. Pollack, "Solute Exclusion and Potential Distribution Near Hydrophilic Surfaces," in *Water and Cell*, eds. Gerald H. Pollack, Ivan L. Cameron, and Denys N. Wheatley (Dordrecht: Springer Netherlands, 2016), 165-74.

22. Mina Rohani and Gerald H. Pollack, "Flow through Horizontal Tubes Submerged in Water in the Absence of a Pressure Gradient: Mechanistic Considerations," *Langmuir* 29, no. 22 (June 2013): 6556-61, https://doi.org/10.1021/la4001945.

23. Binghua Chai, Hyok Yoo, and Gerald H. Pollock, "Effect of Radiant Energy on Near-Surface Water," *The Journal of Physical Chemistry* B 113, no. 42 (September 2009): 13953-8.

24. Arthur Yu, Peter Carlson, and Gerald H. Pollack, "Unexpected Axial Flow Through Hydrophilic Tubes: Implications for Energetics of Water," *The European Physical Journal Special Topics* 223, no. 5 (2014): 947-58.

25. Zheng Li and Gerald H. Pollack, "Surface-Induced Flow: A Natural Microscopic Engine Using Infrared Energy as Fuel," *Science Advances* 6, no. 19 (May 2020): eaba0941.

26. Lee and Lee, "Hemodynamics of the Omphalo-Mesenteric Arteries."

27. Fatma Vatansever and Michael R. Hamblin, "Far infrared Radiation (FIR): Its Biological Effects and Medical Applications," *Photonics and Lasers in Medicine* 1, no. 4 (November 2012): 255-66.

28. Le and Pollack, "On the Driver of Blood Circulation Beyond the Heart."

29 "Brain Amplified MP4," Osteopathy's Promise to Children, posted March 27, 2023, on Vimeo, https://vimeo.com/812217885

30. Schauberger, *Our Senseless Toil*, 34.

31. Michael J. Lopez and Carrie A. Hall, "Physiology, Osmosis," in StatPearls (Treasure Island, FL: StatPearls Publishing, 2023), last updated March 13, 2023, https://www.ncbi.nlm.nih.gov/books/NBK557609/.

32. Lopez and Hall, "Physiology, Osmosis."

33. Aleksandr Goncharenko and Svetlana Goncharenko, "Extrasensory Powers of the Heart," *Technology to the Youth*, No. 5 (2005).

34. Goncharenko and Goncharenko, "Extrasensory Powers of the Heart."

35. L.V. Beloussov, V.L. Voeikov, and V.S. Martynyuk, *Biophotons and Coherent Systems in Biology* (Springer, 2007).

36. Goncharenko and Goncharenko, "Extrasensory Powers of the Heart," 3.

37. František Baluška and Michael Levin, "On Having No Head: Cognition throughout Biological Systems," *Frontiers in Psychology* 7 (June 2016): 902.

38. W. Ross Adey, Testimony before the Ad Hoc Subcommittee on Consumer and Environmental Issues of the Committee on Governmental Affairs, United States Senate, August 10, 1992.

39. W. Grundler and F. Kaiser. "Experimental Evidence for Coherent Excitations Correlated With Cell Growth." *Nanobiology* 1 (1992): 163–76.

40. Robert O. Becker and Gary Seldon. *The Body Electric*. (New York, NY: William Morrow, 1998)

41. H. Frenzel and H. Schultes, "Luminescenz im ultraschallbeschickten Wasser," *Zeitschrift für Physikalische Chemie* B27 (1934): 421–4.

42. Sascha Hilgenfeldt, Siegfried Grossmann, and Detlef Lohse, "A Simple Explanation of Light Emission in Sonoluminescence," *Nature* 389, no. 6726 (1999): 402–5.

43. Michael P. Brenner, Sascha Hilgenfeldt, and Detlef Lohse, "Single Bubble Sonoluminescence," *Reviews of Modern Physics* 74, no. 2 (May 2002): 425–48.

44. Zoran Stankovic et al., "4D Flow Imaging With MRI," *Cardiovascular Diagnosis & Therapy*, 4, no. 2 (April 2014): 173-192, https://doi.org/10.3978/j.issn.2223-3652.2014.01.02.

45. Michael Markl et al., "Time-Resolved Three-Dimensional Magnetic Resonance Velocity Mapping of Cardiovascular Flow Paths in Volunteers and Patients With Fontan Circulation," *European Journal of Cardiothoracic Surgery* 39, no. 2 (February 2011): 206–12.

46. H.G. Bogren and M.H. Buonocore, "4D Magnetic Resonance Velocity Mapping of Blood Flow Patterns in the Aorta in Young vs. Elderly Normal Subjects," *Journal of Magnetic Resonance Imaging* 10, no. 5 (November 1999): 861–9.

47. Peter A. Stonebridge, "Three-Dimensional Blood Flow Dynamics: Spiral/Helical Laminar Flow," *DeBakey Cardiovascular Journal* 7, no. 1 (2011): 21–6.

48. Kenneth E. Nelson et al., "Cranial Rhythmic Impulse Related to the Traube-Hering-Mayer Oscillation: Comparing Laser-Doppler Flowmetry and Palpation," *The Journal of the American Osteopathic Association* 101, no. 3 (March 2001): 163–73.

49. Penaz J. Mayer, "Waves: History and Methodology," *Automedica* 2 (1978): 135-41.

50. Charles Herbert Best, *Best and Taylor's Phsiological Basis of Medical Practice*, 12th ed. (Baltimore, MD: Williams & Wilkins, 1990).

51. K.M. Bykov, *Textbook of Physiology* (Moscow: Foreign Languages Publishing House, 1958), 142.

52. *Guyton and Hall Textbook of Medical Physiology*, 12th ed. (Philadelphia, PA: W.B. Saunders Co., 2006). 210.

53. B.W. Hyndman, "The Role of Rhythms in Homeostasis," *Biological Cybernetics* 15 (1974): 227-36.

54. S. Akselrod et al., "Power Spectral Analysis of Heart Rate Fluctuation: A Quantitative Probe of Beat to Beat Cardiovascular Control," *Science* 213, no. 4504 (July 1981): 220-2.

55.S. Akselrod et al., "Hemodynamics Regulation: Investigation by Spectral Analysis," *American Journal of Physiology* 249, no. 4, part 2 (1985): H867-75

56. *Guyton and Hall Textbook of Medical Physiology*, 210.

57. Kenneth E. Nelson et al., "Cranial Rhythmic Impulse Related to the Traube-Hering-Mayer Oscillation: Comparing Laser-Doppler Flowmetry and Palpation," *The Journal of the American Osteopathic Association* 101, no. 3 (March 2001): 163–73.

58. Nicette Surgeef, Kenneth E. Nelson, and Thomas Glonek, "Changes in the Traube-Hering Wave Following Cranial Manipulation," *American Academy of Osteopathy Journal* 11, no. 1 (Spring 2001): 17.

59. András Varga, *Elektrosmog and Health* (Heidelberg, 2002).

60. Personal communication, May 11, 2024, from David Spencer, D.O.

61. Robert M. Davidson and Stephanie Seneff, "The Initial Common Pathway of Inflammation, Disease, and Sudden Death," *Entropy* 14, no. 8 (August 2012): 1399–442.

62. Davidson and Seneff, "The Initial Common Pathway."

63. Abimael González-Hernández et al., "Heteroreceptors Modulating CGRP Release at Neurovascular Junction: Potential Therapeutic Implications on Some Vascular-Related Diseases," *BioMed Research International* 2016 (2016): 2056786.

64. Cornielia Hahn and Martin A. Schwartz, "Mechanotransduction in Vascular Physiology and Atherogenesis," *Nature Reviews: Molecular Cell Biology* 10, no. 1 (January 2009): 53–62.

65. Jeng-Jiann Chiu and Shu Chien, "Effects of Disturbed Flow on Vascular Endothelium: Pathophysiological Basis and Clinical Perspectives," *Physiological Reviews* 91, no. 1 (January 2011): 327-87.

66. Cornelia Hahn and Martin A. Schwartz, "Mechanotransduction in Vasular Physiology and Artherogenesis," *Nature Reviews Molecular Cell Biology* 10, no. 1 (January 2009): 53-62.

67. Luca Carnevali et al., "Exploring the Effects of Osteopathic Manipulative Treatment on Autonomic Function Throuh the Lens of Heart Rate Variability," *Frontiers in Neuroscience* 14 (October 2020): 579365, https://doi.org/10.3389/fnins.2020.579365.

68. Francesco Cerritelli et al., "Does Osteopathic Manipulative Treatment Induce Autonomic Changes in Healthy Participants? A Thermal Imaging Study," *Frontiers in Neuroscience* 14 (August 2020): 887, https://doi.org/10.3389/fnins.2020.00887.

69. Brian Budgell and Barbara Polus, "The Effects of Thoracic Manipulation on Heart Rate Variability: A Controlled Crossover Trial," *Journal of Manipulative Physiological Therapeutics* 29, no. 8 (October 2006): 603–10, https://doi.org/10.1016/j.jmpt.2006.08.011.

70. Charles E. Henley et al., "Osteopathic Manipulative Treatment and Its Relationship to Autonomic Nervous System Activity as Demonstrated by Heart Rate Variability: A Repeated Measure Study," *Osteopathic Medicine and Primary Care* 2 (June 2008): 7, https://doi.org/10.1186/1750-4732-2-7.

71. Björn E.W. Nordenström, "Impact of Biologically Closed Electric Circuits (BCEC) on Structure and Function," *Integrative Physiology and Behavioral Science* 27, no. 4 (October 1992): 285–303, https://doi.org/10.1007/BF02691165.

72. Andrew Taylor Still, *The Philosophy and Mechanical Principles of Osteopathy* (Kansas City, MO: Hudson-Kimberly Pub. Co., 1902), 60.

73. Craig Holdrege, *The Dynamic Heart and Circulation* (Fair Oaks, CA: The Association of Waldorf Schools of North America, 2002).

74. Myriam Peyrounette et al., "Multiscale Modelling of Blood Flow in Cerebral Microcirculation: Details at Capillary Scale Control Accuracy at the Level of the Cortex," *PLoS One* 13, no. 1 (January 2018): e0189474, doi:10.1371/journal.pone.0189474.

75. James L. Oschman, *Energy Medicine in Therapeutics and Human Performance* (Butterworth Heinemann, 2003).

76. Oschman, *Energy Medicine in Therapeutics and Human Performance.*

77. Andrew Taylor Still. *The Philosophy and Mechanical Principles of Osteopathy* (Kansas City, MO: Hudson-Kimberly Pub. co.: 1902)

78. Aleksandr I. Goncharenko, "Heartspace as the Basis of Superconsciousness," *Consciousness and Physical Reality* 2, no. 3 (1997; translated 2017): 25–35.

79. Konstantin Korotkov, *Energy Fields Electrophotonic Analysis in Humans and Nature* (eBookIt.com, 2013).

80. Irvin Korr, *The Physiological Basis of Osteopathic Medicine* (San Rafael, CA: Insight Publishing Company, 1982).*See Ch 3 pg 18*

81. Davidson and Seneff, "The Initial Common Pathway."

82. Luca Carnevali et al., "Exploring the Effects of Osteopathic Manipulative Treatment on Autonomic Function Through the Lens of Heart Rate Variability," *Frontiers in Neuroscience* 14 (October 2020): 579365, https://doi.org/10.3389/fnins.2020.579365.

83. Francesco Cerritelli et al., "Does Osteopathic Manipulative Treatment Induce Autonomic Changes in Healthy Participants? A Thermal Imaging Study," *Frontiers in Neuroscience* 14 (August 2020): 887, https://doi.org/10.3389/fnins.2020.00887.

84. Brian Budgell and Barbara Polus, "The Effects of Thoracic Manipulation on Heart Rate Variability: A Controlled Crossover Trial," *Journal of Manipulative Physiological Therapeutics* 29, no. 8 (October 2006): 603–10, https://doi.org/10.1016/j.jmpt.2006.08.011.

85. Charles E. Henley et al., "Osteopathic Manipulative Treatment and Its Relationship to Autonomic Nervous System Activity as Demonstrated by Heart Rate Variability: A Repeated Measure Study," *Osteopathic Medicine and Primary Care* 2 (June 2008): 7, https://doi.org/10.1186/1750-4732-2-7.

# Chapter Fourteen

# A Vasculature Description of the Motion of the Primary Respiratory Mechanism

*"All parts in the whole obey the one eternal law of life and motion."*[1]

– Andrew Taylor Still

Dr Sutherland proposed a model to describe the cranial primary respiratory mechanism (PRM), which has engendered debate since its inception: its validity as a model for clinical practice on the one hand and its generation on the other.

Sutherland's insight began with the cranial sutures, recognising anatomical details and features that revealed a mechanism for movement between the cranial bones. He believed these cranial movements were subtle and essential to normal and healthy physiology and biomechanics.[2]

Movement and overlap of the sutures allow the human cranium the malleability to traverse the birth canal and accommodate the growth movements from conception to adulthood. Sutherland described the axes of motion of the cranial bones (Figure 14.1), the reciprocal tension membrane and the neural structures.

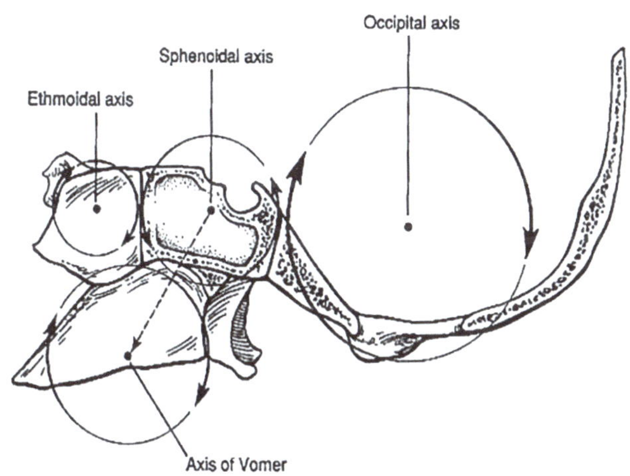


**Figure 14.1 – The Cranial Base in Flexion.** This illustration demonstrates the rotation that takes place around the parallel transverse axis. Reprinted from Sutherland.[3]

Sutherland's model of the PRM correlates with the biomechanics of the vasculature, and we (the authors) propose that these physiological axes of motion and functions represent the expression of biomechanical tensions provided by the vasculature.

Ongoing explorations into the role of the vasculature have developed into an explanation of the motion of the bones of the cranium, as described by Sutherland's model, from a vasculature perspective. What we attempt to do in this chapter is take the motion of the cranial base and relate it to the architecture of the vascular system.

## Biotensegrity of the Vasculature Membranes

As osteopaths, we begin with the motion of the bones of the cranial base. These motions can be seen as a result of embryologic dynamics that persist into adulthood. Now we expand on the implications of a neurovascular model and explore the biomechanical functions of vascular membranes contributing to the biotensegrity of the bony architecture and extending to the whole organism.

Vascular membranes in major vessels are strong, muscular and collagenous structures which have previously not been recognised as lines of tension that exert significant forces on the tissues they supply (Figure 14.2).

The reader is asked to broaden their understanding of biomechanics as the forces of life exerted by living organisms. The neuromuscular model does not account for the growth movements observed in embryonic development.

Cell mechanobiology is an area of research investigating cellular forces that shape our form and function. Cells are shown to sense and respond to external forces in a process called mechanotransduction. Cells sense mechanical forces and respond by changing shape and converting the biomechanical signals into biochemical and biophysical responses.

## A Model to Describe the Morphogenetic and Morphokinetic Functions of the Heart and Vessels

The heart and vessels maintain a reciprocal tension with the tissues they traverse, cleanse and nourish.

Vascular tensions organise the growth movements of the embryo biosculpting human form and function.

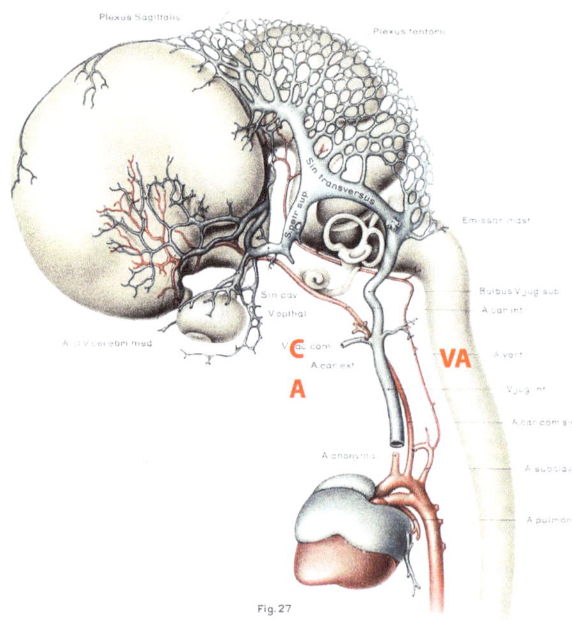


**Figure 14.2 – Vascular Fulcra in Cranial Base Function: A Proposed Model.**[4]

Tens of thousands of capillary rootlets are physiologically cohesive with trillions of cells. We see this as cohesion by metabolism.

The larger vascular branches exert biomechanical forces on the tissue beds and, in the context of the whole vascular tree, these forces are formative. The vascular tensions shape human form and function as dynamic fulcra by bridling the growth dynamics. The heart is the biophysical fulcrum at the centre of autonomic functions utilising thousands of neurons in coordination with the brain. Kaplan, Chow and Gu found that:

"The brain is a highly vascularized organ, with every neuron positioned within 150 μm of a blood vessel. This proximity allows for ready exchange of nutrients and waste products, enabling the high metabolic activity of the brain despite its limited intrinsic energy storage."[5]

This cell-vascular proximity and the cohesive metabolic connection that results explains why tissue ensembles are shaped by their vascular fulcra.

The forces of mechanobiology are exerted by cells as they grow and expand and contract. These growth movements help to shape complex organisms and utilise vascular fulcra for ontogenetic development.

## Suspended From Bregma and the Vascular Midline

The notochord serves as a dynamic midline for the growth of the embryo. This is a functional midline that recognises a null point around which the growth occurs.

In this model, vascular orientation is described in relation to the midline of the interventricular septum of the heart. The vasculature separates into right and left, anterior and posterior territories and will be described in relation to the heart.

In Chapter 4, the interventricular septum (IVS) was introduced as a shifting, suspended fulcrum with fascial connections to the whole body. This septum functions as the vascular midline of the whole and the body will be considered as suspended from bregma.

The continuity between the IVS vascular and periosteal membranes is described in reference to Figure 14.11. This continuity between the jugular vein and the periosteal and dural membranes was established when the embryo was only a few millimetres long and the vascular rootlets were established to their target tissues. The vascular model requires appreciation for the living continuity of all tissues.

In Chapter 6, we explored Blechschmidt and Gasser's book *Biokinetics and Biodynamics of Human Differentiation,* which describes the restraining action of the vasculature on the developing central nervous system (CNS).[6]

As a general concept, the action of flexion by the developing neural tissues can be seen as a reorientation towards the heart and the source of nutrition, whereas the movement of extension can be seen as the resultant growth movement away from the heart. This growth movement is limited purely by the difference of nutrition that exists as a result of the permeative access to nutrition of the CNS versus the parmeative* access available to the conduits of that nutrition.

The relationship between the heart, the CNS and the tissues generally can be described as source and sink with respect to nutrition, with the vessels being the conduit. The sink (the body's 35 trillion cells) readily absorbs nutrition into the tissue and growth is consequently rapid. The access to nutrition for the vessel walls is significantly less because it is parmeative, and so growth rates are significantly lower, and a fluctuant physiologic motion tension consequently develops between source/heart and sink/CNS and tissues. This dynamic around nutrition is the basis of the flexion/extension pattern.

In the classic description of cranial base motion, the movement of the bones is described as occurring around various axes—transverse, vertical and anteroposterior—in health and dysfunction. This description, while useful in teaching the palpatory experience of base motion, fails to adequately explain the compound movement of the sphenoid

*For a discussion of parmeation and permeation, see Chapter 2 and Chapter 6.

and occiput even in the simplest expression of cranial bone motion.

Understanding and working with the vasculature as the primary axis creates an opportunity, when coupled with an understanding of the importance of the associated functional vascular dynamics, to describe the movement of the base and vault, as well as how that movement relates to embryologic development and adult motion expressed.

In this light, the rotatory and lateral motion of the sphenoid and occiput can be integrated with the vertical motion of shortening and lengthening when we understand that the whole mechanism is orientated to the heart (and T4).

Blechschmidt and Gasser[9] state:

> "The anlagen of the umbilical arteries being part of the body stalk cause it to arch convexly into the chorionic cavity. This demonstrates that arteries, with their higher pressure, lengthen at a faster rate than do the weaker, low-pressure veins. This observation is in accordance with a rule for the development of blood vessels. It is believed that the bending of the body stalk is caused by the restraining function of the unpaired umbilical vein against the umbilical arteries in the stalk. If this were not true, then one would expect the arteries to be straight because of their higher blood pressure."

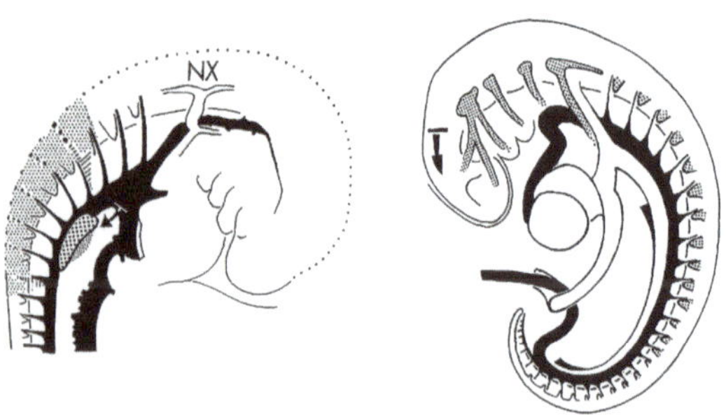


**Figure 14.3 – Vascular Tensions and Growth Fulcra.** The embryo bends as a result of the tension and resistance offered by the dorsal aortae forming the pharyngeal arches. Aortic arch arteries form in response to metabolic fluid gradients that develop from the heart. Reprinted from Blechschmidt.[8]

From this we understand that the flexion of the neural tube is consequent to the differential of growth rates between the neural tube and the anterior embryonic structures (Figure 14.3).

> "These dorsal branches of the aortae function, as do all blood vessels, as restraining structures. They hold on to the growing neural tube just as though they were cords, so that the embryo bends forward as it grows."[10]

Within that dynamic another growth differential phenomenon takes place in the vasculature itself. The veins, with their reduced nutritional supply compared to the arteries, become the growth-limiting factor for the mushrooming nervous system, resulting in a bending of the embryo (Figure 14.4). The arteries, with their access to more nutrition, could keep abreast of the CNS development, but

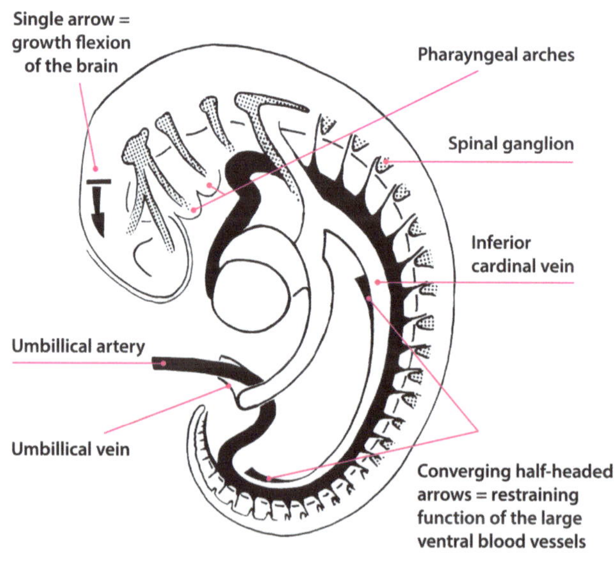


**Figure 14.4 – Embryonic Flexion and Extension.** The neural tube of the embryo flexes towards its nutrient source, swells after assimilating nutrients, then extends away from the nutrient source. These growth movements represent metabolic movements and the future adult functions of flexing and extending in relation to the dominant side of the vasculature. Reprinted from Blechschmidt.[11]

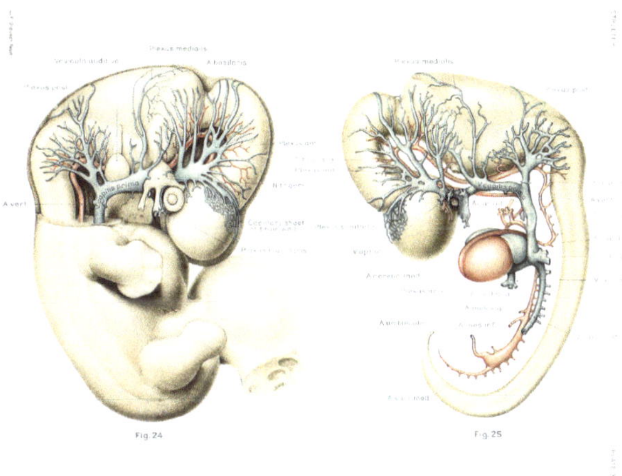

**Figure 14.5 – Right and Left Profile Views of the Blood Vessels of the Brain in a Human Embryo 11.5 mm Long.** The embryo bends on the side of the dominant vasculature. Reprinted from Streeter.[12]

the veins cannot. The dynamic of access to nutrition also plays out in the differential of growth between the CNS and the surrounding mesenchyme with the tissue that will become the face not developing as quickly as the neural tube.

## Vascular Biotensegrity and Dr Sutherland's Model

In Chapter 2 of *Teachings in the Science of Osteopathy*, which is dedicated to the primary respiratory mechanism (PRM), Dr Sutherland describes the features and tissues that give expression to the PRM. These include:

- the fluctuation of the cerebrospinal fluid, which is an expression of the potency of the **Tide**.
- the reciprocal tension membrane, which includes a shifting tension and a fulcrum
- the motility of the neural tube
- the articular mobility of the bones of the cranium at the sutures and the involuntary mobility of the sacrum between the ilia (the pelvic bones).[13]

Sutherland goes on to say:

> "I have been giving you a description of the material mechanism, that mechanism man utilizes in his walk about on earth. I call your attention to the location of the physiologic centers in the floor of the fourth ventricle that regulate the secondary mechanisms of the living body. The location of these vital primary centers points out my reason for naming the primary respiratory mechanism primary. That great battery, the Tide, functions through that region. Realize that the 'highest known element' is transmuted to these physiologic centers. The cranial nerve nuclei also receive the transmutation from that 'highest known element,' from the battery that contains the 'juice.'"[14]

As an extension of Dr Sutherland's insight, in our study of the embryological process, we have recognised the metabolic respiratory movements of all cells and tissues demonstrate a biphasic pattern that represents the assimilation and dissimilation of nutrients and byproducts.

In a healthy embryo, this is a whole-body wave of respiratory metabolism that precedes and prepares for thoracic respiration when the lungs breathe air.

During the flexion phase of primary respiration, the body coils towards the fulcrum of the heart.

The vascular membranes are continuous with dural membranes and these living connections orientate the sacrum, sphenoid and occiput towards the heart.

As a result, the heart and vessels function as morphogenetic fulcra during development and morphokinetic fulcra for later functions.

### Vascular Biotensegrity

The sphenobasilar synchondrosis functions as the fulcrum for cranial base motion, and Dr Sutherland investigated and described the axes of bony motion.

The vectors of cranial base motion share vascular fulcra which relate to the heart (Figure 14.6–10).

Consider this dynamic as we look at cranial base motion. It becomes apparent that the motion described of the sphenoid around its transverse axis relates to the mechanical and physiologic restraint of the vasculature anterior to the tip of the notochord (the ophthalmic and external jugular veins and the internal and external carotid arteries). The vasculature of the cranium behind the tip of the notochord determines the motion of the occiput.

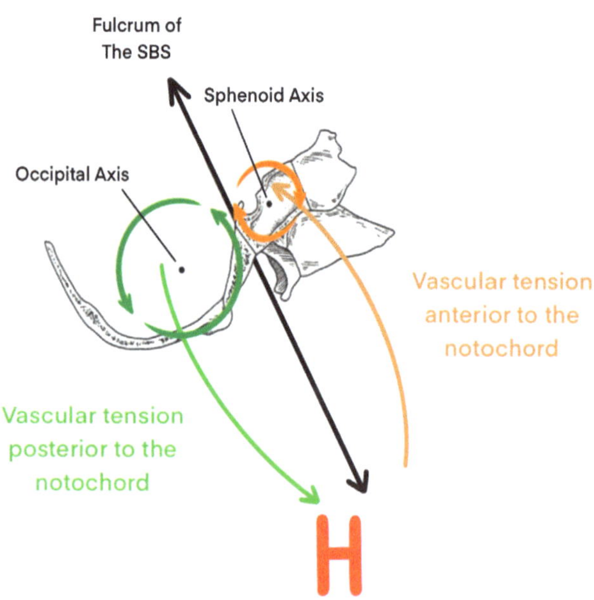


**Figure 14.6 – Arterial Tension During Flexion-Inspiration of the Primary Respiratory Mechanism.**

The occiput rotates posteriorly because the vascular tensions are predominantly posterior to the axes of motion. The sphenoid rotates anteriorly because the vessels woven into the tissue are predominantly anterior to the sphenobasilar synchondrosis.

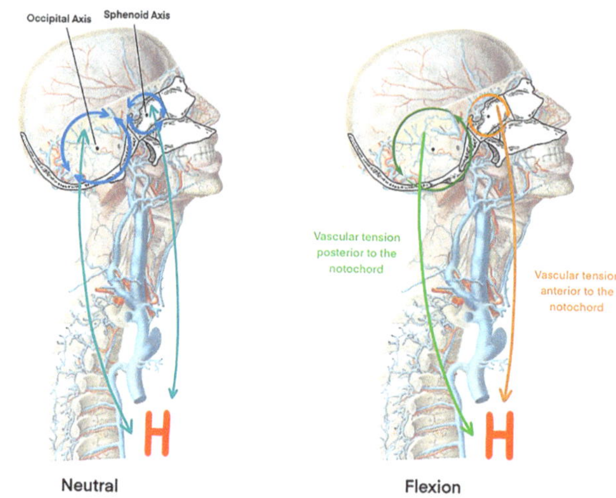


**Figure 14.7 – Lateral View of Cranial Base Motion and Vascular Fulcra in Flexion.**

The neutral image represents the biphasic movements and vectors for metabolic respiration. There is reciprocal vascular tension between the inspiratory-expiratory phases.

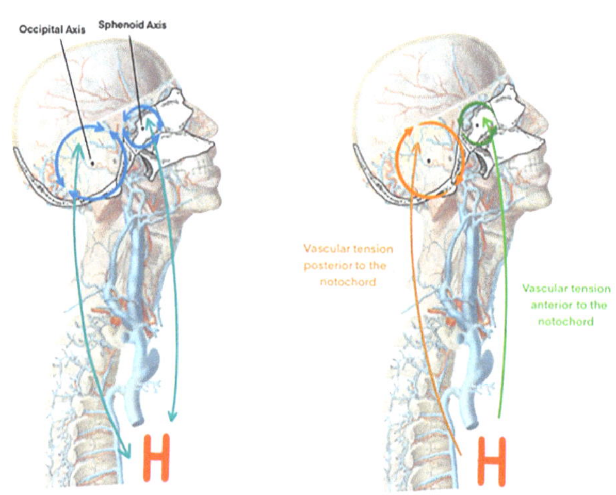


**Figure 14.8 – Lateral View of Cranial Base Motion and Vascular Fulcra in Extension.**

The extension phase of primary respiration involves an arterial spiral that bridles tissues away from the heart. This involves a narrowing and lengthening of the whole organism as it inspires. The axes of motion are opposite to those expressing flexion.

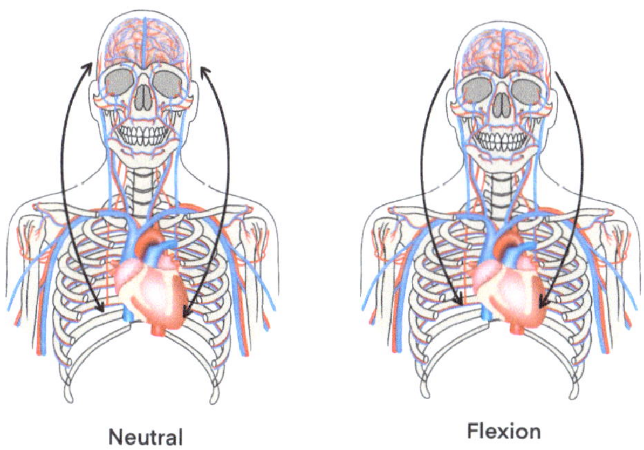


**Figure 14.9 – Anterior View of Cranial Base Motion and Vascular Fulcra During Flexion.**

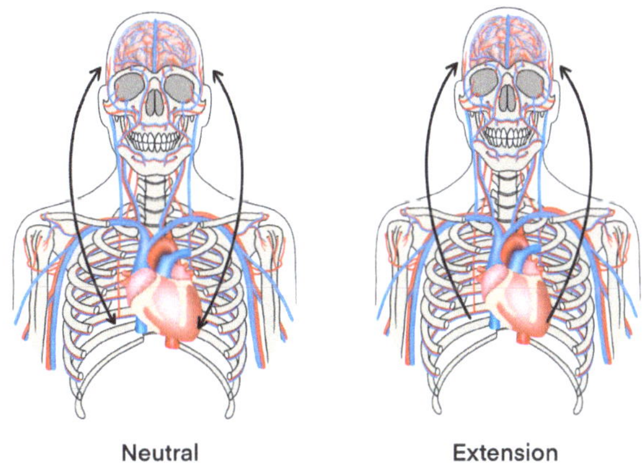


**Figure 14.10 – Anterior View of Cranial Base Motion and Vascular Fulcra During Extension.**

The vessels lateral to the anterior midline tense the tissues in opposite directions, a lateral and anteroposterior growth tugging toward the heart. This serves many functions.

Arteries lateral to bregma (Figure 14.11) are in reciprocal tension with their venous connections via the capillary beds. As tissues respire metabolically, the lateral branches of the arteries and veins are the lateral guy ropes which tether the head and neck in balance with the anterior vasculature to maintain bipedal functions.

Veins exert more restraint than arteries on the tissues they drain because developmentally they grew more slowly. As a result, venous structures exert a widening and shortening of the whole organism during inpiration of the whole body.

The venous sinuses and plexi form a continuous venous organ that adapts to the demands of growth

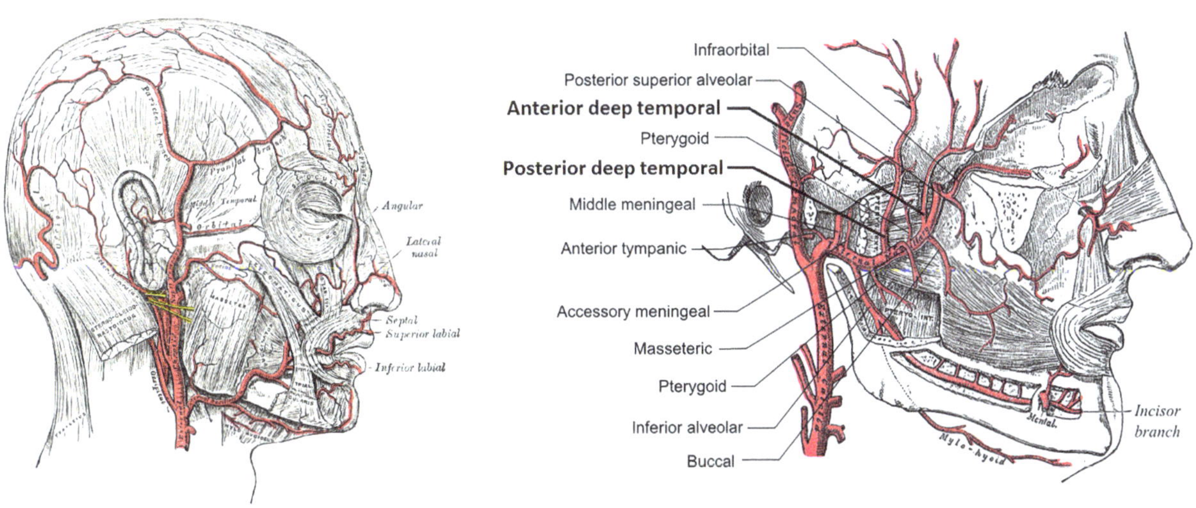


**Figure 14.11 – Lateral Arteries and Veins and Their Deep Temporal Counterparts.**[15,16]

and locomotion. The venous and arterial structures extend to every cell, nourishing and shaping their form and organising their functions (Figure 14.12).

The motion and function of the temporal bone, which has been erroneously described as the troublemaker in the cranial bone mobility model, can more accurately be seen for the role that it fills: the resolution in the bone of the balance between vascularity anterior and posterior to the notochord tip. Any dysfunction between the two fields of vascular influence must necessarily create an adaptive dynamic in temporal bone motion.

### Temporal Bone Mechanics and Vascular Tensions

The axes of rotation for temporal bone motion and the temporal lobe relate to the lateral branches of the Circle of Willis, which develop in response to the coiled growth of the neural tube.

As the cranial mechanism begins a flexion cycle, the combined tensions of the vessels can be interpreted. The temporal bones and membranes are tensed anteriorly, laterally and posteriorly in flexion, which is predominantly an effect of the bridling of the venous membranes, which exert more restraint than the arterial membranes. There is reciprocal tension between the vasculature lateral to the sagittal midline.

Sutherland described the motion of the temporal bones as a 'wobbling wheel'.[18] There is an oblique axis in each temporal bone that functions as a physiological fulcrum. The mechanism flexes and widens as the temporal "wheel" tilts slightly more laterally.

Magoun described the temporal bone axis going through the roughened quadrilateral surface on the underside of the temporal bone and going to the petrous apex beside the petrobasilar articulation.[19] This is what makes the wobbly wheel.

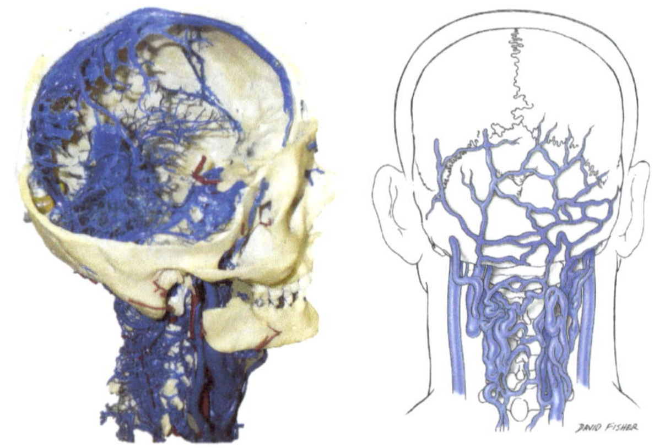

**Figure 14.12 – Venous Drainage is Considerable and Capacious.**[17]

The petrojugular influences the sigmoid sinus and internal jugular and the petrobasilar influences the inferior petrosal sinus, and both are sites for "haltefunktion" (first discussed in Chapter 6).

In flexion, the superior sagittal sinus widens and orientates the dural veins to augment venous drainage. This combines with lateral tensions of the vessels to produce a wobbly wheel where the fulcrum for bony movements follows the axis.[20]

## Bridling of the Vasculature

Professor Blechschmidt used the German term, "*haltefunktion*" or "bridling" to describe how the heart and vessels guide and protect the growing tissues. A similar concept is the bridle of the horse, which describes the tensions used to steer the horse, restrain it and permit it the freedom to gallop.

The heart and vessels perform similar functions to the embryonic tissues. Signaling by nitric oxide or vascular endothelial growth factor guides the direction of flow and the arterial pulse represents the gallop of the spiraling flow. The restraining functions are venous tissues that represent the limits of the resources.

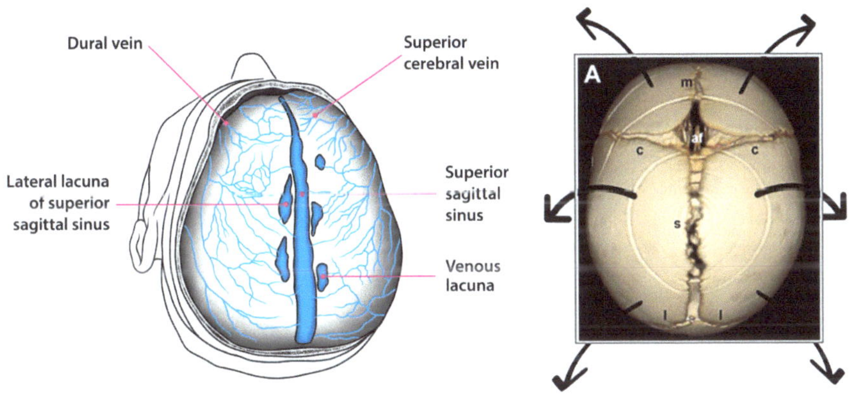


**Figure 14.13 – Sagittal Sinus and Lacunae as Part of "Haltefunktion" or "Bridling".** Arrows indicate the bridling effect of the vessels.

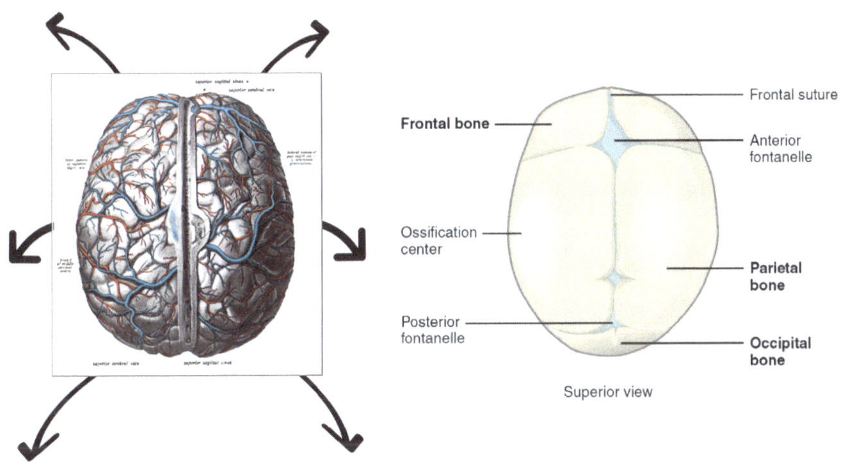


**Fig 14.14 – The Guiding, Supporting, Restraining and Reporting Function of the Veins Operating Anterior and Posterior to the Temporal Bones.**

The function of the superior sagittal suture is a consequence of the bridling of the vessels on the left and right of the sagittal midline (Figure 14.13).

There is a physiological, rhythmic, cohesion of competing tensions. The anterior vessels, predominantly the carotid arteries and jugular veins, are responsible for the coronal suture. Combinations of vascular bridling of the vessels anterior and lateral to bregma with vessels lateral to bregma and the function of the fontanelles is explained.

The motion of the occiput around its transverse axis is dominated by its relationship to the jugular veins and the vertebral venous plexus (vertebral arteries). The motion of the temporal bone around its oblique axis is dominated by the superior and inferior petrosal veins draining into the internal jugular veins and the basilar plexus draining into the vertebral venous plexus.

It is also integrating the position of the carotid running transversely along the anterior border of the petrous portion (The carotid artery is also resolving the restraint of the vertebral arteries.) The resolution of the dynamic between arterial and venous influences generates a balanced tension between the components of the temporal vasculature.

The motion of the temporal bone can be seen to be the result of trying to resolve the relationship with the carotid artery (and its horizontal course along the anterior margin of the petrous) with the drainage of the inferior and superior petrosal veins into the jugular system (Figure 14.14).

This balance of tension between the arteries and

veins can be perceived throughout the cranium and is a major part of the dynamic of the craniofacial suture development that remains as patent as mobile joints. The motion that the sutures accommodate is the remnant of the movement of the embryo toward the heart for nutrition and away in growth, with the mesenchyme differentiating into the tissues as described in Sutherland's phenomena.[22]

The motion persists throughout life as we never resolve the need to return to mother heart for nutrition while we extend into the world in all our activities.

Because growth of the mesenchyme and CNS are both dependent on the vasculature, the resultant **axis of movement for the temporal bone relates to the growth direction of the internal carotid** plus the mechanical forces resulting from the motion and motility of the other phenomena. The axis is not related to the temporal bone but rather to the sum of the forces responding to the need to minimally impact the vasculature (ie, **the artery is the prime reference**) (Figure 14.15).

When we understand the embryology as described by Blechschmidt, it becomes apparent that Blechschmidt's work supports the position that movement persists in the skull, as can be seen in the amplified motion related to circulatory function. The motion of the face (Figure 14.16), including the mandible, is orientated to the restraining effect of the ophthalmic, retromandibular and external jugular veins (external and internal carotids).

The anatomy expresses the pattern of the vascular bundle to any particular structure running along the path of least potential for motion to disrupt the delivery of blood to the target tissue. Thus, the axis of motion for the mandible is seen to commence at the mandibular foramen, which is the point of entry for the inferior alveolar artery and vein. The resultant lines of tension created by the vasculature are consistent with the axes of motion proposed by Sutherland.

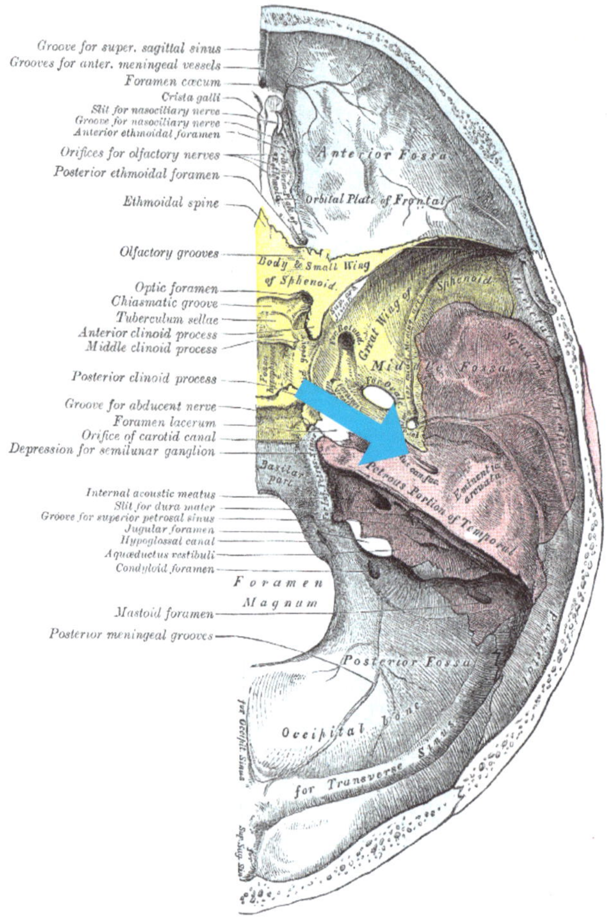


**Figure 14.15 – Base of the Skull Direction of Growth.**[21] The blue arrow shows the direction of growth as the mesenchyme responds to central nervous system development. The most medial portion of the carotid represents the earlier embryologic position and coordinates with the lateral growth of the cervicis. Reprinted from Gray.

These relationships begin embryologically, and the development of the reciprocal tension membrane can be seen to be not only a product of the developing CNS but also the resolution of the growth forces by the mesenchyme associated with the developing hemispheres (Figure 14.17). This mesenchyme is dependent on a supply of nutrition equal to that of the CNS in order to match the growth rate. As the volume of blood flow to the CNS is significantly higher, the mesenchyme cannot match the growth rates. It condenses in order to restrain, and in so doing, it determines CNS growth parameters through the development of the anterior and posterior dural girdles.

The development of the venous sinuses within the reciprocal tension membrane point to the balance between the arterial and venous components of the vasculature and the reciprocal tension between Sutherland's described phenomena. This vasculature description identifies the intracranial membranes as the extension of the venous system into the cranium and validates the role of the membranes in cranial motion physiology.

The close correlation between intracranial venous drainage and the membranous system can be seen in George Streeter's image in Figure 14.18.

There is histological continuity between all of the different layers of the neural membranous and bony structures. Histology reveals a continuity of all tissues and fluids.

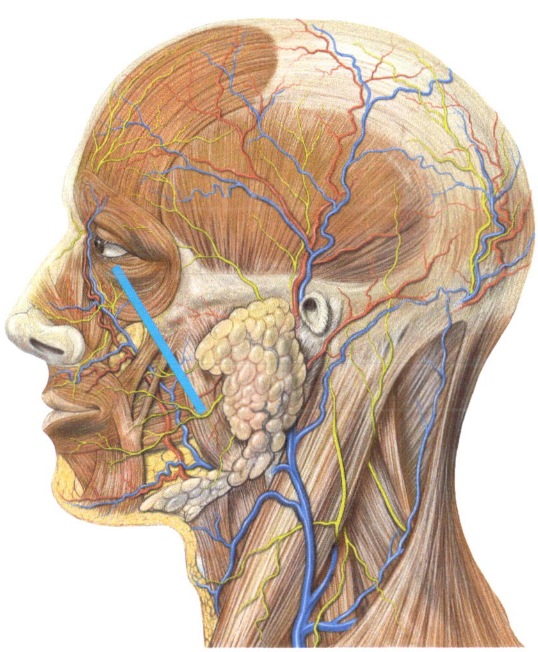

**Figure 14.16 – Axis of Motion of the Face.**[23] The facial vein. The blue line (added to the original image) indicates the axis. Illustration by Patrick J. Lynch, CC BY 2.5.

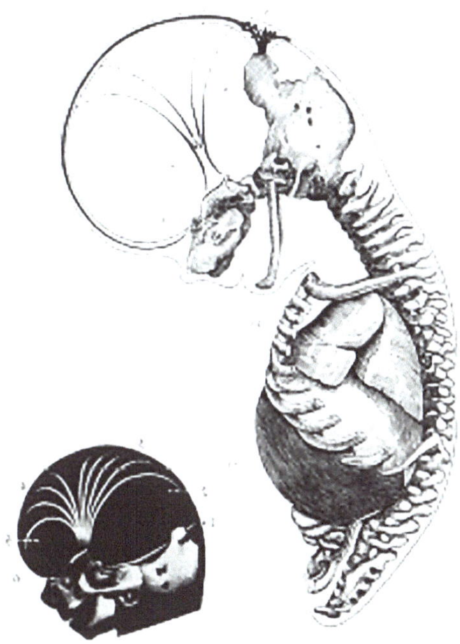

**Figure 14.17 – Vascular Fulcra in Cranial Base Function: Proposed Model.** Reprinted from Blechschmidt.

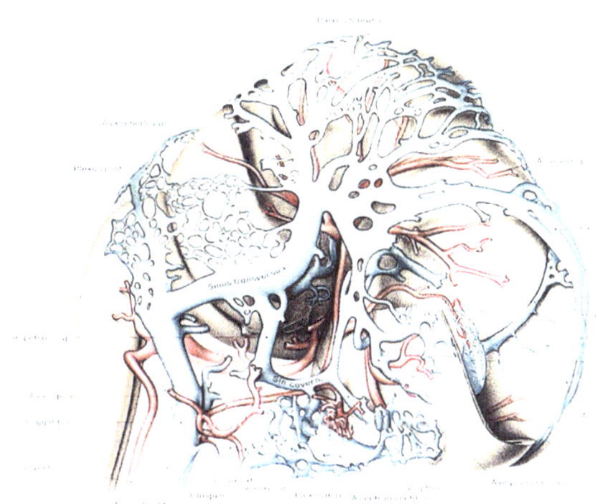

**Figure 14.18 – Blood Vessels of the Brain in a 21-mm Embryo.** Reprinted from George Streeter.

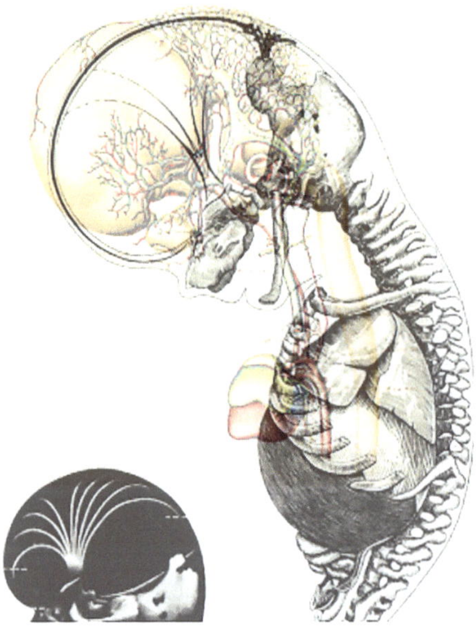

**Figure 14.19 – Left Profile of Blood Vessels of the Brain in 43-mm Embryo.** The anterior dural girdle resolves tensions between the middle cerebral artery and the growing brain. These are restraining and guiding functions for the development of the neural tube.

The periosteal membranes are continuous with the dural membranes and blend into the meninges and neural structures (Figure 14.19). There is fluid compartment continuity between the cerebrospinal fluid in the lymphatics and, most importantly, the directly continuous dural membranes before the venous structures.

Anatomic and physiologic asymmetry in both embryologic as well as adult presentation contributes to the morphology and functioning of all the sutures, down to and including the beveling seen within the vault. It is well understood that the beveling and associated changes that generate the pivot points are related to the growth dynamics of the CNS, with the pivots and axes of motion tracing the growth of the underlying CNS.

The pattern of growth itself is determined by the nutritional dynamic associated with the arterial and venous development generating the axes of motion that relate to the vascular restraint that the veins generate.

There is a mechanical view of bones and human movement that uses pulleys and levers to understand human functions. The neuromuscular model has limitations.

To make sense of the neurovascular model, the reader is asked to review their understanding of bones and mechanics and biomechanics.

Humans do not stand on their bones; the bones support weight and locomotion, but in reality, weight bearing is organised by dense columns of water. In health, weight-bearing bones do not touch each other. There is synovial fluid in joints that lubricates and nourishes the hyaline cartilage and covers and separates the bones.

Hyaline cartilage is a water-dense living sponge that covers these surfaces and uses electromagnetic repulsion between negatively charged proteoglycans to resist and respond to mechanical forces. Humans walk on water.

Human bodies are water, pressurised in a living, semipermeable membrane, encased by an atmosphere that presses on the human body at almost 1 kilogram per square centimeter at sea level.

The neurovascular model views the pressurised flow in vessels as columns of hydraulic tensions which assist movement and structure the organism.

## Morphokinetic Connections

This vascular model introduces the biomechanical and biophysical forces responsible for human functions.

Living tissues maintain physiological connections with their resources, the vessels which nourish and cleanse the cells and their surroundings and function within 100 –150 microns to maintain their viability. The connection between cells and vessels is physiological, and because they interact metabolically, they are cohesive by metabolism.

Human vessels are 60 to 80 thousand kilometers in length, and 90% are the unseen microscopic capillary meshes.

The visible arteries and veins are organs, many with muscular walls. The larger vessels push and pull on their capillary beds and their cellular ensembles.

The importance of the living connections between cells and their nutrient sources is investigated by research in neuronal and vascular coupling.

## Paradigm: The Heart Is Much More Than a "Pump"

Metabolically active tissue release vasodilators to increase their access to nearby blood flows. Nitric oxide was awarded molecule of the year when its function as a short-acting neurotransmitter was discovered. Cells release more NO when they are respiring metabolically and need more oxygen.

Circulation is organised locally and the heart responds. The blood is not pumped into the active areas, it is sucked there by metabolic and osmotic gradients. The cells turn on the tap and drink. The blood wasn't pushed there.

Cells increase their access to the blood flows nearby. When more blood returns to the heart, its output increases to match the increasing demands because cardiac output is proportional to venous return.

Dr Still exhorted us to "dig on" and we have done so in a spirit of profound appreciation for his work and that of Dr Sutherland. We believe the model of function we have proposed in these last two chapters explains the genesis for the inherent or electromotive force that drives fluids and their interface with all tissues. In turn, the biodynamic and biokinetic response of the developing tissues of the embryo interface with the fluids in a dynamic pattern of growth movements, which include twisting, stretching, flexing and extending, the recognition and understanding of which can provide vital clues for the osteopath seeking to promote a tissue response that is focused on health.

Both Dr Still and Dr Sutherland were not convinced that the heart is just a pump. The realisation that Dr Sutherland said as much in *The Cranial Bowl* came almost at the end of writing this book. At the same time, the understanding that the heart both provides and receives information/feedback has led us back to the core of Dr Still's osteopathic philosophy and a part of the practice of early osteopaths.

The last word is given to Dr Still:

*"From the heart as the center of force, electricity carries on the process of delivering blood by way of the arteries and other fluids and gasses by way of the excretories."*[24]

## Chapter 14 Endnotes

1. A.T. Still, *Autobiography of Andrew Taylor Still* (Kirkville, MO: A.T. Still, 1908), 149.

2. William Garner Sutherland, *Teachings in the Science of Osteopathy,* (Fort Worth, TX: Sutherland Cranial Teaching Foundation, Inc., 1990).

3. Sutherland, *Teachings in the Science of Osteopathy.*

4. G.L. Streeter, "The development alterations in the vascular system of the brain of the human embryo," *Contributions in Embryology* 8 (1921): Fig. 27, republished in Mark A. Hill, Embryology, Streeter1921 fig27.jpeg, accessed September 21, 2024. Retrieved from https://embryology.med.unsw.edu.au/embryology/index.php/File:Streeter1921_fig27.jpg.

5. Luke Kaplan, Brian W Chow, and Chenghua Gu, "Neuronal Regulation of the Blood-Brain Barrier and Neurovascular Coupling," *Nature Reviews Neuroscience* 21, no. 8 (August 2020): 416-32, https://doi.org/10.1038/s41583-020-0322-2.

6. Erich Blechschmidt and Raymond F. Gasser, "Axial Process," *Biokinetics and Biodynamics of Human Differentiation: Principles and Applications* (Springfield, IL: Charles Thomas Publishing, 1978).

7. See footnote on page 239.

8. Erich Blechschmidt, *The Ontogenetic Basis of Human Anatomy: A Biodynamic Approach to Development From Conception to Birth* (Berkeley, CA: North Atlantic Books, 2004), 104.

9. Blechschmidt and Gasser, "Axial Process."

10. Erich Blechschmidt, *The Ontogenetic Basis of Human Anatomy: A Biodynamic Approach to Development From Conception to Birth* (Berkeley, CA: North Atlantic Books, 2004), 102.

11. Blechschmidt, *The Ontogenetic Basis of Human Anatomy,* 102.

12. George L. Streeter, "The development alterations in the vascular system of the brain of the human embryo," *Contributions in Embryology* 8 (1921): plate 3, republished in Mark A. Hill, Embryology, Streeter-plate03.jpeg, accessed August 23, 2024, https://embryology.med.unsw.edu.au/embryology/index.php?title=File:Streeter-plate03.jpg

13. Sutherland, *Teachings in the Science of Osteopathy,* 13-30.

14. Sutherland, *Teachings in the Science of Osteopathy*, 22.

15. Henry Gray, "Plate 508," *Anatomy of the Human Body.* https://commons.wikimedia.org/wiki/File:Gray508.png.

16. Henry Gray, "Deep Temporal Arteries, Plate 510," *Anatomy of the Human Body.* https://commons.wikimedia.org/wiki/File:Deep_temporal_arteries.png.

17. Kennedy Carpenter,et al., "Revisiting the Vertebral Venous Plexus–A Comprehensive Review of the Literature," *World Neurosurgery* 145 (January 2021): 381-95, https://doi.org/10.1016/j.wneu.2020.10.004.

18. Sutherland, *Teachings in the Science of Osteopathy,* 123.

19. Harlod Ives Magoun, *Osteopathy in the Cranial Field,* 3rd ed. (The Cranial Academy, 1976), 148.

20. Carpenter, "Revisiting the Vertebral Venous Plexus."

21. Henry Gray, "Base of the Skull: inner cerebral surface," *Gray's Anatomy* (20th edition). https://commons.wikimedia.org/wiki/File: Gray193.png.

22. Ann L. Wales, "The Work of William Garner Sutherland," *The Journal of the American Osteopathic Association* 71 (May 1972): 788-793.

23. Patrick Lynch, "Lateral Head Anatomy Detail," Creative Commons Attribution 2.5 License 2006 "Wikimedia Commons. https://en.wikipedia.org/wiki/Angular_vein#/media/File:Lateral_head_anatomy_detail.jpg.

24. A.T. Still, *Osteopathy Research and Practice* (Kirksville, MO: The Journal Printing Co, 1910), 328–30.

Appendix

# The Interstitium and the Transfer of Information: A Brief Synopsis

**By R. Paul Lee**

*This brief presentation provides background information that will help readers in understanding the material presented in Chapter 5.*

The hypothesis I first expressed in my book *Interface*[1] is that extracellular fluids actively convey *life* from the capillaries to otherwise inert structures, such as connective tissue fibres involved in extracellular structural support and physiological functions, as well as cell membranes and intracellular proteins that determine the rate of cellular metabolism.[2] These fibrous constituents of tissue would be inanimate without the life-giving interstitial fluids that bathe them and the extracellular fluids not found in the interstitium—blood and cerebrospinal fluid—that distribute them. Lymph, the other vitalising vascular liquid, generates from the interstitial fluids.

In 2018, Benias et al declared the interstitium to be a newly discovered "organ."[3] These histologists realised that they had been overlooking this "organ" because of fixation techniques that turned this fluid-filled space into what appeared to be a tight collagen band under the light microscope. Using advanced in vivo technology (probe-based confocal laser endomicroscopy), they discovered that the interstitium is indeed fluidic and vital. In their article, Benias et al commented that the interstitium has multiple functions that they previously didn't recognise in both health and disease. They indicated that the interstitium serves cells by delivering nutrients, cell-signaling molecules, cytokines, hormones, etc, as well as by providing the fluid to form lymph. It also may play a role in metastasis of cancer and could contribute to disease in general.[4]

As osteopaths, we have a fundamental understanding about fascia from the founder of our profession, A.T. Still, because it is philosophically formative and basic to our manual methods. And we are happy to have others confirm fascia's seminal contribution to the structure and function of the organism. Since the time of Dr. Still's teachings, we have endorsed the concepts that these modern histologists have only recently recognised. Osteopaths refer to the tissue in the interstices between the cells as the interstitium or the extracellular matrix, which connects everything to everything.[5]

Extracellular fluids deliver an energy that Dr. Still called "life"[6] and Dr. Sutherland called the "Breath of Life."[7] Life is the gift, delivered by water, the essential medium. The resulting "Tide," expressed throughout the body by extracellular fluids, enlivens the fluids and fibres not only outside but also inside the cells via Potency, which is represented in the interstitium by waves of calcium ions. Calcium ions repetitively gather where the capillary contributes substance and fluids to the interstitium. The ions coalesce under the influence of cyclical waves of electromagnetic information in the blood known as the Traube-Hering waves.[8]

Calcium waves create a periodic electromotive force that travels from the capillary through the interstitium. This is palpably observed in the tissues as the "Tide"[9] of the primary respiratory mechanism. As the calcium waves move through the gel-like matrix, they locally change the charge of the components of the matrix and depolymerise the long fibrous elements (the glycosaminoglycans), thereby freeing water that has been bound to the strong negative charge of the polymerised matrix. These calcium waves thus enable the temporarily less viscous matrix to permit a watery interstitial fluid to momentarily carry information, such as life, oxygen, and glucose, before the matrix resumes its negatively charged, more organised, and gel-like character. In the fluid phase, information travels with the moving calcium wave that is now attracted to the greatest proximate negative charge, which is the cell membrane.

Once the calcium wave reaches the plasma membrane of the parenchymal cell, calcium ions interact with cell membrane receptors classified as integrins. This interaction produces mechanotransduction,[10] a transmission of chemical or mechanical information from outside the cell through the action of integrins in the membrane that affect the cytoskeleton. From the cytoskeleton within the cell, the information is transferred into the organelles, such as the mitochondria, and on into the nucleus. This outside information changes the structure (shape and size) and function (metabolic activity) on the inside of the cell. Thus, the informational transfer from the heart is completed.

Life is in the fluids. As osteopaths, we understand that fluids express the Potency and Intelligence of the Breath of Life. Importantly, we engage both Potency and Intelligence in osteopathic treatment. The calcium wave, an electromotive force, takes the baton of potency from the Traube-Hering wave within the vessel to finish the race started by the firing of the sinoatrial node. That firing initiates the contraction of the heart, which then produces the largest electromagnetic field in the body. The calcium wave carries the information from the flowing blood across the no-man's land of the extracellular matrix and reconfigures the interior of the parenchymal cell, thereby cyclically regulating metabolic activity.

Further study in the coming years will clarify the details of this hypothesis.

## Endnotes

1. R. Paul Lee, *Interface: Mechanisms of Spirit in Osteopathy* (Portland: Stillness Press, 2005).

2. R. Paul Lee, "The Living Matrix: A Model for the Primary Respiratory Mechanism," *Explore* 4 (2008): 374–8, https://cranialosteopathy.com/wp-content/uploads/2017/03/livingmatrix.pdf

3. Petros C. Benias et al, "Structure and Distribution of an Unrecognized Interstitium in Human Tissue," *Scientific Reports* 8 (2018): 4947.

4. R. Paul Lee, "The Interstitium," *R. Paul Lee, DO, FAAO, FCA* (blog), posted March 25, 2024, https://cranialosteopathy.com/2024/03/25/the-interstitium/.

5. Lee, "The Interstitium."

6. A.T. Still, *Philosophy and Mechanical Principles of Osteopathy* (Kansas City, MO: Hudson-Kimberly Publishing Co., 1902), 82.

7. William Garner Sutherland, *Teachings in the Science of Osteopathy* (Sutherland Cranial Teaching Foundation, 1990), 32.

8. W.D. Halliburton, "Traube Waves and Mayer Waves," *Quarterly Journal of Experimental Physiology* 12, no. 3 (October 1919): 227-9.

9. Sutherland, *Teachings in the Science of Osteopathy*, 31.

10. Ning Wang, James P. Butler, and Donald E. Ingber, "Mechanotransduction Across the Cell Surface and Through the Cytoskeleton," *Science* 260, no. 5111 (May 1993): 1124–7.

# Index

Note: *Italic* page numbers refer to figures.

# About the Author

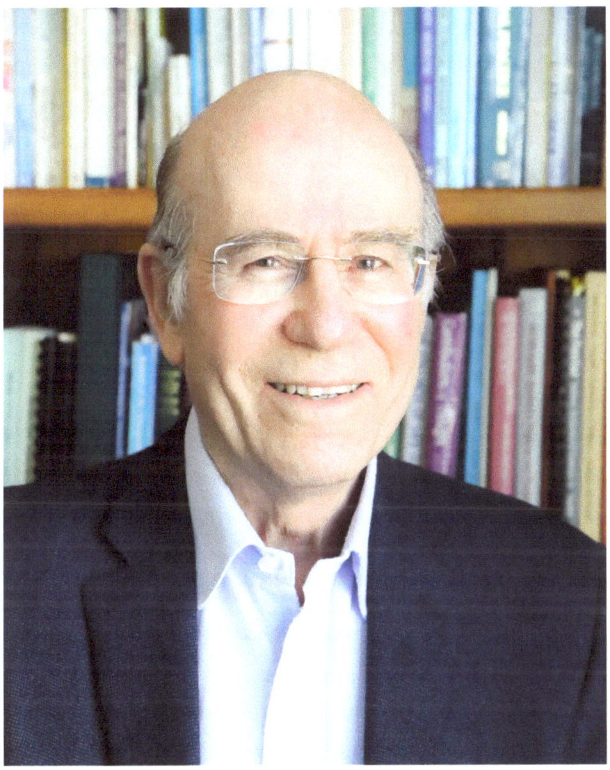

**Maxwell Fraval,** LLB, DO, MOsteoSc(Paed)

**Maxwell Fraval** came to osteopathy via a significant career change inspired by inner guidance. Later, when he was in practice, he developed a particular dedication to the treatment of babies and children after successfully treating his baby son, who had projectile vomiting. Witnessing the success of osteopathic care in young patients is, for Maxwell, an ongoing source of wonder at the strength of the response that can be achieved with osteopathy. He has been on a continuing journey of discovery into the benefits of osteopathic treatment throughout his long career.

Maxwell trained at the British School of Osteopathy and subsequently joined its Board of Governors. He also served on the board of the General Council of Registered Osteopaths in the United Kingdom (UK) before moving to Australia in 1983.

Maxwell has taught and mentored generations of osteopathic practitioners. He began teaching undergraduates in the UK in 1979, and in 1985, after relocating to Australia, he joined the Royal Melbourne Institute of Technology (RMIT) as a part-time lecturer. RMIT was the first university in Australia to run an osteopathic degree course.

Maxwell is a founding member of the Sutherland Cranial Teaching Foundation of Australia and New Zealand, which was established in 1990 as a vehicle for teaching postgraduate courses. In 1993, he pioneered the first osteopathic paediatrics program (leading to a master's degree) in Australia at RMIT. Since 2001, Maxwell has taught Rule of the Artery courses in Australia, New Zealand, the United States of America, UK and several European countries.

# About the Contributors

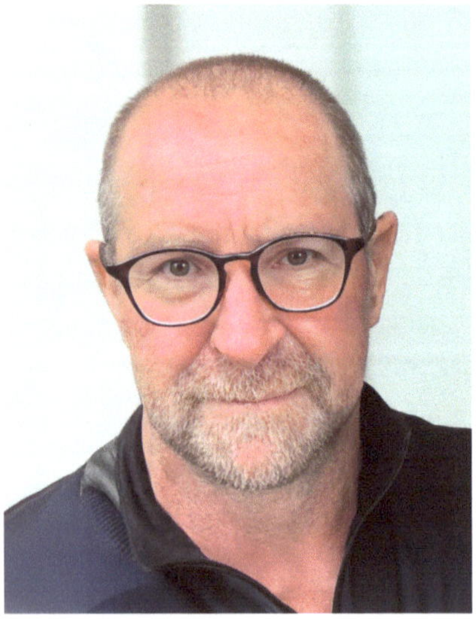

## Michael Solano, BAppSc(Osteo), DipEd(Sec), BSc(HM)

Michael Solano graduated as an osteopath from the Royal Melbourne Institute of Technology University in 1992. His previous studies include a Bachelor of Science from Melbourne University, where he majored in psychology and human movement, and a Diploma of Education. Michael has been in general osteopathic practice for 32 years.

In 2005, Michael began his deeply impactful studies with the anatomist-embryologist Dr Brian Freeman. He later went on to organise and teach international seminars on the biodynamic approach to embryology.

Michael has been involved in undergraduate teaching in the university setting and at the Osteopathic Summer School held by the Australian Research College of Osteopathic Medicine, an educational organization. He has taught postgraduate students through the Sutherland Cranial Teaching Foundation of Australia and New Zealand, Osteopathy Australia, and the Rule of the Artery program.

Michael's passion for exploring the therapeutic implications of embryological dynamics results from his understanding that the biomechanics of the embryo are also the construction and repair manuals for human form and function.

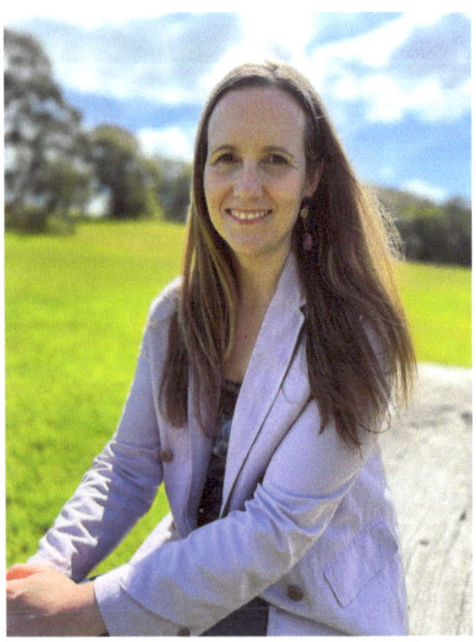

## Prue Eddie, MOsteo, BAppSc(CompMed), GradCertNeoInfPaedManThpy

Prue Eddie attained both bachelor's and master's degrees in osteopathic studies from the Royal Melbourne Institute of Technology University. Upon completion of her training, Prue moved to New Zealand and received valuable mentorship from Anthony Norrie and Pili Munoz. After returning to Australia, she obtained a Graduate Certificate of Neonatal and Infant Paediatric Manual Therapy from Victoria University.

In 2012, Prue began tutoring at the Osteopathic Summer School, a mentoring program for osteopathic university students, and she began assisting at the Rule of the Artery program. She has continued to be a faculty member on the Rule of the Artery programs in Australia and Europe. In addition, she is a faculty member of the Sutherland Cranial Teaching Foundation of Australia and New Zealand.

Prue enjoys balancing private practice with ongoing learning and lecturing. She sees that teaching expands the positive ripple effect beyond one's own patients to support and enhance the health of many more.

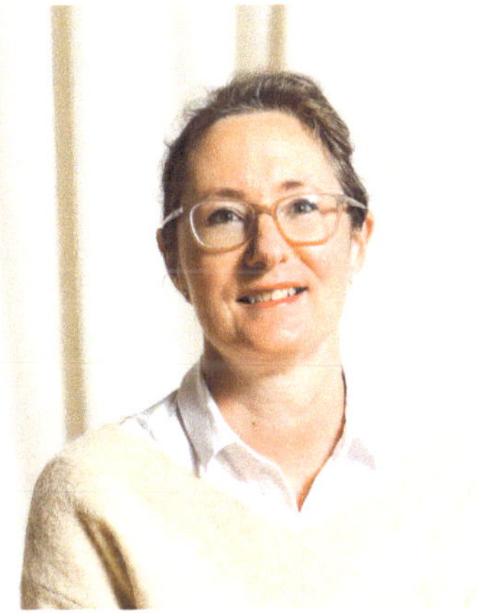

## Cate McDonald, BAppSc(Osteo), BAppSc(ClinSc), GradCertNeoInfPaedManThpy

Cate McDonald graduated from the Royal Melbourne Institute of Technology University in 1995 with a double bachelor's degree in applied science (osteopathic science) and clinical science. She always had a special interest in paediatrics, and this led Cate to also complete a Graduate Certificate in Neonatal and Infant Paediatric Manual Therapy. She completed her first Sutherland Cranial Teaching Foundation of Australia and New Zealand cranial course in 1995, and since then, she has worked primarily with the techniques she learned in that course.

Cate has served on the Australian Osteopathic Association's ethics and continuing professional development committees. She is a long-standing faculty and board member of the Sutherland Cranial Teaching Foundation of Australia and New Zealand and is currently the vice-president. She is grateful for her 10 years of mentoring from Maxwell Fraval and for her years tutoring and lecturing with the Rule of the Artery faculty. Teaching hand to hand is her passion.

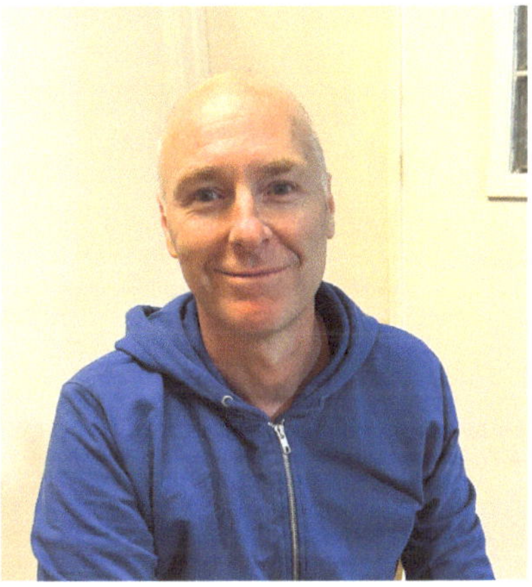

## Alistair Moresi, BAppSc(Osteo)

Alistair Moresi has been practising traditional hands-on osteopathy since graduating from the Royal Melbourne Institute of Technology in 1992.

Alistair has immersed himself in the continuing study and teaching of osteopathy, maintaining a full-time, hands-on osteopathic practice for more than 30 years and lecturing at local, national, and international conferences. In the United States of America, where he resides, he has taught many courses, including Dr Viola Frymann's Expanded Osteopathic Concepts, Dr Eliot Blackman's Embryonic Midline/Mesoderm, and Dr Jim Jealous's BioBasic Studies. Alistair currently directs and lectures at the Rule of the Artery courses in the United States along with his mentors and colleagues from Australia.

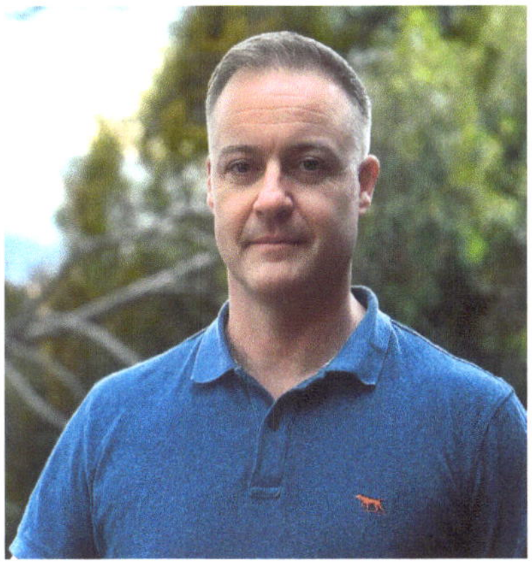

## Ben Stringer, MHSc (Osteo), BSc(ClinSc), BDA(NIDA)

Ben Stringer graduated from Victoria University in 2012 with a Bachelor of Science (Clinical Science) and Master of Health Science (Osteopathy). Ben also holds a Bachelor of Dramatic Arts from Australia's National Institute of Dramatic Art.

Ben's particular focus is osteopathy in the cranial field, and he continues to pursue study in this discipline. Ben has been a board member and teaching faculty member of the Sutherland Cranial Teaching Foundation of Australia and New Zealand, as well as a teacher on the Rule of the Artery courses, since 2015.

# Praise for *Osteopathy Is in the Blood*

Inspired by the axiom "The Rule of the Artery is Absolute," *Osteopathy Is in the Blood* is a quantum leap forward in osteopathic philosophy and practice. This groundbreaking book presents current cardiovascular research, embryologic perspectives, and physiologic understanding that underlies and explains A.T. Still's insights 120 years ago. It also opens doors to far-reaching clinical applications. The reader will find the scholarship definitive and the book to be one of the most valuable to appear in the past 50 years of osteopathy.

*– Prof Hollis King, DO, PhD (USA)*

Perfused with osteopathic wisdom, this important work presents new and perhaps unexpected knowledge about the blood and vascular system. Drawing upon cutting-edge science, biodynamic embryology, and perceptive insight, it presents a wealth of information to guide new approaches to treatment. A true "digging on" along the lines of A.T. Still's and W.G. Sutherland's philosophy.

*– John Lewis, DO (UK), Author of* A.T. Still: From the Dry Bone to the Living Man.

An invaluable reference text for all osteopaths, this book contains extensive research demonstrating that the founding principles of osteopathy are fully backed up by modern scientific research. Studying these concepts will challenge osteopaths to think more deeply and work more effectively with the blood and circulation, which is fundamental to exploring the full potential of osteopathy to enhance our patients' health.

*– Liz Hayden, DO (UK)*

I highly recommend this book, which utilizes extensive visual aids and research to explain the interconnected relationship between embryology, anatomy, and physics in osteopathic practice.

*– Christiane Topf, DO (Germany)*

This book offers a much-needed explanation of what we as osteopaths feel in our work but have not always been able to put into words. The inspiring thoughts and theories presented reveal completely new therapeutic possibilities for osteopaths to work with the circulatory system. A very interesting and highly recommended book.

*– Noori Mitha, DO, FSSCO (Germany)*

We have been waiting for this book like waiting for the sunrise!

*– Veikko Toivainen, DO (Finland)*

Understanding that osteopathy *is* indeed in the blood, as this book so eloquently lays out, will transform how you think and practice in your daily work with patients. It did for me.

*– Rachel Brooks, MD (USA), Editor of the works of Rollin E. Becker, DO.*

These teachers are among those leading the way in a rapidly growing current of thought that is elevating osteopathic understanding. Attending their courses has enlarged my whole osteopathic perspective, both microscopically and universally. This book is an expansive source of instruction and insight for the subtle and profound work of future osteopaths.

*– R. Paul Lee, DO, (USA), Author of* Interface: Mechanisms of Spirit in Osteopathy.

The teachings in *Osteopathy Is in the Blood* have been pivotal in deepening my work with patients. They have allowed me to bring about tremendous restorations of health, especially in those who are seriously ill. The restoration of a powerful primary respiratory mechanism expression in the vascular function has remarkable value, especially in situations such as long COVID.

This osteopathic work applies the fundamental cranial concept knowledge, which I have taught for decades with the Osteopathic Cranial Academy, into very real and successful clinical applications. I encourage all osteopaths to explore this work and reap these benefits. The founders of the Rule of the Artery approach are dedicated, insightful thinkers, and they have graced our profession and patients with a precious gift.

*– Ilene M. Spector, DO, FCA (USA)*

This book, with its in-depth knowledge of cardiovascular biomechanics and bioenergetics, is an excellent theory companion to the practical Rule of the Artery courses taught around the world. Anyone who endeavours to broaden their appreciation of working with structure and function will love this book.

*– Julie Streckfuss, B.App.Sci (Osteo), Grad Cert Higher Ed (Australia)*

www.ingramcontent.com/pod-product-compliance
Lightning Source LLC
LaVergne TN
LVHW070934210926
848482LV00003B/237
*9798991742009*